Emerging Viruses in Human Populations

PERSPECTIVES IN MEDICAL VIROLOGY

Volume 16

Series Editors

A.J. Zuckerman

Royal Free and University College Medical School
University College London
London, UK

I.K. Mushahwar

Abbott Laboratories
Viral Discovery Group
Abbott Park, IL, USA

Emerging Viruses in Human Populations

Editor

Edward Tabor

Rockville, MD, USA

ELSEVIER

Amsterdam – Boston – Heidelberg – London – New York – Oxford – Paris
San Diego – San Francisco – Singapore – Sydney – Tokyo

Elsevier
Radarweg 29, PO Box 211, 1000 AE Amsterdam, The Netherlands
The Boulevard, Langford Lane, Kidlington, Oxford OX5 1GB, UK

First edition 2007

Library of Congress Cataloguing-in-Publication Data
A catalog record for this book is available from the Library of Congress

British Library Cataloguing in Publication Data
A catalogue record for this book is available from the British Library

ISBN-13: 978-0-444-52074-6
ISBN-10: 0-444-52074-0
ISSN: 0168-7069

For information on all Elsevier publications
visit our website at books.elsevier.com

Printed and bound in The Netherlands

07 08 09 10 11 10 9 8 7 6 5 4 3 2 1

Working together to grow
libraries in developing countries

www.elsevier.com | www.bookaid.org | www.sabre.org

ELSEVIER   BOOK AID
International   Sabre Foundation

Contents

Introduction
Edward Tabor 1

History of Emerging Viruses in the Late 20th Century and the
Paradigm Observed in an Emerging Prion Disease
Brian W.J. Mahy 5

Zoonoses in the Emergence of Human Viral Diseases
Birgitta Åsjö, Hilde Kruse 15

Severe Acute Respiratory Syndrome Coronavirus (SARS-CoV)
Tommy R. Tong 43

The Pandemic Threat of Avian Influenza Viruses
Amorsolo L. Suguitan Jr., Kanta Subbarao 97

The Emerging West Nile Virus: From the Old World to the New
Theresa L. Smith. 133

Monkeypox Virus Infections
Kurt D. Reed 149

Hantavirus in the Old and New World
J. Clement, P. Maes, M. Van Ranst. 161

Nipah and Hendra Viruses
Vincent P. Hsu. 179

Japanese Encephalitis Virus: The Geographic Distribution, Incidence and
Spread of a Virus with a Propensity to Emerge in New Areas
John S. Mackenzie, David T. Williams, David W. Smith 201

Dengue and the Dengue Viruses
Ching-Juh Lai, Robert Putnak 269

Crimean-Congo Hemorrhagic Fever Virus
Pierre Nabeth. 299

Surveillance for Newly Emerging Viruses
David Buckeridge, Geneviève Cadieux. 325

Colour Section. 345

List of Contributors. 359

Index. 363

Emerging Viruses in Human Populations
Edward Tabor (Editor)
© 2007 Elsevier B.V. All rights reserved
DOI 10.1016/S0168-7069(06)16001-2

1

Introduction: The Emergence of Pathogenic Viruses

Edward Tabor

Quintiles, Inc., 1801 Rockville Pike, Suite 300, Rockville, MD 20852 USA

Diseases caused by emerging viruses are a permanent part of the human condition. In fact, there is a current but controversial theory that all DNA, including that in the cells of humans, originated when RNA viruses underwent adaptive changes to avoid host defenses (Zimmer, 2006). The genes of viruses are prone to changes that allow the viruses to adapt easily to new hosts. The relatively simple structure of viruses allows mutations to occur easily; the explosive replication of viruses magnifies the mutations. RNA viruses are particularly prone to these modifications, since they lack molecular "proofreading" mechanisms to correct mutations and errors in replication.

The emergence of pathogenic viruses must be defined from the point-of-view of the susceptible population. For instance, the emergence of smallpox virus (variola virus) during the settlement of North America should be defined in terms of the susceptible native populations, not in terms of the partially immune populations migrating from Europe where the virus was endemic. Smallpox virus, sometimes called "the invisible pioneer" of North America, arrived in New England on the ships of explorers even before the arrival of the settlers, and a wave of infections caused by the smallpox virus moved westward across North America among the previously unexposed native populations a few decades ahead of the frontier of European settlement (Davidson and Lee, 1992). In many native populations, the mortality from the spreading smallpox virus (perhaps combined with the mortality from other emerging viruses such as varicella zoster virus and measles virus) approached 90%. To the Europeans migrating across North America, smallpox virus was an endemic virus. From the point-of-view of the native peoples of North America, smallpox virus was a devastating emerging virus.

Viruses can emerge because of changes in the host, the environment, or the vector. Changes in the host population can include cultural changes such as the acquisition of new customs, new diets, or new living conditions. When a virus emerges by transfer to a susceptible population from a population in which it is endemic, the emergence can result from cultural changes in either host population. Changes in the host population caused by other diseases such as cancer and immunodeficiency virus infections can also lead to emergence of other pathogenic viruses. Changes in the environment can result from travel, and major political changes such as war and conquest can lead to the emergence of pathogenic viruses due to migrations of armies and displaced civilians, crowding, deterioration of hygiene, and famine.

Changes in the habitat of the vector can lead to emergence of viruses in humans. For instance, when new areas of irrigation are opened they may provide new breeding grounds for mosquito vectors; this happened in Southeast Asia, leading to expansion of the areas with Japanese encephalitis virus. In another example, adaptation of the West Nile virus to new mosquito species in the eastern US, or the mere availability of additional mosquito species capable of carrying the virus, contributed to the emergence of West Nile virus there.

A new pathogenic virus can emerge in humans from among existing human viruses or from animal viruses. Mutations in a nonpathogenic virus of humans can create a pathogenic virus of humans. A virus of animals can mutate or recombine with a virus of humans (with "reassortment" of the genome, in the case of viruses with segmented genomes, such as influenza virus) to create a virus that is highly pathogenic for humans.

Viruses can emerge from animal viruses when mutation(s) of the virus and/or increased accessibility to humans enables the virus to make the "cross-species jump" to infect humans. Agriculture, meatpacking, pet ownership, and hunting of animals (and preparing the killed animals for food or other commercial use) have all enabled viruses to emerge among humans. Changes in the habitats of animal hosts such as rodents, livestock, poultry, and animals kept as pets, also can lead to viruses emerging among humans. In the most noteworthy of these instances in the late 20th century, close contact between nonhuman primates and humans in Africa, resulting in part from habitat changes, may have been responsible for the emergence of human immunodeficiency virus from simian immunodeficiency virus, and human T-lymphotropic virus from simian T-lymphotropic virus.

Active surveillance of disease patterns in animals sometimes can provide advance warning of emerging viruses in humans. Widespread deaths among wild birds in the Eastern US served as a warning of the future emergence of West Nile virus in humans in the US. Deaths due to the H5N1 strain of avian influenza virus among poultry in Asia are considered an indication that future reassortment of this virus with the genome of human influenza virus could lead to a virulent strain emerging in humans. Monitoring recurring veterinary syndromes can detect unknown emerging agents; monitoring atypical cases of known veterinary diseases (atypical clinical characteristics, severity, species, or geographic regions) can detect emerging variants of known agents (Vourc'h [sic] et al., 2006).

Re-emergence of viruses can also be a serious public health problem. In Singapore, a campaign to reduce the population of the A. aegypti vector mosquito population resulted in a 15-year decrease in the incidence of dengue virus infections, but a resurgence occurred in the 1990s. This was due to a variety of factors, including decreasing "herd immunity" and the arrival of imported dengue virus from neighboring countries that did not themselves have good vector control programs (Ooi et al., 2006). Because of the extent of global travel today, the control of emerging viruses requires a global effort in order to ensure sustained control. *Re-emergence* of viruses can also occur when fear of vaccination becomes a regional political issue, as happened when polio vaccination was suspended due to fear and politics in parts of Nigeria in 2003; within 18 months, poliovirus had spread and caused disease in 16 nearby countries from which it previously had been eradicated (Rosenstein and Garrett, 2006).

Research and preparation for dealing with emerging viruses have been intensified due to concerns about bioterrorism. An emerging virus of high virulence and with other characteristics that could lead to panic in an affected community might be used as a weapon of bioterrorism. Furthermore, the detection of an apparently emerging virus could be the first indication that a bioterrorist attack has taken place. Perfection of methods of surveillance, detection, containment, and quarantine of emerging viruses can be applicable to outbreaks resulting from bioterrorism, and vice versa. The public health infrastructure for responding to emerging viruses can be useful for responding to attacks of bioterrorism.

This book addresses viruses that are emerging or that threaten to emerge among human populations in the 21st century. Some viruses that emerged in the late 20th century are discussed in an historical context; many of the experiences faced in the 20th century with viruses such as human immunodeficiency virus and human T-lymphotropic virus provide models for developing programs to monitor and counteract emerging viruses in the 21st century.

References

Davidson JW, Lee MH. The invisible pioneers. In: After the Fact: The Art of Historical Detection (Davidson JW, Lee MH). New York: McGraw-Hill; 1992; pp. 95–121.

Ooi E-E, Goh K-T, Gubler DJ. Dengue prevention and 35 years of vector control in Singapore. Emerg Infect Dis 2006; 12: 887–893.

Rosenstein S, Garrett L. Polio's return: a WHO-done-it? The American Interest, Spring 2006; pp. 19–27.

Vourc'h G, Bridges VE, Gibbens J, De Groot BD, McIntyre L, Poland R, Barnouin J. Detecting emerging diseases in farm animals through clinical observations. Emerg Infect Dis 2006; 12: 204–210.

Zimmer C. Did DNA come from viruses? Science 2006; 312: 870–872.

Emerging Viruses in Human Populations
Edward Tabor (Editor)
© 2007 Elsevier B.V. All rights reserved
DOI 10.1016/S0168-7069(06)16002-4

History of Emerging Viruses in the Late 20th Century and the Paradigm Observed in an Emerging Prion Disease

Brian W.J. Mahy

National Center for Infectious Diseases, Centers for Disease Control and Prevention, Atlanta, GA 30333, USA

Introduction

The concept of emerging infectious diseases became established in the 1980s, and it was given formal authority by the creation in 1991 of a 19-member multidisciplinary Committee on Emerging Microbial Threats to Health of the Institute of Medicine of the National Academy of Sciences, USA (Lederberg et al., 1992). In the report of this committee, many factors contributing to the emergence of new microbial threats were noted. These included genetic and other biological microbial changes, physical environmental changes, and especially individual and collective changes in human behavior.

In this overview, I will consider the history of some of the most serious viruses to emerge in the late 20th century.

Human behavior and herpes simplex virus, type 2 (HSV-2)

Undoubtedly, the most important virus to emerge in the early 1980s was human immunodeficiency virus (HIV), which has since become the fourth leading cause of death worldwide. This is a prime example of a virus infection introduced into the human population from animal hosts; this virus, however, depended on human behavior patterns for its subsequent spread among the human population. In contrast, at least two decades before the emergence of HIV, HSV-2 emerged within the human population, but not from an animal host. In this case, changes in human behavior caused an alarming increase in cases of HSV-2 infection, correlated with increases in promiscuous sexual behavior and increased intravenous drug use in the 1960s.

HSV-2 is transmitted primarily by sexual contact. This is illustrated by the observation that antibodies to HSV-2 are almost never found in nuns, but are found in the majority of prostitutes, and by the observation that the appearance of antibodies to HSV-2 in humans correlates with the onset of sexual activity.

Current surveillance suggests that as many as 25% of the adult population are infected with HSV-2 in the USA and the UK (Ades et al., 1989; Leone, 2005). HSV-2 infection is associated with a threefold risk of HIV infection among the general population (Freeman et al., 2006). Yet this disease could be controlled by changes in human behavior, for instance by modification of "high risk" sexual behavior (Wald et al., 2005). In addition, the development of specific antiviral drugs based on the nucleoside analogue acycloguanosine (Elion, 1989) has played an important role in treating and controlling this and other herpes virus infections.

Human immunodeficiency virus, type 1 (HIV-1)

The early history of the emergence of HIV is unknown, but a number of facts have been inferred by analysis of viral phylogenetic data. It is now believed that HIV entered the human population from a simian reservoir, but early recognition was confounded by the length of the incubation period, which averages 8–10 years in humans. As a result, the extent of the epidemic was initially underestimated.

The disease caused by HIV-1, acquired immunodeficiency syndrome (AIDS), was first recognized in the early 1980s by physicians caring for patients with sexually transmitted diseases in young male homosexuals. (In retrospect, isolated cases of AIDS had been observed and described as early as 1979.) The first detailed published study of AIDS described four young men who presented with *Pneumocystis carinii* pneumonia, esophageal candidiasis, and multiple opportunistic viral infections, including cytomegalovirus infection (Gottlieb et al., 1981). By 1983 it had become clear that AIDS was an infectious disease and that a retrovirus was the causative agent. However, there was disagreement as to which retrovirus was involved. Scientists in the US claimed that human T-cell lymphotropic virus, type III (HTLV-III) was the causative agent (Essex et al., 1983; Gallo et al., 1983), whereas scientists in France claimed that a lentivirus called lymphadenopathy-associated virus (LAV) was the causative agent (Barre-Sinoussi et al., 1983; Klatzmann et al., 1984). Despite ongoing controversy for several years, including evidence that both isolates actually were derived from the French isolate, (Barre-Sinoussi et al., 1985) in 1986 the causative agent of AIDS was officially named HIV by the International Committee on Taxonomy of Viruses.

Various methods have been used to attempt to reconstruct the history of the emergence of HIV-1 as an important cause of human disease. Retrospective studies of stored serum samples revealed that earliest documented case of HIV infection recognized by the presence of antibodies occurred in 1958 in Zaire. Retrospective analysis of clinical reports revealed that the first clinically recognized case of AIDS occurred in Norway, in a sailor who probably became infected in the 1960s after visiting an African port (and later shown to be infected with HIV), who then infected his wife, pregnant with their third child, and all three died of AIDS (Froland et al., 1988). Subsequently, HIV as a cause of AIDS became known as HIV-1 when a related virus, designated HIV-2, was found in persons connected with West Africa. Genetic analysis revealed that HIV-1 probably entered the human population by "species jumping" from the chimpanzee, and HIV-2 entered the human population by "species jumping" from sooty-mangabey monkeys in West Africa (Hahn et al., 2000). HIV-2 is in fact more closely related to simian immunodeficiency virus than it is to HIV-1. The process of "molecular dating analysis" suggests that HIV-1 entered the human population around 1931 (Korber et al., 2000) and HIV-2 entered the human population around 1940 (Lemey et al., 2003).

The growing number of people living with AIDS (more than 40 million at the end of 2005) and the action of HIV-1 in incapacitating the human immune system contributes to the emergence of other new virus infections. Examples include viruses that cause malignancies in the AIDS-infected host, such as Kaposi's sarcoma caused by human herpes virus 8, and anal and cervical cancers due to human papillomavirus (Karpas, 2004). In addition, other serious infectious diseases such as tuberculosis that had previously been rare or subject to successful control measures have emerged in HIV-infected populations as significant diseases (Mukadi et al., 2001).

Human T-lymphotropic viruses

Leukemia was the first malignancy to be shown to be caused by a virus, albeit in chickens (Ellermann and Bang, 1908), and soon after a solid malignancy—sarcoma in chickens—was also found to be transmitted by a virus (Rous, 1911). Then, in the early 1950s leukemia in mice was also shown to be transmitted by a virus (Gross, 1951), and this discovery prompted a great deal of research into possible viral etiologies for leukemia in other animals and in man.

The first reports of a virus associated with human adult T-cell leukemia, human T-lymphotropic virus (later designated HTLV-1), appeared in 1981 (Hinuma et al., 1982; Kalyanaraman et al., 1981), and reports of a subtype of HTLV, designated HTLV-2, found in association with hairy cell leukemia, appeared in 1982 (Kalyanaraman et al., 1982). These C-type retroviruses probably originated from separate "species-jumping" transmissions from simian species to humans. The viruses found in simian hosts are so closely related to the human viruses that they are classified as single species, simian T-lymphotropic virus, type 1 and simian T-lymphotropic virus, type 2 (STLV-1, STLV-2) within the genus *Deltaretrovirus* (Fauquet et al., 2005). The two species share 65% genetic identity, and isolates from different geographical regions show very little genetic variation.

The HTLV viruses are endemic in southwest Japan; they are also found in Africa and the Caribbean, and in emigrants from these areas (Proietti et al., 2005). These viruses are commonly transmitted from mother to infant through infected milk (Kaplan and Khabbaz, 1993). Fewer than 1% of HTLV-infected persons develop clinically apparent disease. Even in those who eventually develop leukemia, it takes many years before symptoms are recognized. HTLV infection also can cause HTLV-associated myelopathy or tropical spastic paraparesis (HAM/TSP), but this is rarely seen in the same patients who develop HTLV-associated leukemia. The reasons for the different disease manifestations are unknown. HTLV infection may be associated with immunosuppression, and there is some evidence that infected persons may have an increased susceptibility to other infectious diseases (Murphy et al., 1999).

Hepatitis C virus

The possible existence of a virus that caused post-transfusion hepatitis and was distinct from hepatitis A and hepatitis B viruses was first noted in the 1970s (Alter et al., 1975; Feinstone et al., 1975), and this virus was usually referred to as non-A, non-B hepatitis virus. The virus was transmitted to chimpanzees (Tabor et al., 1978), establishing it as a transmissible agent, and some of its characteristics were delineated even without its having been isolated or grown in cell culture (Bradley et al., 1979).

It became clear that the non-A, non-B hepatitis virus was an important cause of chronic liver disease, including cirrhosis. Since the disease was clearly being transmitted by blood transfusion, it became extremely important to develop a diagnostic test for the virus, which was accomplished as a result of collaborative research between Bradley et al. at CDC and Choo et al. at chiron corporation. RNA extracted from the blood of a chimpanzee infected with the virus was reverse transcribed using random primers to make cDNAs, which were then cloned into a lambda-gt-11 bacteriophage expression vector. The resulting clones were expressed in *Escherichia coli* and screened with serum from a patient with non-A, non-B hepatitis. After screening thousands of plaques, one immunoreactive clone (designated 5-1-1) was detected (Choo et al., 1989). This clone expressed a non-structural protein that was recognized by the sera of patients with non-A, non-B hepatitis, but not by control sera (Kuo et al., 1989), and was the basis of an early ELISA test for the virus. Clone 5-1-1 was then used to search for overlapping sequences in the lambda-gt-11 library and this led to the assembly of most of the sequence of the virus (Choo et al., 1991). The determination of the genome sequence and organization led to the designation of the virus as "hepatitis C virus," sole member of the newly designated genus *Hepacivirus* within the family *Flaviviridae.*

The complete nucleotide sequence of the virus also allowed the development of a better ELISA test, which showed that the virus was present in more people than previously recognized (Alter, 1995). It is now estimated that 3% of the world population (i.e. about 180 million people) are infected with hepatitis C virus. It has also become clear that the virus is a major cause of hepatocellular carcinoma (Tabor and Kobayashi, 1992; Hoofnagle, 2002).

Although there is only one species of hepatitis C virus, molecular genotyping indicates the existence of six major genetic groups (called HCV Clades 1–6). These clades differ from each other by > 30%, but each contains one or more genotypes that differ in nucleotide sequence by 20%. Worldwide, the commonest genotypes are 1a, 1b, and 3a, which are common in the USA and Europe. The existence of many genotypes in west Africa (all within Clade 2) (Candotti et al., 2003) and in Asia (within Clades 3 and 6) (Mellor et al., 1995,1996) has led to the suggestion that hepatitis C virus has been endemic in sub-Saharan Africa and Southeast Asia for a long time, and that the appearance of hepatitis C in western countries may represent relatively recent emergence of this infection (Simmonds and Mutimer, 2005).

Variant Creutzfeldt-Jakob disease (vCJD)

vCJD is not caused by a virus, but any discussion of emerging viruses should address this disease as well, because the history of its emergence from a disease of animals bred for food provides a paradigm for the emergence of diseases caused by viruses. vCJD is caused by prions, small proteinaceous infectious particles that are resistant to most procedures that can inactivate other infectious agents by modifying nucleic acids (Prusiner, 1982). They lack nucleic acid, which would be found in all viruses; their principal component is a modified protein, encoded by a cellular gene, existing as an isoform that is highly resistant to inactivation with protease enzymes. It is possible that human vCJD arises by conversion of the cellular prion protein into the protease-resistant isoform as a result of exposure to the variant isoform.

CJD has been recognized for decades as a sporadic and fatal encephalopathy that occurs worldwide with an incidence of one case per million population per year. The exact cause was unknown, but instances of iatrogenic transmission of CJD through corneal transplantation, contaminated EEG electrode implantation, and the use of contaminated instruments during surgical operations (Brown et al., 1994) was considered evidence of it having an infectious etiology. Other transmissible spongiform encephalopathies (TSEs) have long been known to occur in a variety of animals (Aguzzi et al., 2001).

The emergence of a previously unknown disease, bovine spongiform encephalopathy (BSE), appeared as an epidemic in cattle in the United Kingdom in 1986 (Wells et al., 1987). The epidemic was traced to a food made from meat and bone meal prepared from sheep and cattle offal that was fed to dairy calves. A change in the process of preparing this supplement in the late 1970s was linked to the appearance of BSE, and since 1988 the use of such dietary supplements for cattle was forbidden in the United Kingdom (Wilesmith and Wells, 1991). However, from 1986 to 2003 more than 186,000 cases of BSE in cattle were recorded in the United Kingdom. The disease subsequently spread to several other European countries, and later to countries in other parts of the world.

In 1996, the first cases of a CJD-like disease were observed in humans. This was soon called "vCJD," and it was linked to BSE (Will et al., 1996; Weissmann and

Aguzzi, 1997; Almond, 1998). Several clinical features distinguish vCJD from the classical CJD, most notably the younger age of vCJD patients (19–39 years, compared to 55–70 years in classical CJD), but also distinct pathological features in the brain, including "florid plaques." The exact mechanism by which humans become infected with vCJD is unknown, although it has been assumed to be due to eating meat from BSE-infected cattle. However such purported transmission of a prion disease to humans by ingestion of infected meat has never been seen with scrapie, a TSE of sheep, despite many investigational studies (Harries-Jones et al., 1988). Experimental infection of cynomolgus macaques with brain extracts of BSE-infected cows produced a disease in the monkeys with the characteristic pathological changes of vCJD in humans including florid plaques in the brain (Lasmezas et al., 1996). From an epidemiological point of view, the occurrence of BSE over a wide area of Europe might be expected to cause a large-scale epidemic of vCJD (Valleron et al., 2001), but the annual number of vCJD cases in the UK reached a peak of 28 in 2000, and since then has been declining, with only five reported cases in 2005. At the beginning of 2006 there had been an overall total of 159 definite or probable recorded cases of vCJD in the UK since the beginning of the epidemic, of whom six were still alive (Department of Health, 2006). Elsewhere, there had been 16 cases of vCJD in France, three in Ireland, two in the US, and one each in Canada, Japan, the Netherlands, Portugal, Saudi Arabia, and Spain, for a grand total of 186 recognized cases of vCJD worldwide. It appears that all cases of vCJD that occurred outside of Europe were in people who had spent some time in the UK, where they are presumed to have acquired the infection.

Conclusions

Several virus diseases that emerged in the last two decades of the 20th century have now become entrenched in human populations worldwide, and unfortunately the methodological advances that led to their detection have not been matched by similar advances in our ability to prevent and control them. Attempts to develop vaccines for these have in most cases eluded all efforts. There have been improvements in antiviral therapy, but these are not effective in all cases, often resulting in control rather than cure of the disease, and they remain out of the reach of many patients in poor and underdeveloped countries.

In 2001, the Institute of Medicine of the National Academy of Sciences issued a new report on "Microbial Threats to Health in the 21st Century" (Smolinski et al., 2003), which concluded that one of the "bright spots on the global scene" was the containment of H5N1 flu in Hong Kong in 1997. The fact that the H5N1 influenza virus has since re-emerged to become a major worldwide public health threat in 2006 shows that we cannot afford to be complacent. We must redouble our efforts in surveillance, prevention, and control measures as we continue to face new emerging virus diseases.

References

Ades AE, Peckam CS, Dale GE, Best JM, Jeansson S. Prevalence of antibodies to herpes simplex virus type 1 and 2 in pregnant women and estimated rates of infection. J Epidemiol Commun Health 1989; 43: 53–60.

Aguzzi A, Montrasio F, Kaeser PS. Prions: health scare and biological challenge. Nat Rev Mol Cell Biol 2001; 2: 118–126.

Almond JW. Bovine spongiform encephalopathy and new variant Creutzfeldt-Jakob diseases. Br Med Bull 1998; 54: 749–759.

Alter HJ, Holland PV, Morrow AG, Purcell RH, Feinstone SH, Moritsugu Y. Clinical and serological analysis of transfusion-associated hepatitis. Lancet 1975; II: 838–841.

Alter MJ. Epidemiology of hepatitis C in the west. Seminar Liv Dis 1995; 15: 5–14.

Barre-Sinoussi F, Chermann JC, Rey F, Nugeyre MT, Chamret S, Gruest J, Dauguet C, Axler-Blin C, Vezinet-Brun F, Rouzioux C, Rozenbaum W, Montagnier L. Isolation of a T-lymphotropic retrovirus from a patient at risk for acquired immunodeficiency syndrome (AIDS). Science 1983; 220: 868–871.

Barre-Sinoussi F, Mather-Wagh U, Rey F, Brun Vezinet F, Yancovitz SR, Rouzioux C, Montagnier L, Mildvan D, Chermann JC. Isolation of lymphadenopathy-associated virus (LAV) and detection of LAV antibodies from US patients with AIDS. JAMA 1985; 253: 1737–1739.

Bradley DW, Cook EH, Maynard JE, McCaustland KA, Ebert JW, Dolana GH, Petzel RA, Kantor RJ, Heilbrunn A, Fields HA, Murphy BL. Experimental infection of chimpanzees with antihemophilic (Factor VIII) materials: recovery of virus-like particles associated with non-A, non-B hepatitis. J Med Virol 1979; 3: 253–269.

Brown P, Cervenakova L, Goldfarb LG, McCombie WR, Rubenstein R, Will RG, Pocchari M, Martinez-Lage JF, Scalici C, Masullo C. Iatrogenic Creutzfeldt-Jakob disease: an example of the interplay between ancient genes and modern medicine. Neurology 1994; 44: 291–293.

Candotti D, Temple J, Sarkodie F, Allain JP. Frequent recovery and broad genotype 2 diversity characterize hepatitis C virus infection in Ghana, West Africa. J Virol 2003; 77: 7914–7923.

Choo QL, Kuo G, Weiner AJ, Overby LR, Bradley DW, Houghton M. Isolation of a cDNA derived from a blood-borne non-A, non-B hepatitis genome. Science 1989; 244: 359–362.

Choo QL, Richman KH, Han JH, Berger K, Lee C, Dong C, Gallegos C, Coit D, Medina-Selby R, Barr PJ, Weiner AJ, Bradley DW, Kuo G, Houghton M. Genetic organization and diversity of the hepatitis C virus. Proc Natl Acad Sci USA 1991; 88: 2451–2455.

Department of Health. Monthly Creutzfeldt-Jakob Disease Statistics, at http://www.dh.gov.uk/PublicationsAndStatistics/PressReleases/PressReleasesNotices/fs/en?CONTENT_ID = 4126119&chk = joOCEs 2006.

Elion GB. The purine path to chemotherapy. Science 1989; 244: 41–47.

Ellermann V, Bang O. Experimentelle leukaemie bei Huehnern. Zentbl Bakt ParasitKde Abt 1 Orig 1908; 46: 595–609.

Essex M, McLane MF, Lee TH, Falk L, Howe CW, Mullins JI, Cabradilla C, Francis DP. Antibodies to cell membrane antigens associated with T-cell leukemia virus in patients with AIDS. Science 1983; 220: 859–862.

Fauquet CM, Mayo MA, Maniloff J, Desselberger U, Ball LA. Virus Taxonomy. Eighth Report of the International Committee on Taxonomy of Viruses. London: Elsevier Academic Press; 2005.

Feinstone SM, Kapikian AZ, Purcell RH. Transfusion-associated hepatitis not due to viral hepatitis A or B. N Engl J Med 1975; 292: 767–770.

Freeman EE, Weiss HA, Glynn JR, Cross PL, Whitworth JA, Hayes RJ. Herpes simplex virus 2 infection increases HIV acquisition in men and women: systematic review and meta-analysis of longitudinal studies. AIDS 2006; 20: 73–83.

Froland SS, Jenum P, Lindboe CF, Wefring KW, Linnestad PJ, Bohmer T. HIV-1 infection in Norwegian family before 1970. Lancet 1988; I: 344–345.

Gallo RC, Sarin PC, Gelmann EP, Robert-Guroff M, Richardson E, Kalyanaraman VS, Mann D, Sidhu GD, Stahl RE, Zolla-Pazner S, Leibowitch J, Popovic M. Isolation of human T-cell leukemia virus in acquired immune deficiency syndrome (AIDS). Science 1983; 220: 865–867.

Gottlieb MS, Schroff R, Schanker HM, Weisman JD, Fan PT, Wolf RA, Saxon A. *Pneumocystis carinii* pneumonia and mucosal candidiasis in previously healthy homosexual men: evidence of a new acquired cellular immunodeficiency. N Engl J Med 1981; 305: 1425–1431.

Gross L. "Spontaneous" leukemia developing in C3H mice following inoculation, in infancy, with AK-leukemic extracts or AK-embryos. Proc Soc Exp Biol Med 1951; 76: 27–32.

Hahn BH, Shaw GM, De Cock KM, Sharp PM. AIDS as a zoonosis: scientific and public health implications. Science 2000; 287: 607–614.

Harries-Jones R, Knight R, Will RG, Cousens S, Smith PG, Matthews WB. Creutzfeldt-Jakob disease in England and Wales, 1980–1984: a case–control study of potential risk factors. J Neurol Neurosurg Psychiatry 1988; 51: 1113–1119.

Hinuma Y, Komoda H, Chosa T, Kondo T, Kohakura M, Takenaka T, Kikuchi M, Ichimaru M, Yunoki K, Sato I, Matsuo R, Takiuchi Y, Uchino H, Hanaoka M. Antibodies to adult T-cell leukemia-virus-associated antigen (ATLA) in sera from patients with ATL and controls in Japan: a nationwide sero-epidemiologic study. Int J Cancer 1982; 9: 631–635.

Hoofnagle JH. Course and outcome of hepatitis C. Hepatology 2002; 36: S21–S29.

Kalyanaraman VS, Sarngadharan MG, Robert-Guroff M, Miyoshi I, Golde D, Gallo RC. A new subtype of human T-cell leukemia virus (HTLV-II) associated with a T-cell variant of hairy cell leukemia. Science 1982; 218: 571–573.

Kalyanaraman VS, Sarngadharan MG, Bunn PA, Minna JD, Gallo RC. Antibodies in human sera reactive against an internal structural protein of human T-cell lymphoma virus. Nature 1981; 294: 271–273.

Kaplan JE, Khabbaz RF. The epidemiology of human T-lymphotropic virus types I and II. Rev Med Virol 1993; 3: 137–148.

Karpas A. Human retroviruses in leukaemia and AIDS: reflections on their discovery, biology and epidemiology. Biol Rev Camb Philos Soc 2004; 79: 911–933.

Klatzmann D, Barre-Sinoussi F, Nugeyre MT, Danquet C, Vilmer E, Griscelli C, Brun-Veziret F, Rouzioux C, Gluckman JC, Chermann JC. Selective tropism of lymphadenopathy associated virus (LAV) for helper-inducer T lymphocytes. Science 1984; 225: 59–63.

Korber B, Muldoon M, Theiler J, Gao F, Lapedes A, Hahn BH, Wolinsky S, Bhattacharya T. Timing the ancestor of the HIV-1 pandemic strains. Science 2000; 288: 1789–1796.

Kuo G, Choo QL, Alter HJ, Gitnick GL, Redeker AG, Purcell RH, Miyamura T, Dienstag JL, Alter MG, Stevens CE. An assay for circulating antibodies to a major etiologic virus of human non-A, non-B hepatitis. Science 1989; 244: 362–364.

Lasmezas CL, Deslys JP, Demaimay R, Adjou KT, Lamoury F, Dormont D, Robain O, Ironside J, Hauw JJ. BSE transmission to macaques. Nature 1996; 381: 743–744.

Lederberg J, Shope RE, Oaks SC. Emerging Infections: Microbial Threats to Health in the United States. Washington: National Academy Press; 1992.

Lemey P, Pybus OG, Wang B, Saksena NK, Salemi M, Vandamme AM. Tracing the origin and history of the HIV-2 epidemic. Proc Natl Acad Sci USA 2003; 100: 6588–6592.

Leone P. Reducing the risk of transmitting genital herpes: advances in understanding and therapy. Curr Med Res Opin 2005; 21: 1577–1582.

Mellor J, Holmes EC, Jarvis LM, Yap PL, Simmonds P. Investigation of the pattern of hepatitis C virus sequence diversity in different geographical regions: implications for virus classification. J Gen Virol 1995; 76: 2493–2507.

Mellor J, Walsh EA, Prescott LE, Jarvis LM, Davidson F, Yap PL, Simmonds P. Survey of type 6 group variants of hepatitis C virus in southeast Asia by using a core-based genotyping assay. J Clin Microbiol 1996; 34: 417–423.

Mukadi YD, Maher D, Harries A. Tuberculosis case fatality rates in high HIV prevalence populations in sub-Saharan Africa. AIDS 2001; 15: 143–152.

Murphy EL, Glynn SA, Fridey J, Smith JW, Sacher RA, Nass CC, Ownby HE, Wright DJ, Nemo GJ. Increased incidence of infectious diseases during prospective follow-up of human T-lymphotropic virus type II- and I-infected blood donors. Retrovirus Epidemiology Donor Study. Arch Intern Med 1999; 159: 1485–1491.

Proietti FA, Carnero-Proietti AB, Catalan BC, Murphy EL. Global epidemiology of HTLV-I infection and associated diseases. Oncogene 2005; 24: 6058–6068.

Prusiner SB. Novel proteinaceous infectious particles cause scrapie. Science 1982; 216: 136–144.

Rous P. Transmission of a malignant new growth by means of a cell-free filtrate. J Am Med Ass 1911; 56: 198.

Simmonds P, Mutimer D. Hepatitis C virus . In: Topley and Wilson: Microbiology and Microbial Infections (BWJ Mahy, V ter Meulen, editors). 10th ed. London: Hodder Arnold, 2005; vol. 2 (Virology): 1189–1225.

Smolinski MS, Hamburg MA, Lederberg J, editors. Microbial Threats to Health: Emergence, Detection and Response. Washington: The National Academies Press; 2003.

Tabor E, Gerety RJ, Drucker JA, Seeff LB, Hoofnagle JH, Jackson DR, April M, Barker LF, Pineda-Tamondong G. Transmission of non-A, non-B hepatitis from man to chimpanzees. Lancet 1978; 1: 463–466.

Tabor E, Kobayashi K. Hepatitis C virus, a causative infectious agent of non-A, non-B hepatitis: Prevalence and structure-summary of a conference on hepatitis C virus as a cause of hepatocellular carcinoma. J. Natl Cancer Inst 1992; 84: 86–90.

Valleron AJ, Boelle PY, Will R, Cesbron JY. Estimation of epidemic size and incubation time based on age characteristics of vCJD in the United Kingdom. Science 2001; 294: 1726–1728.

Wald A, Langeberg AG, Krantz E, Douglas Jr. JM, Handsfield HH, DiCarlo RP, Adimora AA, Izu AE, Morrow RA, Corey L. The relationship between condom use and herpes simplex virus acquisition. Ann Intern Med 2005; 143: 707–713.

Weissmann C, Aguzzi A. Bovine spongiform encephalopathy and early onset variant Creutzfeldt-Jakob disease. Curr Opin Neurobiol 1997; 7: 695–700.

Wells GA, Scott AC, Johnson CT, Gunning RF, Hancock RD, Jeffrey M, Dawson M, Bradley R. A novel progressive spongiform encephalopathy in cattle. Vet Rec 1987; 121: 419–420.

Wilesmith JW, Wells GA. Bovine spongiform encephalopathy. Curr Top Microbiol Immunol 1991; 172: 21–38.

Will RG, Ironside JW, Zeidler M, Cousens SN, Estibeiro K, Alperovitch A, Poser S, Pocchiari M, Hofman A, Smith PG. A new variant of Creutzfeldt-Jakob disease in the UK. Lancet 1996; 347: 921–925.

Emerging Viruses in Human Populations
Edward Tabor (Editor)
© 2007 Elsevier B.V. All rights reserved
DOI 10.1016/S0168-7069(06)16003-6

Zoonoses in the Emergence of Human Viral Diseases

Birgitta Åsjö[a], Hilde Kruse[b]

[a]*Center for Research in Virology, The Gade Institute, University of Bergen, The Bio-Building 5th floor, Jonas Lies vei 91, Bergen N-5009, Norway*
[b]*National Veterinary Institute, Department for Health Surveillance, Oslo, Norway*

Viral zoonoses have represented a significant public health problem throughout history, affecting all continents. Furthermore, many viral zoonoses have emerged or reemerged in recent years, highlighting the importance of such diseases. Emerging viral zoonoses encompass a vast number of different viruses and many different transmission modes. There are many factors influencing the epidemiology of the various zoonoses, such as ecological changes, changes in agriculture and food production, the movement of pathogens, including via travel and trade, human behavior and demographical factors, and microbial changes and adaptation. Cost-effective prevention and control of emerging viral zoonoses necessitates an interdisciplinary and holistic approach and international cooperation. Surveillance, laboratory capability, research, training and education, and last but not least, information and communication are key elements.

Introduction

Throughout the history of mankind, animals have been an important source of infectious diseases transmissible to humans. Such diseases were formerly called anthropozoonoses (Greek "anthrópos" = man, "zoon" = animal, "nosos" = disease), whereas the diseases transmissible from humans to animals were called zoo-anthroponoses (Hubálek, 2003). Today, the term zoonoses is commonly used for infectious diseases that are naturally transmitted between vertebrate animals and man (WHO/FAO, 1959). The total number of zoonoses is unknown, but according to Taylor et al. (2001), who in 2001 cataloged 1415 known human pathogens, including 217 viruses and prions, 538 bacteria and rickettsia, 307 fungi, 66 protozoa, and 287 helminths, 61% were zoonotic. With time, more and more human pathogens are found to be of animal origin. Interestingly, wild animals seem to be involved in the epidemiology of most zoonoses and serve as significant reservoirs for transmission of zoonotic agents to domestic animals and man.

Many infectious diseases have emerged in the human population in recent years. According to Lederberg et al. (1992), emerging infectious diseases include those whose incidences in humans have increased within the past two decades or threaten to increase in the near future. Emerging infections also include those that have newly appeared in a population or that have been known for some time, but are rapidly increasing in incidence or geographic range.

Most emerging infectious diseases in humans are zoonoses. The WHO/FAO/ OIE joint consultation on emerging zoonotic diseases held in Geneva in 2004 (whqlibdoc.who.int/hq/2004/WHO_CDS_CPE_ZFK_2004.9.pdf)   defined   an emerging zoonosis as "a zoonosis that is newly recognized or newly evolved, or that has occurred previously but shows an increase in incidence or expansion in geographical, host or vector range". At this consultation it was stated that emerging zoonotic diseases have potentially serious human health and economic impacts and that their current increasing incidences are likely to continue. Avian influenza was used as an example; events since that time have shown that these predictions were unfortunately correct.

Of the 1415 known human pathogens, 175 (12%) are associated with an emerging disease (Taylor et al., 2001), and can be designated emerging pathogens. Of these emerging pathogens, 75% are zoonotic. Overall, zoonotic pathogens are twice as likely to be associated with emerging diseases, compared to non-zoonotic pathogens. However, the result varies among taxa, with viruses and protozoa particularly likely to emerge, and helminths particularly unlikely to do so, regardless of their zoonotic status. Interestingly, no association between transmission route and emergence was found (Taylor et al., 2001).

Historical aspects of zoonoses

Throughout history, wild animals have always played a role in viral zoonoses. Rabies is one of the most feared viral zoonoses. It is an ancient disease; the origin of the word dates to 3000 BC from Sanskrit, meaning "to do violence". Rabies was described in hunting dogs in Mesopotamia as early as 2300 BC. Recognizable descriptions of rabies can also be found in early Chinese, Egyptian, Greek, and Roman records (Blancou, 2003). In medieval Europe, rabies occurred in both domestic and wild animals. Rabid foxes, wolves, badgers, and bears were described in literature as well as in figurative art. Although rabies is an ancient disease that is endemic in many areas, the zoonosis has also been emerging in some regions in recent years.

Ancient accounts and modern hypotheses suggest that Alexander the Great died of West Nile virus (WNV) encephalitis in Babylon 323 BC (Marr and Calisher, 2003). It was reported that "as he entered Babylon a flock of ravens exhibiting unusual behavior died at his feet" (Marr and Calisher, 2003). In 1999, WNV was introduced into the United States causing an epizootic in birds with spillover infections to man and equine animals.

A major human epidemic of influenza was recorded by Hippocrates in 412 BC. Influenza viruses have different hosts, both birds and different mammals including humans, and have a zoonotic potential. An antigenic shift in influenza A virus can cause the sudden emergence of a new subtype of the virus. Although this shift occurs only occasionally, large numbers of people, and sometimes the entire population, have no antibody protection against the new subtype of virus, resulting in a worldwide epidemic ("pandemic"). Three major influenza A pandemics emerged during the 20th century. Of these, the Spanish flu in 1918–1919 (subtype H1N1) was the most severe with an estimated 50 million deaths worldwide (Taubenberger and Morens, 2006). The Asian flu in 1957–1958 (H2N2) and the Hong Kong flu in 1968–1969 (H3N2) caused less serious pandemics. The latter two are known to be the result of a reassortment between an avian influenza strain from wild waterfowl and a human strain of influenza A, with the introduction of a new hemagglutinin protein in the human strain.

The avian influenza A subtype H5N1 epidemic that emerged in birds in Asia in 2002 has caused substantial death and economic losses in poultry. This strain can also infect humans, although rarely, but with a high degree of lethality. There is no evidence so far of human-to-human transmission of the H5N1 virus. The public health concern is that genetic reassortment of this avian strain with a human strain could cause the emergence of a new pandemic with the high degree of lethality seen in the sporadic zoonotic cases to date (http://www.cdc.gov/flu/avian/gen-info/avian-flu-humans).

An epidemic of hantavirus infections emerged in the southwestern US in 1993. Healthy adults sickened and died suddenly of an unknown disease. Navajo leaders gave public health scientists clues; that year had seen a particularly bountiful harvest of piñon nuts accompanied by a large population of deer mice. The years 1918 and 1936 had also seen large harvests and large deer mouse populations as well as unexplained epidemics. Serological analyses of the blood of the victims revealed antibodies to the Haantan virus family, and as CDC scientists isolated and amplified viral DNA from victims' blood, trappers caught deer mice in the area, which proved to carry hantavirus.

Transmission modes

Zoonotic viruses replicate in the reservoir animal host and are usually transmitted to humans by direct contact (a bite by the infected reservoir animal or handling of the animal's tissues or materials contaminated by the animal's body fluids) or the bite of a hematophagous arthropod. For example, rabies virus is transmitted by the saliva from a bite of a rabid animal, and simian foamy virus (SFV) can be transmitted by bites from an infected monkey. Hantaviruses like Puumala and Sin Nombre viruses are typically spread from rodents to humans by aerosols of dust containing rodent excreta. Transmission of simian immunodeficiency virus (SIV) and SFV can occur when hunters and butchers handle the meat of infected monkeys. Ebola virus transmission has been reported after preparation of dead chimpanzees and gorillas for food.

Most viral zoonoses require a blood-sucking arthropod for transmission to humans. Mosquitoes are the most important arthropod vectors (examples of viral zoonoses transmitted by mosquitoes are Rift Valley fever, WNV, and Japanese encephalitis), followed by ticks, sandflies, and midges. Arthropod vector-borne viruses are called arboviruses and are maintained in complex life cycles involving a non-human vertebrate primary host and a primary arthropod vector. The arthropod vector becomes infected when it ingests virus while feeding on the blood of a viremic animal. Virus replicates in the arthropod tissues, ultimately infecting the salivary glands. The arthropod then transmits the virus to a new host when it injects infectious salivary fluid while taking a blood meal. Arthropod-borne viruses generally remain undetected until the virus escapes the primary cycle via a secondary vector or secondary vertebrate host, such as when humans enter the enzootic cycle. Although humans may become ill as a result of these viruses, they are generally considered dead-end hosts for many of the viruses because they do not develop sufficient viremia to infect feeding vectors and thus do not contribute to the transmission cycle. Notable exceptions include dengue, yellow fever, chikungunya, and Ross River virus infections (www.acpmedicine.com/sample2/ch0731s.htm).

Zoonotic viruses may also be spread from wild animals to humans indirectly by contaminated food and water. An unusual and unexpected example of zoonotic transmission of this type has been suggested for hepatitis E virus (HEV) infection. In an outbreak of HEV infection among people who had eaten uncooked deer meat 6–7 weeks before, a leftover portion of the deer meat, kept frozen for a future meal, was positive for HEV RNA, and the nucleotide sequence was identical to sequences of virus from the patients. Patients' family members who ate little or none of the deer meat remained uninfected. These findings provide direct evidence that HEV infection may be a zoonosis (Tei et al., 2003).

Human noroviruses are a common cause of gastrointestinal infection and are spread between humans by contact, or indirectly via food and water. Other noroviruses can be found in animals. Although noroviruses are not considered zoonotic, new research raises questions of whether pigs may be reservoirs for emergence of new human noroviruses or if porcine/human genogroup II recombinants could emerge (Wang Q.-H. et al., 2005).

Factors influencing the epidemiology of viral zoonoses

Ecological changes

Ecological changes of natural or human origin can have a profound impact on the epidemiology and the emergence of viral zoonoses. These include, but are not limited to, human population expansion and encroachment, de-forestation and reforestation, other habitat changes, pollution, and climatic changes. The opening of isolated ecosystems to human activity has contributed to the emergence of viral diseases. One classic example is the emergence of yellow fever when humans entered the Central American jungle to build the Panama Canal (Murphy, 1998).

Unprecedented population growth, mostly in developing countries, has resulted in major movements of people into urban centers. This unplanned and uncontrolled urbanization with inadequate housing, deteriorating water, sewage, and waste management systems, produces ideal conditions for increased transmission of mosquito- and rodent-borne diseases (Gubler, 1998). Meteorological factors such as temperature, rainfall, and humidity can influence the dynamics of vector-borne diseases. Climate changes with milder winters and early arrival of spring has been suggested as an explanation for the increased incidence of tick-borne encephalitis in Sweden (Lindgren and Gustafson, 2001). There are indications that warmer temperatures aid dengue virus transmission by accelerating development of the larvae of the mosquito vector, *Aedes egypti*, whose range is limited by cold weather. Yet another climate-related threat comes from the Asian tiger mosquito (*Aedes albopictus*), which transmits dengue virus and yellow fever virus and is able to tolerate cold weather (Ward and Burgess, 1993).

Hantavirus

Wild rodents constitute a reservoir of hantaviruses (virus family *Bunyaviridae*) (Schmaljohn and Hjelle, 1997). Each of the known hantaviruses appear to have one unique, natural, species-specific rodent reservoir. The rodents are chronically infected without any visible symptoms. The viruses are shed in urine, excretory droppings, and saliva, and humans are mainly infected by inhaling aerosols containing the virus. Human-to-human transmission of the viruses has not been reported.

A non-fatal form of hantavirus infection was described in Sweden in 1934 as nephropathia epidemica (NE), a hemorrhagic fever with renal disease syndrome (Niklasson and Le Duc, 1984). It is endemic in northern Sweden, Finland, western Russia, and some other areas in Europe. The causative agent, Puumala virus, is transmitted from excreta of the bank vole (*Clethrionomys glareolus*). Typically, infection occurs by inhalation of contaminated dust in relation to activities in forests or cleaning of sheds, barns, or huts.

Hantavirus infections first received serious attention in the western world when more than 3000 soldiers in the Korean War developed a disease with a fatality rate of approximately 10%, which became known as Korean hemorrhagic fever. The etiological agent, the Hantaan virus, is carried by the field mouse (*Apodemus agrarius*).

Critical environmental factors that can affect rodent population dynamics as well as viral transmission between animals, and from animals to humans, include the amount of precipitation, habitat structure, and food availability. In 1993, a previously unknown infectious disease was recognized in humans in New Mexico,

Colorado, and Nevada. The infection mainly affected the lungs, with a fatality rate of around 60%. The causative agent, a previously unknown hantavirus, subsequently was named Sin Nombre virus and the disease was named Hantavirus pulmonary syndrome (HPS). The principal animal host of Sin Nombre virus is the common deer mouse (*Peromyscus maniculatus*), which lives on pine kernels. The El Nino weather event of 1991–1992, with its unusually heavy summer rains, led to abundant crops that greatly increased the local mouse populations. The deer mouse population was 10–15 fold higher in that period than the seasonal average during the previous 20-year period (McMichael, 2004).

Arenaviruses

Deforestation with fragmentation of habitat increases the "edge effect", a phenomenon at the edge of a forest that promotes pathogen–vector–host interactions. The expansion of the world population, which perturbs ecosystems that were stable a few decades ago, has contributed in recent years to the emergence of hemorrhagic fevers in South America. These are caused by various members of the Arenavirus family, and wild rodents are their natural hosts. Human outbreaks have mostly occurred in rural populations. Clearing of forested land in Bolivia in the early 1960s was accompanied by blanket spraying of DDT to control malaria-bearing mosquitoes, and incidentally killed many village cats leading to decreased control of mice near human populations. Large areas with maize supported huge populations of *Calomys* mice carrying Machupo virus; this resulted in the appearance of the Bolivian hemorrhagic fever with a high fatality rate (McMichael, 2004). In addition, aerosols of mouse blood, urine, and feces were generated during harvests that infected the workers. A new outbreak occurred in the same place in 1994, killing seven members of one family.

Ebola virus

Ebola hemorrhagic fever is one of the most virulent and contagious viral diseases known, with a fatality rate of 50–90%. The virus belongs to the family *Filoviridae* and occurs in four distinct subtypes (Zaire, Sudan, Côte d'Ivoire, and Reston subtypes). Ebola virus was first identified in 1976 after significant epidemics in Yambuku, Zaire (now the Democratic Republic of Congo, DRC) and in Nzara, Sudan. Since its first discovery in 1976, there was a second Ebola outbreak in Nzara in 1979, then an outbreak 15 years later in Gabon in1994, and a major epidemic in Kikwit, DRC, in 1995 (with 315 cases and 250 deaths). Since then, new outbreaks have occurred almost each year. The largest outbreak ever occurred in Uganda in 2000–2001 with a total of 425 cases and a fatality rate of 53% (WHO, 2000).

The natural animal reservoir of the Ebola virus is unknown despite extensive studies. The reservoir animal seems to reside in the rain forests of Africa and the western Pacific. Humans as well as other primates are severely affected by Ebola virus, which is transmitted by direct contact with the blood, secretions, organs, or other body fluids of infected individuals. Infection of humans has also been documented to have occurred as a result of handling infected chimpanzees and gorillas found dead in the rainforests, which suggests that they are not a reservoir since they die from the infection. Interestingly, bats experimentally infected with Ebola virus do not die. Furthermore, evidence of asymptomatic Ebola virus infection was found in three species of fruit bats collected during Ebola outbreaks in humans and great apes between 2001 and 2003 in Gabon and DRC. This evidence that fruit bats may be acting as reservoirs for Ebola virus supports previous evidence suggesting bats as candidate reservoirs for Ebola virus and the closely related Marburg virus (Leroy et al., 2005). If this is correct, humans coming into greater contact with bats because of encroaching agriculture may be at increasing risk for outbreaks of Ebola virus infection.

The Ebola-Reston subtype was detected in 1989 in Virginia, USA, in a colony of cynomolgus monkeys imported from the Philippines, illustrating the risk for spread of viral zoonoses through trade in animals. Several monkeys died and four people were infected, although none of the humans were symptomatic (WHO, 2000).

Changes in agriculture and food production

Over the past 50 years, changes in agricultural practices, including livestock handling and food production, directly or in combination with ecological factors, have influenced the emergence of viral zoonoses. Unprecedented human population growth has increased the demand for highly efficient and mechanized farming. Operators of agricultural machinery in some areas are likely to be exposed to hantaviruses. Combine harvesters suspend clouds of infective dust and create aerosols of infective blood when they accidentally crush the animals that are living among the crops.

Economic factors have resulted in dramatic changes in food animal production. Under such crowded animal conditions, rapid pathogen transmission can occur and lead to an epidemic situation. For instance, pig farms in many countries have grown recently from small family operations with fewer than 20 animals to huge facilities with thousands of animals.

Paramyxoviruses

During the 1990s three zoonotic paramyxoviruses, known to cross species barriers, have emerged from a wildlife reservoir. Hendravirus emerged in Australia in 1994 and was responsible for an outbreak of acute fatal respiratory disease that killed 14 racehorses and two humans (O'Sullivan et al., 1997). Menangle-virus was described in Australia in 1996, where it caused reproductive disorders in pigs and a flu-like disease in humans. Nipah virus emerged in Malaysia in 1998–1999 and caused a massive outbreak of a serious respiratory disease among pigs and spread to humans who were in close contact with pigs. Most patients presented with severe febrile encephalitis with a fatality rate of 40% (Wong et al., 2002). The natural reservoirs for Hendra, Menangle, and Nipah viruses are bats, in particular large fruit bats, also called flying foxes (Daszak et al., 2004).

Bat Hendra virus isolates have shown a rather conservative genetic past, as shown by sequencing studies, not having undergone major mutational changes prior to their emergence. The concurrent appearance of several bat-associated viruses implies that changes in the ecology of fruit bats, as opposed to evolution of the pathogen itself, is the likely explanation for the spillover to new hosts (Daszak et al., 2004). The ecological trigger for the Nipah virus outbreak appears to have been a complex series of alterations to the fruit bat habitat caused by human activities including agriculture, in combination with a period of drought. The fruit bat's habitat was largely replaced in peninsular Malaysia by oil palm plantations. Deforestation in Sumatra, coupled with a serious drought and fires caused by a major El Nino-event in 1997, led to significant air-pollution haze that covered large areas in Malaysia and parts of Southeast Asia. This reduced the flowering of forest trees and caused a marked decline in forest fruit production, resulting in the encroachment of bats into fruit plantations where pig farms were also maintained (Chua et al., 2002). The culling of hundreds of thousands of pigs probably stopped the Nipah virus epidemic; human-to-human transmission has not been demonstrated.

Japanese encephalitis virus

Japanese encephalitis is a zoonosis caused by a flavivirus transmitted by Culex mosquitos that breed in wet rice fields. Intensification and expansion of irrigated rice production systems over the past 20 years in south Asia and Southeast Asia have had an important impact on the disease burden. The flooding of the fields by irrigation at the start of each cropping cycle leads to an explosive buildup of the mosquito population. The virus circulates in birds with pigs as amplifying hosts. Because of the critical role of pigs, its presence in Muslim countries is negligible. The distribution of Japanese encephalitis is significantly linked to irrigated rice production combined with pig farming (www.who.int/water_sanitation_health/diseases/encephalitis/).

Movements of pathogens; travel and trade

The movements of pathogens, vectors, and animal hosts are additional factors influencing the epidemiology of viral zoonoses. Such movements can occur via human travel and trade, by natural movement of wild animals including migratory birds, and by anthropogenic movements of animals. Wherever and whenever we travel and trade, unseen microbes accompany us. The speed, volume, and extent of today's travel and trade are unprecedented in human history and offer multiple potential routes for microbial spread around the globe. For instance, viruses harbored within insects, animals, or humans can travel halfway around the globe in

<24 h by plane; zoonotic viruses can be transported to the farthest land in less time than the incubation times of most diseases.

Rabies

Movement of infected wild and domestic animals is an important factor in the appearance of rabies in new locations. Rabies virus was introduced into North America by infected dogs in the early 18th century, with subsequent spillover to a variety of wild terrestrial mammals. Rabies became established in raccoons in the Mid-Atlantic States in the late 1970s due to translocation of raccoons from the southeastern United States, where rabies was endemic in this species (Smith et al., 1984). Finland experienced an outbreak of rabies linked to raccoon dogs in 1988. The raccoon dog had spread to Finland following the release of this species in western Russia for fur trade. Rabies most probably arrived in Finland with infected wolves migrating from Russia during winter along the ice-packed coast (Sihvonen, 2003). The movement of the arctic fox across ice "bridges" between continents, from the archipelago of Spitzbergen, Norway, to Novaja Zemlja in Siberia, and from Canada to Greenland has been described (Prestrud et al., 1992; Ballard et al., 2001).

West Nile virus

WNV was first isolated from a febrile patient in Uganda in 1937. In 1941, an outbreak occurred in Tel Aviv, Israel. Despite several outbreaks in Israel, WNV was considered a minor arbovirosis in the Old World and until the early 1990s; the virus was mainly confined to Africa and parts of Europe. Mosquitos of the *Culex pipiens* genus are the principal vectors for the virus; birds are amplifying hosts for the virus but were initially considered resistant to disease. However, the occurrence of an abnormal number of deaths in some bird species in Israel in 1998 indicated that a more virulent strain had emerged.

WNV was unknown in North America until it arrived in New York in 1999, via an infected mosquito in an airplane (McMichael, 2004). Apparently there were conditions in New York that were favorable for the virus, such as: (i) seasons of early rains and summer drought that provided ideal conditions for the *Culex* mosquitos; (ii) a high population of susceptible bird species, especially crows; and (iii) urban and suburban ecosystems that were conducive to close interactions of mosquitos, birds, and humans. In 2002, WNV had dramatically expanded its geographical range in the US and caused the largest recognized epidemic of arboviral diseases affecting the CNS (causing encephalitis and meningitis) in the Western Hemisphere.

Monkeypox

During the summer of 2003, an outbreak of monkeypox occurred in the United States with 37 confirmed human cases (Reed et al., 2004). Monkeypox is a rare zoonosis, caused by a poxvirus that typically occurs in Africa. It was first found in monkeys in 1958, and later in other animals, especially rodents. The African squirrel is probably the natural host. Transmission to humans occurs by contact with infected animals or body fluids. The cases in the United States, the first outside Africa, were associated with contact with infected prairie dogs. The outbreak was epidemiologically linked to an import of African rodents from Ghana. It is most likely that infected rodents imported into the United States transmitted the virus to prairie dogs. This illustrates the fact that non-native animal species can create serious public health problems when they introduce a viral disease to native animal and human populations. Thus, the transportation, sale, or distribution of animals, or the release of animals into the environment, can contribute to the spread of zoonoses.

Avian influenza (influenza A; H5N1)

In the fall of 2005, avian influenza subtype H5N1 emerged in Europe; there were outbreaks among poultry in Turkey, Romania, and Ukraine, and in wild migratory birds in Croatia and Romania. In January 2006, the first human cases of H5N1 infection in Europe were confirmed; fatal human cases occurred in Turkey, and were associated with contact with diseased poultry (www.who.int/csr/disease/ avian_influenza/avianinfluenza_factsheetJan2006/en/index.html). It is believed that H5N1 reached Europe from Asia by means of migratory birds. Wild waterfowl are the natural reservoirs of influenza A viruses, but they usually do not get sick from them. H5N1 in its highly pathogenic form has been isolated from dead migratory birds (Liu et al., 2005). This finding may suggest a role for migratory waterfowl in the evolution and maintenance of highly pathogenic H5N1. The role of imported infected wild birds was demonstrated in October 2005, when two smuggled hawk eagles carried on a flight from Thailand to Belgium tested positive for H5N1 (WHO, 2005), and when a parrot imported from Surinam to the United Kingdom was found positive for H5N1 (www.defra.gov.uk/news/latest/2005/animal-1024.htm).

Human behavior and demographic factors

Aspects of human behavior and other demographic factors can influence the epidemiology of viral zoonoses. These include human recreational activities, such as hunting, camping, and hiking as well as eating habits and sexual habits.

Acquired immunodeficiency syndrome (AIDS)

The AIDS pandemic is probably the major example of a zoonosis that emerged in the 20th century; it entered the human population as a result of cross-species transmission of SIVs. Since the initial clinical description of AIDS 25 years ago (Gottlieb et al., 1981), about 30 million persons have died of AIDS worldwide and it is estimated that approximately 40 million people are living and infected with the etiologic agent of AIDS, Human Immunodeficiency Virus, type 1 (HIV-1). It is estimated that there are 6 million new infections per year, which means that an average of about 14,000 persons become infected per day, or 10 persons are newly infected every minute (www.WHO.int/hiv).

The two types of human HIV, HIV-1 and HIV-2, are members of the Retrovirus family and the genus *Lentivirus*. HIV-1 consists of three distinct groups (M, N, and O), with group M being responsible for the majority of HIV infections worldwide. HIV-2 is represented by six subtypes, A–F. Current molecular biological evidence indicates that the SIV counterparts of HIV-1 and HIV-2 have been transmitted into the human population on several occasions from two distinct primate sources: HIV-1 from the chimpanzee *Pan troglodytes troglodytes* (from the virus SIVcpz) and HIV-2 from the sooty mangabey monkey *Cercocebus atys* (virus SIVsm) (Gao et al., 1999; Hahn et al., 2000; Sharp et al., 2001). Since the three groups of HIV-1 (M, N, and O) genetically differ as much from each other as do different SIVcpz genomes, it is believed that they are each derived from a separate zoonotic transmission. Likewise, for HIV-2 there may have been six separate crossover events from sooty mangabeys to humans.

Although the simian lentiviruses are termed immunodeficiency viruses because of their genetic and structural similarities to the human AIDS viruses, the SIVs have not been linked to diseases in their natural hosts (Cichutek and Norley, 1993). SIV infections appear to be common and geographically widespread in African primates; in at least 31 different non-human primate species there has been evidence of SIV infection. In contrast, no Asian primate species has been reported to harbor SIV in the wild (Sharp et al., 2001); for instance, rhesus macaques do not seem to be naturally infected with SIV. However, cross-species transmission of the strain SIVsm from sooty mangabey to an "unnatural host", the macaque, results in immunosuppression and an AIDS-like disease in the macaque. SIVsm infection of macaques now serves as a valuable model for HIV disease in humans and has been used for vaccine development (Letvin, 1992) (Fig. 1).

The timing of SIVcpz cross-species transmission to humans, leading to the HIV-1 pandemic, has been evaluated using stored samples and molecular biological tools. A stored human serum sample from 1959 in Kinshasa, DRC contains the earliest laboratory-proven evidence of HIV-1 group M infection (Zhu et al., 1998). By use of the molecular clock approach, this particular chimpanzee-to-human transmission is estimated to most likely have occurred around 1930 (Korber et al., 2000).

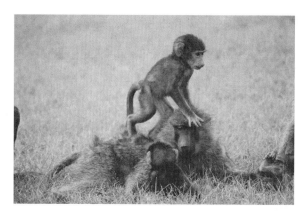

Fig. 1 Non-human primates represent the origin of many important viral zoonoses (For colour version: see Colour Section on page 347).

Group O, was not identified until 1990 and has spread to a much lesser extent than group M. However, the genetic diversity points to an origin in time similar to that of group M. The earliest stored samples shown to contain HIV-1 group O are from a Norwegian sailor and his family, all of whom died in 1976 (Froland et al., 1988; Jonassen et al., 1997). The sailor probably was infected during a visit to Africa in the early 1960s and showed symptoms of AIDS by 1966. The daughter is the first recorded case of pediatric AIDS.

HIV-1 group N seems to have arisen more recently. This is most similar to SIVcpz. The scarcity of group N infections in humans may reflect a recent transmission event or, alternatively, lack of adaptation to the new host.

Sooty mangabey monkeys are the natural host for SIVsm and are infected in the wild at apparently high frequency (Hahn et al., 2000). Sooty mangabey monkeys inhabit forests in West Africa and are often hunted for food and are also kept as pets. HIV-2 is endemic among humans in West Africa and is frequently found in patients in, or originating from, that region. SIVsm and HIV-2 sequences from animals and humans from the same immediate geographic area are most closely related, consistent with the molecular biological evidence of cross-species transmission. Although HIV-2 also is associated with immunodeficiency and development of AIDS, the progression is slower than for HIV-1. HIV-2 also is appears less easily transmitted than HIV-1, with fewer cases of mother-to-child transmission and the lack of a pandemic such as seen with HIV-1 (Pepin et al., 1991; Lemey et al., 2003). HIV-1 group M viruses have spread globally, but HIV-2 subtypes are mainly restricted to West Africa and can be categorized as epidemic subtypes (A and B) and non-epidemic subtypes (C–G).

All primates that naturally carry SIV have been in contact with humans for thousands of years. Yet, despite centuries of opportunity to emerge as infections in humans, there is no evidence to suggest that HIV existed in Africa prior to the 20th century. Moreover, the chimpanzee and the sooty mangabey hosts are not found in the same areas in Africa, but exist in widely separated, non-contiguous regions (Marx et al., 2001). To explain the almost simultaneous emergence of HIV-1 and HIV-2, occurring in different parts of Africa, Marx et al. (2001) suggested that a massive increase in unsterile medical injections may have served to increase the probability of serial transmission of partially adapted SIV infections in humans, particularly as a result of the general availability of penicillin beginning in the early 1950s. According to this theory, serial passage of partially adapted SIV between humans resulted in a cumulative series of mutations and the emergence of epidemic HIV strains.

The AIDS epidemic in Romania is a documented example of the role that unsterile injections can play in the serial transmission of HIV. Before December 1989, 13 AIDS cases were identified in Romania as reported to the WHO. By December 31, 1990, almost 1200 cases were reported, of which 94% occurred in children <13 years of age. Almost 60% of those children had acquired HIV infection from unsterilized medicinal use of needles and syringes (Hersh et al., 1991).

Human T-lymphotropic viruses

Human T-lymphotropic Virus, type 1 (HTLV-1) is associated with adult T-cell leukemia (ATL) and a variety of immune-mediated disorders, including the chronic neurological disease named HTLV-1-associated myelopathy/tropical spastic paraparesis (HAM/TSP) (Barmak et al., 2003; Proietti et al., 2005). ATL was originally described as a particular leukemia, with a striking cluster of cases in Kyushu island, Japan, in 1976, which suggested a unique etiology (Uchiyama et al., 1977). HTLV-1 was first isolated in 1979 (Poiesz et al., 1980). ATL or HAM/TSP occurs among only 1–5% of seropositive individuals. The vast majority of infected individuals remain asymptomatic virus carriers.

A few years later, a virus quite similar to HTLV-1, now called HTLV-2, was isolated from a person with T-cell "hairy cell leukemia". Despite being isolated from a patient with leukemia, there is no convincing role of HTLV-2 in human disease (Feuer and Green, 2005). HTLV-2 is endemic at a low level among the American Indian population in Brazil and among certain tribes in Africa, whereas in Europe and in the US it is mainly associated with intravenous drug abuse, still at a very low level (Alcantara et al., 2003). An interesting question is whether serial passage of this abuse, still at a very low level virus can result in cumulative mutations leading to emergence of a more pathogenic virus.

The simian counterpart of HTLV, STLV (simian T-lymphotropic virus) is endemic in many African and Asian monkeys; it can infect most Old World primate species (Watanabe et al., 1986; Slattery et al., 1999). In some instances, STLV-1 infection has been related to lymphomas and leukemias in monkeys (Sakakibara et al., 1986). STLV-1 sequences have been identified in a wild-caught gorilla and a chimpanzee in Cameroon (Nerrienet et al., 2004) that are similar to the sequence of HTLV-1 of central African subtype B, supporting the suggestion that HTLV-1 subtypes in humans have arisen from separate interspecies transmissions from STLV-1 infected monkeys (Vandamme et al., 1998).

Foamy viruses

Foamy viruses are widely distributed retroviruses and are endemic in most mammals except humans. Virtually all non-human primate species harbor distinct and species-specific clades of SFVs (Heneine et al., 2003). There is so far no clear role for foamy viruses in disease. They appear to be non-pathogenic viruses *in vivo*, in contrast to their strong cytopathic effects *in vitro* (Falcone et al., 2003). In the wild, these viruses are readily spread, most likely via biting. They can be found in all tissues as integrated DNA copies, but the replication has only been demonstrated in oral submucosal cells, which probably explains the natural route of transmission (Falcone et al., 1999).

Humans are susceptible to infection by SFV, as shown by a relatively high frequency of seropositivity (5.3%) among individuals working with primates at research centers and zoos (Switzer et al., 2004). However, all seropositive persons have been reported to be in good health even after longstanding infection (as long as 26 years, documented by an archival serum sample) and there has been no documented secondary transmission to spouses. Thus, these zoonotic infections may represent benign dead-end infections.

Bushmeat—a source for transmission of new viruses

Hunting of wildlife for food is associated with a substantial risk for cross-species transmission of new pathogens. The risk of zoonotic transmission and emergence of new zoonoses is increasing due to an increasing demand for food for the growing human population, and a globalized trade. In Africa, the forest is often referred to as "the bush", and thus, meat derived from it is often called "bushmeat". Non-human primates and other wildlife probably have been killed for food in parts of Africa for generations; it is estimated to account for 50–80% of the protein in the diet in some parts of Africa. Hunting, butchering, and eating bushmeat places people at increased risk of exposure to primate retroviruses and other zoonotic agents. Deforestation of tropical forests also contributes to increased contact with non-human primates and the consumption of bushmeat.

Since SFV is endemic in most non-human primates, the presence of SFV infection among bushmeat hunters can serve as a marker for the risk of acquiring potentially pathogenic simian retroviruses via zoonotic transmission. A study of 1099 individuals in Cameroon identified 10 persons (1%) with serologic evidence of SFV infection. Sequence analysis of samples from human lymphocytes revealed three viruses with known associations with three different non-human primates, associated with individual histories of contact with blood or body fluids from those primates, thus indicating separate zoonotic transmissions from gorilla, mandrill, and Brazza's guenon (Wolfe et al., 2004).

Two new unique HTLVs, designated HTLV-3 and HTLV-4, also have been associated with bushmeat preparation and/or consumption in rural villages in southern Cameroon (Calattini et al., 2005; Wolfe et al., 2005a). Serologic surveys of bushmeat hunters in southern Cameroon (Wolfe et al., 2005a) and among different tribes living in remote villages in the rainforest in Cameroon (Calattini et al., 2005) were performed with the aim of searching for infection of divergent HTLVs. The simian counterpart of HTLV-3, STLV-3, has been identified in wild-caught monkey species from several different ecosystems in Africa (Meertens and Gessain, 2003). So far, HTLV-3 infection has not been linked to disease and it is not known whether it is transmissible between humans. (HTLV-4 was identified in a Cameroonian bushmeat hunter (Wolfe et al., 2005a). The origin of HTLV-4 is unclear because so far no simian counterpart has been identified, although it most likely represents either an ancient or a recent transmission to humans from a non-human primate.)

The naming of HTLV-3 and HTLV-4 may need a word of caution. The strong phylogenetic relationship between the two HTLV-3 isolates and STLV-3 appears to justify calling them HTLV-3. However, the one isolate of HTLV-4 is the only known virus in a previously undescribed group; following the guidelines of the International Committee on Taxonomy of Viruses (Fauquet et al., 2004), it qualifies to be named HTLV-4. However, the term "HTLV-3" was used to refer to the virus now known as HIV-1 before the current nomenclature was agreed on (Gallo et al., 1984), and HIV-2 was referred to as "HTLV-4" during the early years after its discovery (Kanki et al., 1987; Kornfeld et al., 1987). There are thus a number of publications already describing an "HTLV-3" and an "HTLV-4" that have nothing to do with the newly discovered viruses. To avoid confusion and misunderstanding, renaming these new viruses should possibly be considered.

Microbial changes and adaptation

Cross-species infections probably occur quite frequently. However, most of them represent transient or abortive infections with no further human-to-human transmission and are thus deed-ends. Despite frequent exposure to SIV-infected monkeys in Africa only about a dozen known cross-species transmissions have occurred in the past 50 years that have resulted in significant human-to-human transmission of what are now known as HIV-1 and HIV-2. Several infections of humans by SFVs, which will not lead to further human-to-human transmission, have been documented. In the human host, the SFV remains mainly in its integrated proviral form and there is no detectable virus replication. Other zoonotic pathogens have also led to several small human epidemics with little or no evidence of human-to-human transmission. This phenomenon has been termed "viral chatter" and is probably an important mechanism in viral emergence (Wolfe et al., 2005b). High rates of viral chatter increase the diversity of virus sequence variants moving into humans and form a basis for accumulation of genetic changes that may result in adaptation to the new host.

The mechanisms that underlie cross-species transfer through host-range expansion and establishment of viruses in a new host species depend on the accumulation of genetic changes that may result in adaptation to the new host (Kilbourne, 1991). This process can occur by various mechanisms such as mutations, genetic drift, genetic shift, reassortment, and recombination. Most of the genetic changes do not result in altered proteins (silent mutations). Others may result in non-functional proteins or proteins with slightly altered properties that may allow the virus to adapt to a new milieu.

Mutations can occur in the genomes of both RNA and DNA viruses. However, because the genomes in RNA viruses are replicated by RNA polymerases that lack the proofreading function of many DNA polymerases, mistakes made by the polymerase during replication will not be corrected. Mutations can therefore occur much more frequently in RNA viruses than in DNA viruses. As a consequence, RNA viruses generally evolve more rapidly and lead to genetic heterogeneity, which can be seen as the presence of viral quasispecies. This means that, in the infected individual, the virus exists as a population of genetically related but divergent variants, of which the most common variant is a "master sequence". While the master sequence remains the dominant one, the spectrum of mutants may shift in response to selective pressure and any variant may be selectively expanded (Domingo and Holland, 1997). The importance of quasispecies was first recognized in infections with HIV-1 (Meyerhans et al., 1989).

Accumulation of point mutations is regarded as a major mechanism driving the adaptation of viruses to new hosts. However, evolution of the virus also can occur through recombination, leading to the exchange of parts of genomes. For recombination to take place, it is necessary that the cell be co-infected by two different virus variants.

Influenza A

Genetic changes typically influence the epidemiology of influenza viruses. Surveillance and characterization of the circulating strains are important in determining whether an available influenza vaccine will give protection or not. Influenza viruses are classified into types A, B, and C, of which types B and C are specific to humans, whereas type A viruses can have different hosts, both birds and different mammals including humans. There are only three A subtypes of influenza viruses (H1N1, H1N2, and H3N2) known to be currently circulating among humans as seasonal influenza. The seasonal influenza epidemics occur as a result of genetic drift, the accumulation of point mutations that occur due to lack of proofreading (Webster et al., 1992). Antigenic shift, an abrupt change in the hemagglutinin and/or the neuraminidase proteins of the virus, causes the sudden emergence of a new subtype of a type A virus that is antigenically distinct from former circulating influenza A viruses. The new virus is potentially capable of causing an epidemic in an immunologically naïve human population (Webster et al., 1992). Worldwide epidemics, called pandemics, occur only occasionally.

Avian influenza A viruses have caused occasional human infections since 1997. Most incidents have occurred in Asia (H5N1 yearly since 2003), in January 2006 in Turkey (H5N1), in the Netherlands in 2003 (H7N7), and a few instances in Canada in 2004 (H7N3), and in the US in 2002 (H7N2). To date, human infections with avian influenza A have not resulted in sustained human-to-human transmissions, although in certain instances transmission to family members cannot be ruled out (www.cdc.gov/flu/avian/gen-info/avian-flu-humans).

Of the avian influenza A variants infecting humans during the last decade, the 1997 Hong Kong H5N1 epidemic involved the most pathogenic variant. Analysis of the virus genome revealed that a reassorted virus entirely of avian origin had crossed the species barrier without adaptation to a mammalian host (Hatta and Kawaoka, 2002). There is evidence that H5N1 is now endemic in parts of Asia, having established a permanent ecological niche in poultry. As of January 2006, H5N1 has spread to Europe, with outbreaks among wild birds (Croatia and Romania), poultry (Turkey, Romania, and Ukraine), and humans (Turkey). Genomic analyses of H5N1 virus isolates from birds and humans show that the hemagglutinin has undergone significant antigenic drift since 1997 (Horimoto et al., 2004). Moreover, evidence further suggests that H5N1 is expanding its mammalian host range in that an outbreak was documented among captive tigers in Thailand (Keawcharoen et al., 2004).

SARS coronavirus

The severe acute respiratory syndrome coronavirus (SARS-CoV), the agent of SARS, emerged as a new cross-species transmission event in Guandong province, China, in 2002 and caused a serious epidemic in 2003, spreading to a number of other countries. Beijing experienced the largest SARS outbreak, with more than 2000 cases and a close to 10% fatality rate (Liu, 2005). Through a remarkable effort, the infectious agent was rapidly identified.

Coronaviruses closely related to SARS-CoV were discovered in several wild animal species and in live animal markets in Guandong. SARS-CoV isolated from patients during the 2002–2003 epidemic and from sporadic cases in 2003 and 2004 appears to be derived from a nearly identical virus in palm civets and raccoon dogs (Guan et al., 2003) (Fig. 2).

Sequencing of hundreds of SARS virus genomes from humans and animals have identified mutations in the receptor-binding domain (RBD) that distinguish the species-specific strains (Song et al., 2005). (The RBD of coronaviruses is located in the spike protein (S). Trimers of the S-protein bind to the specific cellular receptor, which for the SARS virus is angiotensin-converting enzyme 2 (ACE2); Prabakaran et al., 2004.) Only four amino acids differ between the human and the civet strains, but the human viral S-protein binds the human receptor 1000–10, 000 times more tightly than does its civet S-protein counterpart. The intimate interface between a loop of the S-protein of viruses from the SARS epidemic in 2002–2003 and human ACE2 mediates efficient binding and infection of the cell, which

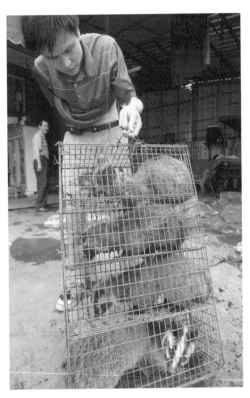

Fig. 2 Animal markets represent a risk factor for transmission of various viral zoonoses, e.g. SARS. *Source*: Reuters/SCANPIX. (For colour version: see Colour Section on page 347).

probably is a key factor in determining the severity and possibly human-to-human transmission (Li F. et al., 2005). In contrast, S-protein from viruses of sporadic SARS cases in 2003 and 2004, each of which was an independent cross-species event with no further human-to-human transmission, had amino acids that more closely resembled the civet virus. The outcome was a reduced binding to human ACE2 and less efficient infection. Epidemiological investigation of the 2003 and 2004 SARS cases showed that SARS-CoV-positive palm civets, kept alive in cages close to the customers while waiting to be prepared as dinners in a restaurant, were the source for transmission to a waitress working in the restaurant and to a customer eating there (Wang M. et al., 2005).

In addition to mutations in the S-protein that resulted in high-affinity binding to the human receptor, molecular epidemiology and phylogenetic studies have identified a series of mutations in the so-called 5-locus motif (Liu, 2005). The mutations that occurred at different times in two geographically separate locations in China suggest a dominant process occurring during viral adaptation to the human host. The mutations observed in Beijing followed the same molecular path as isolates from Guandong and from the epidemic outside China, i.e. an early GACTC motif was followed by transition to GGCTC motif before appearance of the stable TGTTT motif.

The SIVcpz recombination

The origin of the HIV-1 pandemic has been traced to the SIVcpz virus of chimpanzees (identified in two chimpanzee subspecies, *P. troglodytes troglodytes* and *P. troglodyte schweinfurthii,* but not in the third species, *P. troglodytes verus*). Species-specific strains of SIV (like SIVsm and SIVagm) have been identified in more than 30 African primate species, but all except SIVcpz infect monkeys. SIVs seem to be non-pathogenic in the vast majority of natural hosts despite high levels of virus replication (Apetrei et al., 2004). This may be a consequence of the fact that the incubation period of the disease generally exceeds the life span of the host. SIVs also have a high propensity for cross-species transmission. SIV phylogeny is complex and analyses indicate recombination among viruses from different major lineages. Of the identified recombinants, SIVcpz so far represents the most important one, being the source of the HIV-1 pandemic. SIVrcm from red-capped mangabeys and SIVgsn from greater spot-nosed monkeys are most closely related to SIVcpz, but they are similar only in certain regions of the genome that do not overlap. Extensive phylogenetic analyses of subsets of SIV strains comparing the topologies among four regions of the proteome have provided evidence for a more recent origin of SIVcpz than of other strains, being a result of recombination between ancestors of SIVgsn and SIVrcm (Bailes et al., 2003). The geographic region of these two monkey species overlaps that of the chimpanzee and it is known that chimpanzees hunt smaller monkeys for food. The founder chimpanzee most likely was infected by one of the ancestor SIVs and thereafter became superinfected by the other ancestor virus, leading to recombination in a doubly infected cell.

The hybrid origin of SIVcpz, in contrast to SIVsm (from which HIV-2 is derived), has several important implications. First, it provides evidence that, in addition to humans, another primate species can acquire cross-species transmission under natural conditions. Second, the hybrid virus had adapted to the host and established substantial secondary spread within the species. Third, the chimpanzee virus was capable of spreading to humans. Moreover, the chimpanzee most likely acquired SIV-infection relatively recently, subsequent to the split of the chimpanzee into two subspecies, since SIVcpz has not been found in the third chimpanzee subspecies, *P. troglodytes verus.*

Retrovirus superinfection and recombination—potential emergence of new viruses

Two biological properties of retroviruses make them particularly likely candidates for the generation of new emerging viruses. One is the integration of the reversely transcribed provirus into the cellular genome, causing a life-long infection. Another is the potential for superinfection, in which recombination may occur when a cell becomes infected with two genetically distinct viruses. During reverse transcription, the reverse transcriptase can switch from one RNA template to the other, thereby generating a progeny that is a mosaic of the parent viruses (Preston et al., 1988). HIV-1 genomes with this kind of mosaic structure are called circulating recombinant forms (CRFs). There are an increasing number of such CRFs identified; CRF 01_AE is mainly responsible for the HIV epidemic in Southeast Asia (Takebe et al., 2003; Watanaveeradej et al., 2003). These CRFs now constitute 10–20% of newly characterized circulating strains (Perrin et al., 2003).

The recent cross-species transmission of retroviruses like SFV and the recognition of two new HTLV retroviruses (HTLV-3 and HTLV-4) open wider possibilities of superinfection. Concomitant HIV-1 and HIV-2 infections have been documented in Africa, India, and Greece (Georgoulias et al., 1988; Rubsamen-Waigmann et al., 1994; Esteves et al., 2000). However, recombination between HIV-1 and HIV-2 has not been reported so far. Although recombination frequently takes place in HIV-1, certain genetic barriers may exist to recombination with HIV-2 or other retroviruses such as SFV, HTLV, etc.

Prevention and control

Efficient and cost-effective prevention and control of viral zoonoses necessitates an understanding of the nature of zoonoses and their ecology. The emergence of a new viral zoonosis and its further development into a pandemic can be conceptualized as a series of steps leading from initial contact to global spread and depends largely on three factors: (1) The prevalence of a potential zoonotic virus in animal populations and the frequency of human contact with these animal reservoirs. (2) Successful transmission of the zoonotic virus from the animal reservoir to humans, establishment of a productive infection in humans, and further direct transmission between humans. (3) The movement of the zoonotic virus into the global population.

The prevention and control of viral zoonoses share many common aspects, but in all cases the animal reservoir must be considered in the risk-analysis framework. It is thus important to integrate medical, veterinary, ecological, and other sciences in interdisciplinary teams (Daszak et al., 2004, FAO, WHO, and OIE, 2004). The role of bats in the etiology of many viral zoonoses illustrates the challenges of prevention and control (Dobson, 2005). Bats represent a reservoir of rabies, Hendra, Menangle, and Nipah viruses. Furthermore, there is strong evidence that bats may be the wildlife reservoir of Ebola virus and one of the reservoirs of SARS-CoV (Leroy et al., 2005; Li W. et al., 2005). Although SARS-CoV isolated from humans appeared to derive from a nearly identical virus circulating in masked palm civets and racoon dogs (Guan et al., 2003; Song et al., 2005), subsequent studies did not reveal widespread infection in wild or farmed civets, and experimental infection of civets with human SARS-CoV resulted in overt clinical symptoms suggesting that they are not the reservoir. A recent large study of different bat species from four locations in China showed a high prevalence and wide distribution of SARS-CoV-seropositive bats (Lau et al., 2005; Li W. et al., 2005). Although horseshoe bats appear to be the natural reservoir of a SARS-like corona virus (SL-CoV), it is not clear how this virus could have got from the bat or another reservoir to humans. The human and civet isolates of SARS-CoV are phylogenetically located within the spectrum of these SL-CoVs. One possibility is that bats passed the virus to civets or to other animals in the wild or in the live animal markets of southern China.

In the wild, bats can transmit viruses to other species from the fruit they spit out after extracting the juice and sugars. This could explain how gorillas and chimpanzees might acquire Ebola virus during seasonal fruiting events when bats and primates feed among the same fruit-bearing trees. In the near future, zoonotic transmission of viruses from bats to humans must be given greater attention.

In order to increase the capability of recognizing viral zoonoses, there is a need for better national surveillance systems both in humans and animals, and better international sharing of information from such surveillance systems. Improved notification systems and screening programs for human infections, including the application of syndromic surveillance, are warranted in order to detect new and emerging zoonoses. Efficient surveillance is dependent upon a laboratory system that is capable of identifying and characterizing the pathogens in question. More research is needed to understand better the epidemiology and pathogenesis of various zoonoses, to improve diagnostic methods, and to develop cost-effective vaccines and drugs. Training and education are prerequisites in order to enable the personnel involved at the various stages, from field to laboratory personnel, to detect zoonoses. Information and communication are key components in any prevention and control strategy, and this should also involve the general public. The importance of public education and behavioral change are critical factors for successful intervention. The implementation of restrictions of animal movements caused by human activity is another important preventive measure. For vector-borne zoonoses, vector control should be an integral part of any intervention strategy.

Interdisciplinary and international collaboration are crucial for the rapid identification and effective management of viral zoonoses. The pivotal role of international organizations such as the World Health Organization, the Food and Agricultural Organization, and the Office International des Epizooties is exemplified by the response to the current avian influenza outbreak in Asia and Europe. Containment of viral zoonoses relies on efficient national, regional, and international cross-sectional networks to improve data sharing and enable a timely and effective response to disease outbreaks.

References

Alcantara LC, Shindo N, Van Dooren S, Salemi M, Costa MC, Kashima S, Covas DT, Vandamme AM, Galvao-Castro B. Brazilian HTLV type 2a strains from intravenous drug users (IDUs) appear to have originated from two sources: Brazilian Amerindians and European/North American IDUs. AIDS Res Hum Retroviruses 2003; 19: 519.

Apetrei C, Robertson DL, Marx PA. The history of SIVS and AIDS: epidemiology, phylogeny and biology of isolates from naturally SIV infected non-human primates (NHP) in Africa. Front Biosci 2004; 9: 225.

Bailes E, Gao F, Bibollet-Ruche F, Courgnaud V, Peeters M, Marx PA, Hahn BH, Sharp PM. Hybrid origin of SIV in chimpanzees. Science 2003; 300: 1713.

Ballard WB, Follmann EH, Ritter DG, Robards MD, Cronin MA. Rabies and canine distemper in an arctic fox population in Alaska. J Wildl Dis 2001; 37: 133.

Barmak K, Harhaj E, Grant C, Alefantis T, Wigdahl B. Human T cell leukemia virus type I-induced disease: pathways to cancer and neurodegeneration. Virology 2003; 308: 1.

Blancou J. History of the Surveillance and Control of Transmissible Animal Diseases. Paris: Office International des Epizooties; 2003; p. 362.

Calattini S, Chevalier SA, Duprez R, Bassot S, Froment A, Mahieux R, Gessain A. Discovery of a new human T-cell lymphotropic virus (HTLV-3) in Central Africa. Retrovirology 2005; 2: 30.

Chua KB, Chua BH, Wang CW. Anthropogenic deforestation, El Nino and the emergence of Nipah virus in Malaysia. Malays J Pathol 2002; 24: 15.

Cichutek K, Norley S. Lack of immune suppression in SIV-infected natural hosts. AIDS 1993(Suppl 1): S25.

Daszak P, Tabor GM, Kilpatrick AM, Epstein J, Plowright R. Conservation medicine and a new agenda for emerging diseases. Ann N Y Acad Sci 2004; 1026: 1.

Dobson AP. Virology. What links bats to emerging infectious diseases? Science 2005; 310: 628.

Domingo E, Holland JJ. RNA virus mutations and fitness for survival. Annu Rev Microbiol 1997; 51: 151.

Esteves A, Parreira R, Piedade J, Venenno T, Canas-Ferreira WF. Genetic characterization of HIV type 1 and type 2 from Bissau, Guinea-Bissau (West Africa). Virus Res 2000; 68: 51.

Falcone V, Leupold J, Clotten J, Urbanyi E, Herchenroder O, Spatz W, Volk B, Bohm N, Toniolo A, Neumann-Haefelin D, Schweizer M. Sites of simian foamy virus persistence in naturally infected African green monkeys: latent provirus is ubiquitous, whereas viral replication is restricted to the oral mucosa. Virology 1999; 257: 7.

Falcone V, Schweizer M, Neumann-Haefelin D. Replication of primate foamy viruses in natural and experimental hosts. Curr Top Microbiol Immunol 2003; 277: 161.

FAO, WHO, and OIE. Report of the FAO/WHO/OIE Joint Consultation on Emerging Zoonotic Diseases in Collaboration with the Health Council of the Netherlands. Geneva, Switzerland; 2004.

Fauquet CM, Mayo MA, Maniloff J, Desselberger U, Ball LA. Virus Taxonomy, Seventh Report on the International Committee on Taxonomy of Viruses. London: Elsevier; 2004; p. 421.

Feuer G, Green PL. Comparative biology of human T-cell lymphotropic virus type 1 (HTLV-1) and HTLV-2. Oncogene 2005; 24: 5996.

Froland SS, Jenum P, Lindboe CF, Wefring KW, Linnestad PJ, Bohmer T. HIV-1 infection in Norwegian family before 1970. Lancet 1988; 1: 1344.

Gallo RC, Salahuddin SZ, Popovic M, Shearer GM, Kaplan M, Haynes BF, Palker TJ, Redfield R, Oleske J, Safai B. Frequent detection and isolation of cytopathic retroviruses (HTLV-III) from patients with AIDS and at risk for AIDS. Science 1984; 224: 500.

Gao F, Bailes E, Robertson DL, Chen Y, Rodenburg CM, Michael SF, Cummins LB, Arthur LO, Peeters M, Shaw GM, Sharp PM, Hahn BH. Origin of HIV-1 in the chimpanzee *Pan troglodytes troglodytes*. Nature 1999; 397: 436.

Georgoulias V, Fountouli D, Karvela-Agelakis A, Komis G, Malliarakis-Pinetidou E, Antoniadis G, Samakidis K, Kondakis X, Papapetropoulou M, Zoumbos N. HIV-1 and HIV-2 double infection in Greece. Ann Intern Med 1988; 108: 155.

Gottlieb MS, Schroff R, Schanker HM, Weisman JD, Fan PT, Wolf RA, Saxon A. *Pneumocystis carinii* pneumonia and mucosal candidiasis in previously healthy homosexual men: evidence of a new acquired cellular immunodeficiency. N Engl J Med 1981; 305: 1425.

Guan Y, Zheng BJ, He YQ, Liu XL, Zhuang ZX, Cheung CL, Luo SW, Li PH, Zhang LJ, Guan YJ, Butt KM, Wong KL, Chan KW, Lim W, Shortridge KF, Yuen KY, Peiris JS, Poon LL. Isolation and characterization of viruses related to the SARS coronavirus from animals in southern China. Science 2003; 302: 276.

Gubler DJ. Resurgent vector-borne diseases as a global health problem. Emerg Infect Dis 1998; 4: 442.

Hahn BH, Shaw GM, De Cock KM, Sharp PM. AIDS as a zoonosis: scientific and public health implications. Science 2000; 287: 607.

Hatta M, Kawaoka Y. The continued pandemic threat posed by avian influenza viruses in Hong Kong. Trends Microbiol 2002; 10: 340.

Heneine W, Schweizer M, Sandstrom P, Folks T. Human infection with foamy viruses. Curr Top Microbiol Immunol 2003; 277: 181.

Hersh BS, Popovici F, Apetrei RC, Zolotusca L, Beldescu N, Calomfirescu A, Jezek Z, Oxtoby MJ, Gromyko A, Heymann DL. Acquired immunodeficiency syndrome in Romania. Lancet 1991; 338: 645.

Horimoto T, Fukuda N, Iwatsuki-Horimoto K, Guan Y, Lim W, Peiris M, Sugii S, Odagiri T, Tashiro M, Kawaoka Y. Antigenic differences between H5N1 human influenza viruses isolated in 1997 and 2003. J Vet Med Sci 2004; 66: 303.

Hubálek Z. Emerging human infectious diseases: anthroponoses, zoonoses, and sapronoses. Emerg Infect Dis 2003; 9: 403.

Jonassen TO, Stene-Johansen K, Berg ES, Hungnes O, Lindboe CF, Froland SS, Grinde B. Sequence analysis of HIV-1 group O from Norwegian patients infected in the 1960s. Virology 1997; 231: 43.

Kanki PJ, Hopper JR, Essex M. The origins of HIV-1 and HTLV-4/HIV-2. Ann N Y Acad Sci 1987; 511: 370.

Keawcharoen J, Oraveerakul K, Kuiken T, Fouchier RA, Amonsin A, Payungporn S, Noppornpanth S, Wattanodorn S, Theamboonlers A, Tantilertcharoen R, Pattanarangsan R, Arya N, Ratanakorn P, Osterhaus DM, Poovorawan Y. Avian influenza H5N1 in tigers and leopards. Emerg Infect Dis 2004; 10: 2189.

Kilbourne ED. New viruses and new disease: mutation, evolution and ecology. Curr Opin Immunol 1991; 3: 518.

Korber B, Muldoon M, Theiler J, Gao F, Gupta R, Lapedes A, Hahn BH, Wolinsky S, Bhattacharya T. Timing the ancestor of the HIV-1 pandemic strains. Science 2000; 288: 1789.

Kornfeld H, Riedel N, Viglianti GA, Hirsch V, Mullins JI. Cloning of HTLV-4 and its relation to simian and human immunodeficiency viruses. Nature 1987; 326: 610.

Lau SK, Woo PC, Li KS, Huang Y, Tsoi HW, Wong BH, Wong SS, Leung SY, Chan KH, Yuen KY. Severe acute respiratory syndrome coronavirus-like virus in Chinese horseshoe bats. Proc Natl Acad Sci USA 2005; 102: 14040.

Lederberg J, Shope RE, Oaks SC, editors. Emerging Infections: Microbial Threats to Human Health in the United States. Washington, DC: National Academies Press; 1992.

Lemey P, Pybus OG, Wang B, Saksena NK, Salemi M, Vandamme AM. Tracing the origin and history of the HIV-2 epidemic. Proc Natl Acad Sci USA 2003; 100: 6588.

Leroy EM, Kumulungui B, Pourrut X, Rouquet P, Hassanin A, Yaba P, Delicat A, Paweska JT, Gonzalez JP, Swanepoel R. Fruit bats as reservoirs of Ebola virus. Nature 2005; 438: 575.

Letvin NL. Animal models for the study of human immunodeficiency virus infections. Curr Opin Immunol 1992; 4: 481.

Li F, Li W, Farzan M, Harrison SC. Structure of SARS coronavirus spike receptor-binding domain complexed with receptor. Science 2005; 309: 1864.

Li W, Shi Z, Yu M, Ren W, Smith C, Epstein JH, et al. Bats are natural reservoirs of SARS-like coronaviruses. Science 2005; 310: 676.

Lindgren E, Gustafson R. Tick-borne encephalitis in Sweden and climate change. Lancet 2001; 358: 16.

Liu J, Xiao H, Lei F, Zhu Q, Qin K, Zhang XW, Zhang XL, Zhao D, Wang G, Feng Y, Ma J, Liu W, Wang J, Gao GF. Highly pathogenic H5N1 influenza virus infection in migratory birds. Science 2005; 309: 1206.

Liu W, Tang F, Fontanet A, Zhan L, Wang TB, Zhang PH, Luan YH, Cao CY, Qiu-Min Zhao QM, Wu XM, Xin ZT, Zuo SQ, Baril L, Vabret A, Shao YM, Yang H, Cao WC. Molecular Epidemiology of SARS-associated Coronavirus. Beijing. Emerg. Infect. Dis. 2005; 11: 1420.

Marr JS, Calisher CH. Alexander the Great and West Nile Virus encephalitis. Emerg Infect Dis 2003; 9: 1599.

Marx PA, Alcabes PG, Drucker E. Serial human passage of simian immunodeficiency virus by unsterile injections and the emergence of epidemic human immunodeficiency virus in Africa. Philos Trans R Soc Lond B Biol Sci 2001; 356: 911.

McMichael AJ. Environmental and social influences on emerging infectious diseases: past, present and future. Philos Trans R Soc Lond B Biol Sci 2004; 359: 1049.

Meertens L, Gessain A. Divergent simian T-cell lymphotropic virus type 3 (STLV-3) in wild-caught *Papio hamadryas papio* from Senegal: widespread distribution of STLV-3 in Africa. J Virol 2003; 77: 782.

Meyerhans A, Cheynier R, Albert J, Seth M, Kwok S, Sninsky J, Morfeldt-Manson L, Asjo B, Wain-Hobson S. Temporal fluctuations in HIV quasispecies *in vivo* are not reflected by sequential HIV isolations. Cell 1989; 58: 901.

Murphy FA. Emerging zoonoses. Emerg Infect Dis 1998; 4: 429.

Nerrienet E, Meertens L, Kfutwah A, Foupouapouognigni Y, Ayouba A, Gessain A. Simian T cell leukaemia virus type I subtype B in a wild-caught gorilla (*Gorilla gorilla gorilla*) and chimpanzee (*Pan troglodytes vellerosus*) from Cameroon. J Gen Virol 2004; 85: 25.

Niklasson B, Le Duc J. Isolation of the nephropathia epidemica agent in Sweden. Lancet 1984; 1: 1012.

O'Sullivan JD, Allworth AM, Paterson DL, Snow TM, Boots R, Gleeson LJ, Gould AR, Hyatt AD, Bradfield J. Fatal encephalitis due to novel paramyxovirus transmitted from horses. Lancet 1997; 349: 93.

Pepin J, Morgan G, Dunn D, Gevao S, Mendy M, Gaye I, Scollen N, Tedder R, Whittle H. HIV-2-induced immunosuppression among asymptomatic West African prostitutes: evidence that HIV-2 is pathogenic, but less so than HIV-1. AIDS 1991; 5: 1165.

Perrin L, Kaiser L, Yerly S. Travel and the spread of HIV-1 genetic variants. Lancet Infect Dis 2003; 3: 22.

Poiesz BJ, Ruscetti FW, Gazdar AF, Bunn PA, Minna JD, Gallo RC. Detection and isolation of type C retrovirus particles from fresh and cultured lymphocytes of a patient with cutaneous T-cell lymphoma. Proc Natl Acad Sci USA 1980; 77: 7415.

Prabakaran P, Xiao X, Dimitrov DS. A model of the ACE2 structure and function as a SARS-CoV receptor. Biochem Biophys Res Commun 2004; 314: 235.

Preston BD, Poiesz BJ, Loeb LA. Fidelity of HIV-1 reverse transcriptase. Science 1988; 242: 1168.

Prestrud P, Krogsrud J, Gjertz I. The occurrence of rabies in the Svalbard islands of Norway. J Wildl Dis 1992; 28: 57.

Proietti FA, Carneiro-Proietti AB, Catalan-Soares BC, Murphy EL. Global epidemiology of HTLV-I infection and associated diseases. Oncogene 2005; 24: 6058.

Reed KD, Melski JW, Graham MB, Regnery RL, Sotir MJ, Wegner MV, Kazmierczak JJ, Stratman EJ, Li Y, Fairley JA, Swain GR, Olson VA, Sargent EK, Kehl SC, Frace MA, Kline R, Foldy SL, Davis JP, Damon IK. The detection of monkeypox in humans in the western hemisphere. N Engl J Med 2004; 350: 342.

Rubsamen-Waigmann H, Maniar J, Gerte S, Brede HD, Dietrich U, Mahambre G, Pfutzner A. High proportion of HIV-2 and HIV-1/2 double-reactive sera in two Indian states, Maharashtra and Goa: first appearance of an HIV-2 epidemic along with an HIV-1 epidemic outside of Africa. Zentralbl Bakteriol 1994; 280: 398.

Sakakibara I, Sugimoto Y, Sasagawa A, Honjo S, Tsujimoto H, Nakamura H, Hayami M. Spontaneous malignant lymphoma in an African green monkey naturally infected with simian T-lymphotropic virus (STLV). J Med Primatol 1986; 15: 311.

Schmaljohn C, Hjelle B. Hantaviruses: a global disease problem. Epidemiol Infect 1997; 3: 95.

Sharp PM, Bailes E, Chaudhuri RR, Rodenburg CM, Santiago MO, Hahn BH. The origins of acquired immune deficiency syndrome viruses: where and when? Philos Trans R Soc Lond B Biol Sci 2001; 356: 867.

Sihvonen L. Documenting freedom from rabies and minimising the risk of rabies being reintroduced to Finland. Rabies Bull Eur 2003; 27: 5.

Slattery JP, Franchini G, Gessain A. Genomic evolution, patterns of global dissemination, and interspecies transmission of human and simian T-cell leukemia/lymphotropic viruses. Genome Res 1999; 9: 525.

Smith JS, Sumner JW, Roumillat LF, Baer GM, Winkler WG. Antigenic characteristics of isolates associated with a new epizootic of raccoon rabies in the U.S. J Infect Dis 1984; 149: 769.

Song HD, Tu CC, Zhang GW, Wang SY, Zheng K, Lei LC, Chen QX, Gao YW, Zhou HQ, Xiang H, Zheng HJ, Chern SW, Cheng F, Pan CM, Xuan H, Chen SJ, Luo HM, Zhou DH, Liu YF, He JF, Qin PZ, Li LH, Ren YQ, Liang WJ, Yu YD, Anderson L, Wang M, Xu RH, Wu XW, Zheng HY, Chen JD, Liang G, Gao Y, Liao M, Fang L, Jiang LY, Li H, Chen F, Di B, He LJ, Lin JY, Tong S, Kong X, Du L, Hao P, Tang H, Bernini A, Yu XJ, Spiga O, Guo ZM, Pan HY, He WZ, Manuguerra JC, Fontanet A, Danchin A, Niccolai N, Li YX, Wu CI, Zhao GP. Cross-host evolution of severe acute respiratory syndrome coronavirus in palm civet and human. Proc Natl Acad Sci USA 2005; 102: 2430.

Switzer WM, Bhullar V, Shanmugam V, Cong ME, Parekh B, Lerche NW, Yee JL, Ely JJ, Boneva R, Chapman LE, Folks TM, Heneine W. Frequent simian foamy virus infection in persons occupationally exposed to nonhuman primates. J Virol 2004; 78: 2780.

Takebe Y, Motomura K, Tatsumi M, Lwin HH, Zaw M, Kusagawa S. High prevalence of diverse forms of HIV-1 intersubtype recombinants in Central Myanmar: geographical hot spot of extensive recombination. AIDS 2003; 17(14): 2077.

Taubenberger JK, Morens DM. 1918 influenza: the mother of all pandemics. Emerg Infect Dis 2006; 12: 15.

Taylor LH, Latham SM, Woolhouse ME. Risk factors for human disease emergence. Philos Trans R Soc Lond B Biol Sci 2001; 356: 983.

Tei S, Kitajima N, Takahashi K, Mishiro S. Zoonotic transmission of hepatitis E virus from deer to human beings. Lancet 2003; 362: 371.

Uchiyama T, Yodoi J, Sagawa K, Takatsuki K, Uchino H. Adult T-cell leukemia: clinical and hematologic features of 16 cases. Blood 1977; 50: 481.

Vandamme AM, Salemi M, Desmyter J. The simian origins of the pathogenic human T-cell lymphotropic virus type I. Trends Microbiol 1998; 6: 477.

Wang M, Yan M, Xu H, Liang W, Kan B, Zheng B, Chen H, Zheng H, Xu Y, Zhang E, Wang H, Ye J, Li G, Li M, Cui Z, Liu YF, Guo RT, Liu XN, Zhan LH, Zhou DH, Zhao A, Hai R, Yu D, Guan Y, Xu J. SARS-CoV infection in a restaurant from Palm Civet. Emerg Infect Dis 2005; 11: 1860.

Wang Q-H, Han MG, Cheetham S, Souza M, Funk JA, Saif LJ. Porcine noroviruses related to human noroviruses. Emerg Infect Dis 2005; 11: 1874.

Ward MA, Burgess NR. *Aedes albopictus*—a new disease vector for Europe? J R Army Med Corps 1993; 139: 109.

Watanabe T, Seiki M, Hirayama Y, Yoshida M. Human T-cell leukemia virus type I is a member of the African subtype of simian viruses (STLV). Virology 1986; 148: 385.

Watanaveeradej V, DeSouza MS, Benenson MW, Sirisopana N, Nitayaphan S, Chanbancherd P, Brown AE, Sanders-Buell E, Birx DL, McCutchan FE, Carr JK. Subtype C/CRF01_AE recombinant HIV-1 found in Thailand. AIDS 2003; 17: 2138.

Webster RG, Bean WJ, Gorman OT, Chambers TM, Kawaoka Y. Evolution and ecology of influenza A viruses. Microbiol Rev 1992; 56: 152.

WHO. Ebola Haemorrhagic Fever. Fact Sheet No. 103. http://www.who.int//inf-fs/en/fact103.html2000.

WHO. Avian Influenza: Assessing the Pandemic Threat. http://www.who.int/entity/csr/disease/influenza/H5N1-9reduit.pdf2005.

WHO/FAO. Second Report of the Joint WHO/FAO Expert Committee on Zoonoses. WHO Technical Report Series No. 169. Geneva: WHO; 1959.

Wolfe ND, Daszak P, Kilpatrick AM, Burke DS. Bushmeat hunting, deforestation, and prediction of zoonotic disease. Emerg Infect Dis 2005b; 11: 1822.

Wolfe ND, Heneine W, Carr JK, Garcia AD, Shanmugam V, Tamoufe U, Torimiro JN, Prosser AT, Lebreton M, Mpoudi-Ngole E, McCutchan FE, Birx DL, Folks TM, Burke DS, Switzer WM. Emergence of unique primate T-lymphotropic viruses among central African bushmeat hunters. Proc Natl Acad Sci USA 2005a; 102(22): 7994.

Wolfe ND, Switzer WM, Carr JK, Bhullar VB, Shanmugam V, Tamoufe U, Prosser AT, Torimiro JN, Wright A, Mpoudi-Ngole E, McCutchan FE, Birx DL, Folks TM, Burke

DS, Heneine W. Naturally acquired simian retrovirus infections in central African hunters. Lancet 2004; 363: 932.

Wong KT, Shieh WJ, Kumar S, Norain K, Abdullah W, Guarner J, Goldsmith CS, Chua KB, Lam SK, Tan CT, Goh KJ, Chong HT, Jusoh R, Rollin PE, Ksiazek TG, Zaki SR, Nipah Virus Pathology Working Group. Nipah virus infection: pathology and pathogenesis of an emerging paramyxoviral zoonosis. Am J Pathol 2002; 161: 2153.

Zhu T, Korber BT, Nahmias AJ, Hooper E, Sharp PM, Ho DD. An African HIV-1 sequence from 1959 and implications for the origin of the epidemic. Nature 1998; 391: 594.

Emerging Viruses in Human Populations
Edward Tabor (Editor)
© 2007 Elsevier B.V. All rights reserved
DOI 10.1016/S0168-7069(06)16004-8

Severe Acute Respiratory Syndrome Coronavirus (SARS-CoV)

Tommy R. Tong

Department of Pathology, Princess Margaret Hospital, Laichikok, Kowloon, Hong Kong, China

Severe acute respiratory syndrome (SARS) caused by a coronavirus (CoV), SARS-CoV, emerged into human populations in south China (Anon., 2003d; Peiris et al., 2003b,c; Poon et al., 2004a) from bats (Guan et al., 2003; Kan et al., 2005; Lau et al., 2005; Li et al., 2005d; Normile, 2005) in late 2002. Subsequently, SARS-CoV that had adapted to humans caused an epidemic in 29 countries and regions to which it had been carried by airline passengers. The epidemic was controlled by public health measures coordinated by the WHO and on July 5, 2003 it was officially declared to have ended. Because of these public health measures, a pandemic was averted (Enserink, 2003b). Close to 10% of the 8000 persons infected in this epidemic died. Molecular studies dissected the adaptation of this virus as it jumped from an intermediary animal, the civet, to humans, giving us valuable insights into processes of molecular emergence. Global research efforts are continuing to increase our understanding of the virus, the pathogenesis of the disease it causes (SARS), the "heterogeneity of individual infectiousness" (described below) as well as shedding light on how to prepare for other emerging viral diseases. Promising drugs and vaccines have been identified. The milestones achieved have resulted from a truly international effort.

The beginning of the epidemic and the identification of SARS-CoV

The epidemic began in Guangdong province, China, in late 2002. It spread to Hong Kong on February 21, 2003, and from there to other parts of the world. A week later, Carlo Urbani (Reilley et al., 2003), an Italian infectious disease expert working in the Hanoi, Vietnam, office of the WHO, responded to a possible avian influenza alert from French Hospital. That action by one man set into motion the engagement of the WHO, emergency measures by the Vietnamese government, and eventually the attention of the world. In Geneva, WHO team member Klaus Stöhr

(Stafford, 2005) put together and maintained a network of 11 microbiology laboratories in nine countries to respond to the epidemic and to identify the etiologic agent (Anon., 2003b).

Early encounters with SARS in Hong Kong suggested that a virus may have been the cause of the illness (Tsang et al., 2003a). Early candidate agents suggested were a paramyxovirus and a coronavirus, as well as the bacterial agent *Chlamydia pneumoniae* (Stadler et al., 2003). In the last week of March 2003, laboratories in Hong Kong (China), the United States, and Germany isolated a novel coronavirus from clinical material obtained from patients with SARS (Drosten et al., 2003a; Ksiazek et al., 2003; Peiris et al., 2003b). Serological studies and RT-PCR specific for this coronavirus (subsequently called SARS-CoV) were positive in most "probable" SARS patients but not in controls. RT-PCR products of several specimens from different geographical locations had identical nucleotide sequences, supporting the existence of a point-source outbreak. No other potential agent was consistently identified.

SARS-CoV could be grown in cell culture in Vero/African green monkey kidney cells (Drosten et al., 2003b; Ksiazek et al., 2003) and FRhK-4/fetal Rhesus kidney cells (Peiris et al., 2003b). The Hong Kong group led by Malik Peiris (Peiris, 2003) was the first to observe the cytopathic effect of the virus, seen after 2–4 days of incubation, consisting of cell rounding, refractile appearance, and detachment. The initial cytopathic effect was sometimes delayed until 6 days post-inoculation (Drosten et al., 2003a). (More recently, a clone of persistently infected Vero E6 cells has been established [Yamate et al., 2005].)

Work at Hong Kong University and the U.S. Centers for Disease Control and Prevention (CDC) resulted in the identification of the virus causing SARS. The CDC workers were the first to visualize the characteristic morphology of SARS-CoV in infected cells and in culture supernatant using transmission electron microscopy with negative staining (Fig. 1), which they shared with the network laboratories within 24 h (Anderson, 2005). With that information, the CDC successfully probed the virus with group I coronavirus polyclonal antibodies, and employed primers [IN-2(+), IN-4(−)] that targeted a conserved region of the coronavirus polymerase gene (open reading frame [ORF] 1b), thus amplifying the corresponding genomic region of SARS-CoV (Rota et al., 2003). Microarray hybridization further confirmed that the agent was a coronavirus. In Hong Kong, differential display priming (between SARS-CoV infected and uninfected cell cultures) and cloning were used to show that the virus was a coronavirus (Peiris et al., 2003b). German researchers performed random priming utilizing degenerate bases followed by sequencing and translated BLAST search to identify the RT-PCR products as those of a coronavirus (Drosten et al., 2003a).

Definitive proof of SARS-CoV as the etiologic agent of SARS came when Rotterdam virologists led by Albert Osterhaus (Enserink, 2003a) produced data that fulfilled Koch's last postulates. Macaque monkeys (*Macaca fascicularis*) developed a SARS-like illness after experimental infection, yielded the same virus inoculated, and developed a specific antibody response (Fouchier et al., 2003;

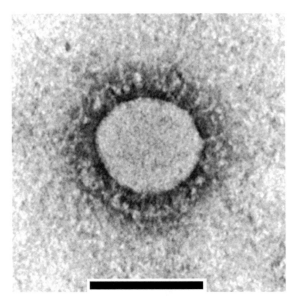

Fig. 1 Electron micrograph of SARS-CoV. The virus measures 60–120 nm in size. See text for description. Image generously provided by CDC/C.D. Humphrey and T.G. Ksiazek (US CDC Website-http://www.cdc.gov/ncidod/sars/lab/images.htm).

Kuiken et al., 2003). Co-infection of macaques with human metapneumovirus (hMPV), a virus that had earlier been a candidate agent for the cause of SARS, was not associated with more severe illness (Fouchier et al., 2003). hMPV infection without SARS-CoV caused only minor upper respiratory illness in adults (Ksiazek et al., 2003), although hMPV alone can cause severe pneumonia in young children (van den Hoogen et al., 2001). SARS-CoV was deemed necessary and sufficient to cause SARS.

On April 16, 2003, David Heymann (2004), Executive Director, WHO Communicable Diseases programs, Klaus Stöhr, and Albert Osterhaus announced that SARS was caused by the novel coronavirus, SARS-CoV (Anon., 2003b), and they dedicated the work to Dr. Urbani, who died from SARS that he had contracted while caring for patients in Vietnam.

The epidemic—timeline and highlights

SARS was notorious for a high incidence of acute respiratory distress and respiratory failure, a significant death rate even in healthy young adults (Lee et al., 2003b; Tsang et al., 2003a), a high rate of nosocomial transmission (Booth et al., 2003), and "superspreading events" (SSE) (Lai et al., 2004; Shen et al., 2004; Lloyd-Smith et al., 2005; Galvani and May, 2005) (Fig. 2). The epidemic in China almost became a pandemic when a physician guest at the Hotel Metropole, Hong Kong, who had been infected while treating SARS patients in Guangzhou, unknowingly

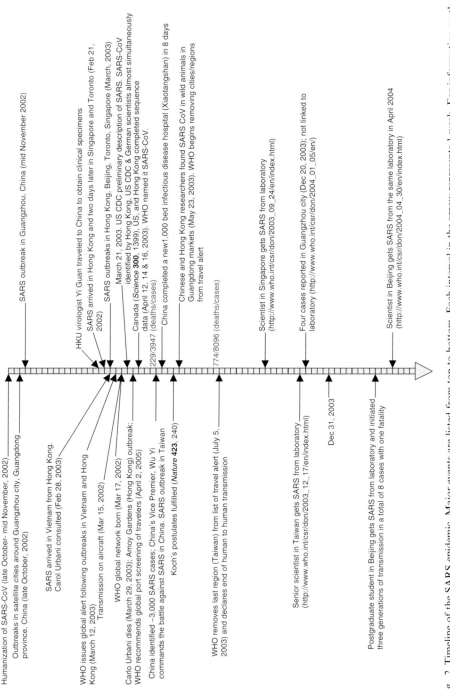

Fig. 2 Timeline of the SARS epidemic. Major events are listed from top to bottom. Each interval in the arrow represents 1 week. For information on the first weeks of the epidemic in China, consult the book by Thomas Abraham, Twenty-First Century Plague. The Story of SARS. The Johns Hopkins University Press. Baltimore, Maryland, 2005. (For colour version: see Colour Section on page 348).

introduced SARS-CoV into Hong Kong on February 21, 2003. He was probably a "superspreader" and Hong Kong became "ground zero."

However, in most other places where SARS-CoV spread, the chain of transmission stopped promptly with the isolation of patients. According to the Basic Reproductive Number (R_0), arrived at by averaging the number of infections produced by infected individuals in susceptible populations, SARS was not as contagious as influenza ($R_0 = 2.7$ [Riley et al., 2003] and 5–25, respectively). However, this simplification ignores a property of certain infectious diseases, including smallpox, influenza, and SARS, called the "heterogeneity of individual infectiousness." Highly variable infectiousness means that some infected individuals may cause explosive transmissions, giving rise to SSEs. During the SARS epidemic, a spectrum of infectiousness was seen that included SSEs, uneventful terminations of transmission chains, and explosive outbreaks (Galvani and May, 2005; Lloyd-Smith et al., 2005).

SSEs likely require high levels of viral shedding and others factors, which together determine the Individual Reproductive Number (Lloyd-Smith et al., 2005). One of these factors might be production of a large amount of bioaerosol by certain individuals (Edwards et al., 2004). Reducing bioaerosol by inhalation of nebulized saline (Edwards et al., 2004) and/or the use of cough suppressants could impact the Individual Reproductive Number and reduce the occurrence of SSEs.

Another cofactor might be a pneumonic phase with airborne dissemination of the virus (Lloyd-Smith et al., 2005). Because infectious disease agents exist as "quanta" and not as "plasma," airborne dissemination is difficult to prove owing to the stochastic process involved in the distribution of viruses by aerosol. During the Toronto portion of the SARS epidemic, investigations using state-of-the-art air sampling devices confirmed the presence of SARS-CoV in the air of a patient's room (Booth et al., 2005). These studies, together with data from investigation of transmission on aircraft (Olsen et al., 2003) and the huge outbreak of SARS in Amoy Gardens, Hong Kong (Yu et al., 2004b), showed that SARS-CoV is an opportunistic airborne pathogen (Roy and Milton, 2004). Having recognized that airborne dissemination of SARS-CoV is the route of transmission, facilities can be upgraded, with impact on other airborne infectious diseases as well.

The high incidence of nosocomial transmission of SARS-CoV during the epidemic exposed a weakness in the infection control procedures in some locations, as medical workers became vectors for SARS-CoV (Meng et al., 2005), but did not occur everywhere (Seto et al., 2003). Multiple layers of defense are needed, as Chowell et al. have suggested, because using their model for R_0, 25% of their R_0 distribution lies at $R_0 > 1$ even with perfect isolation (Chowell et al., 2004). Helpful measures might include the avoidance of crowding in clinics and wards, wearing face masks (Seto et al., 2003), avoiding aerosolizing procedures if possible (Tong et al., 2003; Tong, 2005b), improved ventilation design and rate (Liao et al., 2005a), and making sure that there are no "weak links" in infection control.

Emergence and origin of SARS-CoV

The theory that SARS-CoV came from an animal reservoir gained credence when field investigations by WHO showed that significant numbers of early patients were food-handlers (Anon., 2003c; Normile and Enserink, 2003; Xu et al., 2004c). Yi Guan and others investigated food markets in Guangdong, where a variety of small animals were kept in unhygienic heaped-up cages prior to sale (Guan et al., 2003). SARS-CoV-like coronaviruses were promptly identified in several Himalayan palm civets (*Paguma larvata*) and one raccoon dog (*Nyctereutes procyonoides*). Antibodies against SARS-CoV were also found in market workers. The relationship between these isolates from animals and isolates from humans appeared to be the result of a one-way transmission from animals to humans, because a 29-nucleotide deletion was found in the strain of SARS-CoV isolated from humans compared with civet SARS-CoV (it is easier to lose nucleotides than to gain some) (Chinese, 2004; Kan et al., 2005; Song et al., 2005b). Genomic comparisons further suggested that SARS-CoV was unlikely to be a recombinant between human and animal coronaviruses or between various animal coronaviruses, ruling out natural or laboratory chimerism (Holmes and Rambaut, 2004). Thus, SARS-CoV was probably a zoonotic virus (Holmes, 2003; Zhong et al., 2003b). It was also found that civets make a good amplification reservoir because SARS-CoV genomic RNA persisted in the spleen and lymph nodes of civets for as long as 35 days (Wu et al., 2005b).

Diversity of SARS-CoV genomes among human isolates was greatest in Guangdong, agreeing with animal studies that suggested south China was the site of emergence of the virus (Guan et al., 2004). Moreover, "humanization" likely occurred in a person of recent southern Chinese ancestry, because indigenous Taiwanese, with their distant HLA Class I genes, have been shown to be significantly less susceptible to SARS than residents of Taiwan who are immigrants from mainland China (Lin et al., 2003b). It is believed that the "humanization" of SARS-CoV occurred only a few weeks before the epidemic of SARS in China. The estimated dates of interspecies leap based on mutational analyses in both Singapore and China are in remarkably close agreement, late October 2002 and mid-November 2002, respectively (Chinese, 2004; Vega et al., 2004). The estimated mutation rates were 5.7×10^{-6} nucleotides per site per day in a Singapore isolate and 8.26×10^{-6} in a China isolate, again in remarkable agreement with each other and with the rate of 1.83×10^{-6} in a Taiwan isolate (Yeh et al., 2004). This rate of mutation is among the slowest in RNA viruses.

Retrospective seroepidemiological studies confirmed that SARS-CoV did not begin circulating in humans until recently. Only 1.8% of 938 sera collected in Hong Kong in May 2001 (Zheng et al., 2004b), none of 60 sera collected in Guangdong in early 2003 (Zhong et al., 2003b), and 1 (minimal reactivity on ELISA) of 384 sera from U.S. blood donors contained antibodies against SARS-CoV (Ksiazek et al., 2003; Zheng et al., 2004b). When quantified, titers of antibodies in these early sera were higher against civet SARS-CoV than against human isolates of SARS-CoV (Zheng et al., 2004b).

However, farmed civets elsewhere in China were mostly negative for SARS-CoV (Tu et al., 2004), so the hunt for the natural reservoir continued. Taking clues from other zoonotics, scientists turned to bats as a possible animal reservoir, since bats have been shown to be a reservoir for rabies virus, Ebola virus, Hendra virus, Menangle virus, and Nipah virus (Dobson, 2005; Leroy et al., 2005).

In 2005, two independent groups published definitive findings on the bat as a natural reservoir of SARS-CoV. Kwok-yung Yuen discovered three novel coronaviruses in different species of bat, including one virus with 88% nucleotide identity with SARS-CoV, a virus that they named bat-SARS-CoV (Lau et al., 2005; Poon et al., 2005). Bat-SARS-CoV, found in the insectivorous Chinese horseshoe bat (*Rhinolophus sinicus*), is nearly identical to civet SARS-CoV, including preservation of a 29-nucleotide segment not found in the majority of human isolates of SARS-CoV. Also nearly identical to civet SARS-CoV is SL-CoV Rp3, and perhaps related strains Rp1 and Rp2, found in *Rhinolophus pearsoni* by Li et al. (2005d). Shi, Zhang, and Wang's Sino-Australian cooperative effort, also involving Hong Kong University, produced proof that the bat is the natural reservoir for the SARS-CoV-like coronaviruses. These findings will lead to vaccines and drug treatments for SARS (Dobson, 2005).

Because SARS-CoV appears to jump species easily, more wildlife reservoirs of SARS-CoV may be discovered. Macaques, domestic cats, ferrets, raccoon dogs, pigs, and even mice are known to be susceptible to SARS-CoV infection (Fouchier et al., 2003; Martina et al., 2003; Wentworth et al., 2004; Chen et al., 2005b; Li et al., 2005d). Nevertheless, the fact that bats roost in large colonies makes them ideal reservoirs to maintain viruses and other microorganisms (Normile, 2005). In addition, bats are in the same Mammalia Class as humans, so viruses of bats will not require great changes to infect human cells (Li et al., 2005e).

After the epidemic was declared over, four small subsequent outbreaks occurred. Three were the result of SARS-CoV escaping from the laboratory by infecting personnel, as David Ho had predicted might occur (Enserink, 2003c), and has occurred with Russian influenza in 1977 (Horimoto and Kawaoka, 2005). The fourth case was a form fruste reemergence in the epicenter of the original outbreak, Guangzhou, between December 2003 and January 2004 (Enserink, 2004; Liang et al., 2004; Normile, 2004; Song et al., 2005b). In this reemergence, four people developed SARS and were confirmed to have SARS-CoV by RT-PCR. Three had had direct or indirect contact with palm civets, and one lived near a hospital that earlier admitted many patients with SARS. All recovered and seroconverted. Amplified sequences of the viruses isolated from them were very similar to those of SARS-CoV found in the preceding winter in caged animals (Chinese, 2004; Song et al., 2005b). The one patient in the reemergent outbreak who had had no contact with civets had earlier disposed of a dead rat, leading health officials of Guangdong to trap rodents near his residence; some of the rats (*Rattus rattus*) were found to have SARS-CoV in feces and lung tissue (http://www.egms.de/en/meetings/sars2004/04sars023.shtml), though not overtly ill.

The virus

Taxonomy and phylogeny

SARS-CoV belongs to the family *Coronaviridae*, which are enveloped RNA viruses in the order Nidovirales (Cavanagh, 1997). Coronaviruses are classified into three serogroups. Viruses in groups 1 and 2 are mammalian viruses; group 3 contains only avian viruses. Human coronaviruses (HCoV) are found in both group 1 (HCoV-229E and HCoV-NL63) and group 2 (HCoV-OC43 and CoV-HKU1) and are responsible for 30% or more of generally mild upper respiratory tract illnesses. To position SARS-CoV, Snijder et al. used a rooted phylogenetic tree that included an outgroup, the equine torovirus (EToV) (Snijder et al., 2003). They concluded that SARS-CoV is distantly related to established group 2 coronaviruses, agreeing with Peiris's phylogenetic analysis using the polymerase gene (Peiris et al., 2003b). Most of the genome of SARS-CoV is closely related to group 2 coronaviruses (Magiorkinis et al., 2004). Now SARS-CoV is placed in a new subgroup 2b, with the other group 2 coronaviruses assigned to a new subgroup 2a (Stadler et al., 2003; Gorbalenya et al., 2004). In addition, bat-SARS-CoV was assigned recently to subgroup 2b (Lau et al., 2005).

Ultrastructure of SARS-CoV

SARS-CoV has the characteristic morphology of coronaviruses, with spike (S) protein peplomers, club-shaped projections on the surface, giving the enveloped viral particle a crown-like (hence "corona," Latin for "crown") appearance under the electron microscope (Fig. 1). Atomic force microscopy reveals that each virion has at least 15 spherical spikes, each with a diameter of $7.29 + /-0.73$ nm (Lin et al., 2005a). The center appears amorphous.

SARS-CoV genome, proteome, and replication cycle

Coronaviruses have the largest known non-segmented genome among RNA viruses (27–31 kb). The genome mimics eukaryotic mRNA in being single-stranded positive-sense RNA, capped and methylated at the 5′ end, and polyadenylated at the 3′ end. Consequently, it is more stable than prokaryotic mRNA, and is optimized for translation by eukaryotic translational machinery (i.e. optimized for infectivity). A polymerase is not included in the particle.

The entire genome sequence of SARS-CoV was worked out in <2 months (Leung, 2003; Marra et al., 2003; Rota et al., 2003). The SARS-CoV genome (Fig. 3) begins and ends with untranslated regions (UTR), spanning 192 and 340 nucleotides, respectively. (In the Sabin strain of poliovirus, mutations in the UTR were responsible for the attenuation that permitted vaccine production (Gutierrez et al., 1997). The SARS-CoV genome has 14 predicted open reading frames (ORFs) encoding 28 proteins (Marra et al., 2003; Rota et al., 2003; Snijder et al., 2003).

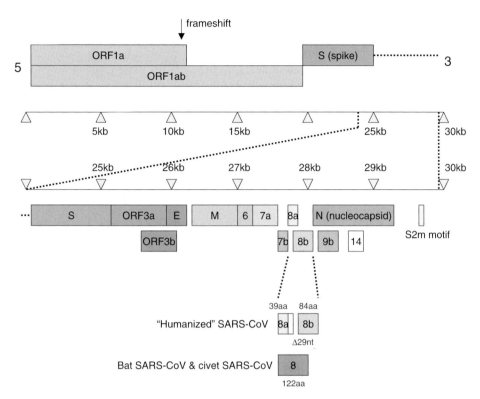

Fig. 3 SARS-CoV genome organization. The genome organization is similar to other coronaviruses with respect to overall size, the relative positions of replicase, spike, envelope, membrane and nucleocapsid genes, and certain other features (see text for details). A 29-nucleotide stretch is deleted in the strain found in human isolates, as illustrated at the bottom. (For colour version: see Colour Section on page 349).

Certain strains lack one ORF (Chinese, 2004), whereas others have 15 ORFs (Groneberg et al., 2005). There are alternative nomenclatures related to this virus, which in this chapter are enclosed within brackets.

A "SARS chip" was offered free to researchers beginning June 23, 2003, by the National Institute of Allergy and Infectious Diseases, NIH (USA), based on the success of the DeRisi "viral discovery microarray" (Wang et al., 2003). Microarray gene expression studies on peripheral blood have been shown to discriminate accurately SARS patients from non-SARS controls (Long et al., 2004; Lee et al., 2005b).

In Shanghai, the proteome of SARS-CoV in Vero cells has been analyzed using conventional proteomic tools and two-dimensional liquid chromatography electrospray ionization tandem mass spectrometry (LC-ESI-MS/MS). In addition, isotope-labeled affinity tag technology coupled with two-dimensional LC-MS/MS has been used to identify and quantify 186 differentially expressed proteins in infected vs. non-infected Vero cells (Zeng et al., 2004b; Jiang et al., 2005b). In Beijing, Kang et al. developed a mass spectrometry decision tree classification algorithm using surface-enhanced laser desorption/ionization time-of-flight mass spectrometry (SE-LDI-TOF MS) and protein array, predicting the virologic diagnosis based on several serum proteomic markers (Kang et al., 2005). Using similar technology, Poon et al. at Chinese University of Hong Kong (CUHK) performed serial analyses of plasma proteomic signatures in pediatric patients with SARS, showing the potential to predict clinical outcome based on its correlation with viral load (Poon et al., 2004c).

Replicase

ORF1a and ORF1b, together spanning two-thirds of the viral genome, are located at the 5′ end and encode replicase polyproteins (pp) 1a and pp1ab. ORF1 is expressed immediately after infection. Translational products can be detected in cell cultures as early as 6 h after infection (Prentice et al., 2004). Like other coronaviruses and many other viruses, the strategy used for translation of pp1ab requires a "slippery sequence" and a structural mRNA element known as a pseudoknot, which causes a 1-ribosomal frameshift just 5′ of the termination codon of ORF1a. The "slippery sequence" is highly conserved and would not function if mutated (Thiel et al., 2003). Another *in cis* element has been discovered, an attenuator 5′ of the slippery sequence that downregulates 1 frameshift efficiency (Su et al., 2005). Transcription attenuation was thought to enable SARS-CoV to synthesize both full-length and subgenomic-length antisense RNA intermediates (Yount et al., 2005).

Sixteen non-structural proteins (nsp) are derived from proteolytic cleavage of pp1a and pp1ab by two, rather than three, viral proteinases (see below) (Snijder et al., 2003). Recently, 12 of the 16 predicted nsp have been identified by immunoblot and their subcellular localization studied by immunofluorescence confocal microscopy (Prentice et al., 2004).

The predicted 20-kD nsp1 has been confirmed, along with immunologically related products of different sizes, and are awaiting further characterization (Prentice et al., 2004). Nsp2 is not essential for viral replication in Vero cells (Graham et al., 2005), which are defective in interferon (IFN) production (Emeny and Morgan, 1979). The two viral proteases, a very specific papain-like cysteine proteinase (nsp3, PL2pro; SARS-CoV does not have PL1pro), and the main chymotrypsin-like protease (nsp5), also known as 3C-like cysteine proteinase (3CLpro), with substrate specificity conserved among coronaviruses, are necessary for co- and post-translational processing of the polyprotein. PL2pro cleaves nsp1, nsp2, and nsp3 from the elongating polypeptide co-translationally, whereas 3CLpro is responsible for the other cleavage sites. The X-domain of nsp3 is homologous to adenosine diphosphate-ribose 1′-phosphatase (ADRP), which is involved in pre-tRNA splicing (Snijder et al., 2003). Its phosphatase activity was recently demonstrated in *in vitro* assays (Saikatendu et al., 2005). Nsp4 is a hydrophobic protein of 35 kDa on SDS-polyacrylamide gel but has a predicted mass of 55 kDa. It is similar to MP1 of murine hepatitis virus (MHV) (Prentice et al., 2004). The use of "artificial neural networks" and SPAAN, a bioinformatics software that has a track record of discovering adhesins, has led to the finding of adhesin-like characteristics in nsp6, a function also ascribed to spike, nsp2, nsp5, and nsp7 (Sachdeva et al., 2005). Nsp7 and nsp8 assemble into a cylindrical hexadecamer with inner positive charges and an internal diameter of 30 Å, thought to confer processivity to RNA-dependent RNA polymerase (RdRp) (Zhai et al., 2005). Other scientists have cloned nsp9, expressed it in *E. coli*, crystallized it, and generated crystallographic data in an effort to facilitate drug design (Campanacci et al., 2003). They further showed that it is a single-stranded RNA-binding protein displaying an oligosaccharide/oligonucleotide fold unique to the world of RNA viruses (Egloff et al., 2004). Nsp12 functions as SARS-CoV RNA-dependent RNA polymerase (RdRp or POL). Nsp13 is a promiscuous helicase (unwinds RNA and DNA) with ATPase activity belonging to the helicase superfamily 1 (Thiel et al., 2003).

The N-terminal domain of nsp14 may play a role in the stability of the SARS-CoV genome. The N-terminal domain of nsp 14 is homologous to 3'–5' exonulcease (ExoN) and it has been speculated that it may perform functions such as RNA proofreading, repair, and/or recombination (Snijder et al., 2003). That SARS-CoV has this genome protection capability may explain the slow estimated mutation rate (Chinese, 2004; Vega et al., 2004; Yeh et al., 2004), the sequence identity between a laboratory-acquired case and a stable laboratory isolate (Vega et al., 2004), and the observed but unexpected resistance to ribavirin, a drug that predisposes other RNA viruses to go into "error catastrophe" (Eigen, 1987; Crotty et al., 2001; Pariente et al., 2001). Nevertheless, preliminary observations suggest that quasispecies do occur with SARS-CoV just as with other RNA viruses, although all patients studied for quasispecies existence had all received ribavirin (Xu et al., 2004a,b), a confounding factor in the experiments.

The C-terminal part of nsp15 is homologous to poly(U)-specific endoribonuclease (XendoU), involved in small nucleolar RNA processing and utilization (Snijder et al., 2003). Nsp15 was further confirmed to have specificity for cleavage at uridylate residues. Structural analysis shows that it is arranged as a dimer or trimer with possible RNA-binding sites (Guarino et al., 2005). Nsp16 shows homology with 2'-*O*-methyltransferase (2'-*O*-MT) (von Grotthuss et al., 2003), and could possibly be used to cap the viral mRNA, disguising it as a eukaryotic mRNA. The cap is recognized by eukaryotic initiation factor eIF4F, which together with other initiation factors, recruit the 43S ribosomal subunit initiation complex that then scans the mRNA for the initiation codon AUG, whereupon the 60S ribosomal subunit docks and begins peptide elongation (Wang et al., 1997). Co-localization studies showed that these enzymes assemble into one or more vesicle membrane-associated replication units (Prentice et al., 2004) and usurp cellular processes for viral replication (without a DNA phase) and mRNA transcription.

Expression of other SARS-CoV genes

Coronaviruses, including SARS-CoV and other viruses in the order Nidovirales, produce a set of 3′ co-terminal mRNA in host cells (Lai and Cavanagh, 1997). For SARS-CoV, the 12 ORFs downstream of the replicase are translated from a nested set of eight subgenomic mRNAs, identified experimentally in infected cells (Snijder et al., 2003; Thiel et al., 2003). Also like other coronaviruses, all of the subgenomic mRNAs can be lined-up with the genome at (are co-terminal with) the 3′ end of the virus. The 5′ ends are also identical. A minimal consensus sequence at the 5′ end, 5′ACGAAC-3′, is sufficient to direct the synthesis of the subgenomic mRNAs (Thiel et al., 2003). This sequence, embedded in a stretch of nucleotides upstream of the ORF(s) of each subgenomic mRNA, is the result of fusion of nucleotides 1–72 of the genome ("leader" transcription regulatory sequence [TRS]) and a unique "body" TRS preceding each ORF. The joining of these two regions is probably achieved in a discontinuous step during minus-strand synthesis (Stadler et al., 2003; Thiel et al., 2003). The TRSs regulate viral transcription and translation.

Spike protein and receptor-based entry

ORF2 encodes a Class I viral membrane-fusion protein, the 1255-amino acid trans-membrane S protein. The precursor, proS, is glycosylated at the Golgi apparatus and proteolytically processed by furin (host membrane-bound proprotein convert-ases), as shown by scientists at the Clinical Research Institute of Montreal (Bergeron et al., 2005). The extracellular domain contains the S1 receptor-binding and the S2 entry-mediating "regions." Breaching the cell membrane barrier is the single most important step in infection (Giroglou et al., 2004; Li et al., 2004a). Neutralizing antibodies against S, especially the receptor-binding region, prevents infection (He et al., 2004b,c).

S binds the host cell membrane protein angiotensin I converting enzyme 2 (ACE2) (Dimitrov, 2003; Li et al., 2003; Kuba et al., 2005), which the newly discovered HCoV-NL63 also employs as its receptor (Hofmann et al., 2005). Civet ACE2 (cACE2) differs from human ACE2 (hACE2), to which human isolates of SARS-CoV are not fully adapted, as shown by increased binding and infection by introduction of residues 90–93 of cACE2 into the human receptor (Li et al., 2005e). As expected, soluble ACE2 (sACE2) but not soluble ACE (sACE), blocks binding of S with Vero E6 cells (Li et al., 2003; Hofmann et al., 2004). However, mutations of the catalytic site of ACE2 have no effect on S-induced syncytia formation, suggesting that existing ACE inhibitors will not block SARS-CoV infection (Dimitrov, 2003).

The receptor-binding region of S has been localized to amino acid residues between 318 and 510 of the S1 "region" (Wong et al., 2004b), in the same neigh-borhood as that of HCoV-229E (Breslin et al., 2003). The avidity of binding (Li et al., 2005e), viral entry (Yi et al., 2005), and immunogenicity (Yi et al., 2005) are affected by single amino acid substitutions within this region, as demonstrated

at 2.9 Å resolution (Holmes, 2005; Li et al., 2005b). Binding is by way of conformational and electrostatic interactions (Yi et al., 2005). The strength differs, depending on the viral strain. Civet S binds cACE2 avidly but hACE2 poorly,
although S from human isolates of SARS-CoV binds strongly with both cACE2
and hACE2 (Li et al., 2005e). Two regions of the S-protein-binding site on ACE2,
and two residues (aa479 and aa487) in the receptor-binding region of S, largely
determine the difference. S from human isolates of SARS-CoV has a small neutral
residue (asparagine) at position 479, replacing a basic residue in civet S, and better
accommodates the lysine at position 31 of hACE2. At position 487, serine in civet S
is replaced by threonine, which has an extra methyl group, in the human isolates.
This residue was absolutely conserved in S evaluated in > 100 isolates during the
epidemic (Li et al., 2005e). These findings suggest that adaptation of S to hACE2
was critical to viral adaptation to humans (Ruan et al., 2003).

After binding to ACE2, S undergoes conformational change mediated by its S2
"region" (Liu et al., 2004; Tripet et al., 2004; Xu et al., 2004d), which presumably
exposes a cleavage site, followed by pH-dependent host endosomal cathepsin
L-mediated proteolysis (Yang et al., 2004a; Simmons et al., 2005). Extracellular
proteases, such as those excreted by neutrophils, facilitate this pathway to a significant degree. Proteases also enable entry into the cell of SARS-CoV adsorbed on
the cell surface (Matsuyama et al., 2005). In a similar way, Ebola virus and Hendra
virus also utilize cathepsin L for the endocytic pathway of cell entry (Chandran
et al., 2005; Pager and Dutch, 2005).

The final step of membrane fusion before viral entry is dependent on the formation of the six-helix bundle by heptad repeats (HR1 and HR2) in the S2 "region" (Liu et al., 2004), also predicted by others using in-silico techniques (Kliger
and Levanon, 2003). Oligomerization of S is required to form the six-helix bundle,
a structure similar to the fusogenic core of HIV-1 gp41 (Liu et al., 2004). The
putative fusion peptide has been located to the region immediately upstream of
HR1 (Bosch et al., 2004) and provided detailed modeling of the fusion core
(Supekar et al., 2004; Xu et al., 2004e; Guillen et al., 2005). This last step of viral
entry appears to be susceptible to inhibition by a component of innate immunity,
mannose-binding lectin (MBL) (Leikina et al., 2005).

Several other cellular proteins are also utilized by S to facilitate entry into the
cell. They include the HIV-attachment factor dendritic cell-specific intercellular
adhesion molecule-grabbing non-integrin (DC-SIGN or CD209), a C-type lectin
expressed on dendritic cells, and CD209L (L-SIGN or DC-SIGNR) (Jeffers et al.,
2004; Marzi et al., 2004). In this way SARS-CoV joins HIV, dengue virus, and
CMV in exploiting dendritic cells as "vehicles" for cell-mediated dissemination
(Yang et al., 2004a). Another lectin (LSECtin) was recently shown to bind to S and
could assist viral entry into the liver and lymph nodes through its expression in
sinusoidal endothelial cells (Gramberg et al., 2005).

In a short period of time, SARS-CoV S has evolved from one that is inefficient
in entering human cells (civet strains) to one that has acquired "keys to both the
front and back doors." This is no less remarkable than influenza virus strains that

have acquired the ability to efficiently enter human cells through mutations of the hemagglutinin cleavage site that became promiscuously cleaved by a wide range of host proteases (Horimoto and Kawaoka, 2005).

Other structural proteins

ORF4 [5] encodes a small envelope (E) protein of 76 amino acids (Shen et al., 2003) that binds to and inactivates the anti-apoptotic protein, Bcl-xL, causing *in vitro* and *in vivo* lymphocytotoxicity (Yang et al., 2005b). E protein was detected in culture supernatant (Hsieh et al., 2005) and could conceivably be taken up *in vivo* by lymphocytes that are not infected by the virus.

ORF5 [6] encodes membrane (M) protein, the most abundant viral glycoprotein (221 amino acids). It is a 3-span transmembrane protein with a short N-terminal ecto- and a long C-terminal interior domain. A 12-amino acid domain of M has been shown to interact with the nucleocapsid, triggering viral encapsidation (He et al., 2004a; Fang et al., 2005).

ORF9a [12] encodes the nucleocapsid (N) protein (422 amino acides). It is a basic protein that binds to viral RNA via its N- and C-terminal regions (Chang et al., 2005; Hsieh et al., 2005). It spontaneously assembles into virus-like particles (VLP) in solution (Azizi et al., 2005). A role in apoptosis has been postulated (Surjit et al., 2005).

Accessory proteins

The functions of the accessory proteins are still unknown (Cai et al., 2005). Systematic deletions of 5 of 8 group-specific ORFs, ORF3a, OF3b, ORF6, ORF7a, and ORF7b, alone or in combinations, did not significantly impair viral viability in cell culture and in mice (Yount et al., 2005). It is possible that they are involved in the struggle between the virus and its natural host, the bat. Deletion of group-specific ORFs from other coronaviruses often leads to attenuation *in vivo* (Yount et al., 2005). Evidence is emerging that some of these deletions might be pathogenic in man. ORF3a [3] and ORF3b [4] encode U274 (sars3a) and U154 (sars3b), respectively, two novel proteins not found in other coronaviruses (Tan et al., 2004b; Yu et al., 2004a; Ito et al., 2005). Both are implicated in triggering apoptosis (Law et al., 2005b; Yuan et al., 2005). U274 (sars3a) co-localizes with S and M and is packaged into virions (Ito et al., 2005). U122 (sars7a) encoded by ORF7a [8] (Snijder et al., 2003) is also localized to the rough endoplasmic reticulum/Golgi compartment. It has been reported to induce apoptosis by a caspase-dependent mechanism (Tan et al., 2004a). It is tempting to associate these apoptosis-inducing activities with lymphopenia, in a "Trojan horse" role. Infection of lymphocytes by SARS-CoV might be needed for survival (Gu et al., 2005); by causing lymphocyte apoptosis, virus with these deletions might permit survival of the virus in other cells that would otherwise be destroyed by the lymphocytes.

Viral assembly and exit

Assembly of viral particles is triggered by the association of membrane-bound M proteins with N proteins that coat the helical viral nucleocapsid (He et al., 2004a). Viral packaging is dependent on viral RNA-binding motifs at the N- and C-terminals of N and a packaging signal in the hypervariable region of ORF1b near the 3′ terminus, similar to that found in MHV and BCoV (Qin et al., 2003; Chang et al., 2005; Hsieh et al., 2005). The virions assemble and bud into vesicles formed in the compartment between the endoplasmic reticulum and the Golgi apparatus, picking up carbohydrate moieties before being released by exocytosis. The entire process of SARS-CoV replication takes from 9 to 24 h (Yount et al., 2003; Prentice et al., 2004), compared with the 5–6 h for influenza virus, as reflected by the slow rise in viral titers in SARS patients (Peiris et al., 2003a; Tsang et al., 2003b; Cheng et al., 2004).

Viral countermeasures

Microarray studies of host gene expression have shown that SARS-CoV elicits a non-specific innate inflammatory reaction rather than an antiviral response (Reghunathan et al., 2005). SARS-CoV in a sense "edits" the responses of dendritic cells and macrophages, resulting in induction of non-specific inflammatory chemokines, a low-level pro-inflammatory cytokine production, and a muted anti-viral cytokine response (including IFN and IL-12p40). Data have suggested that in fact SARS-CoV avoids activating dendritic cells and macrophages (Ziegler et al., 2005). A suppressed Th-2 response, which would otherwise orchestrate the humoral immune response, could also result (Wong et al., 2004a).

In search of an explanation for the absent IFN-β response, it has been found that SARS-CoV blocks a step after the early nuclear transport of IRF-3, a key IFN-β gene transcription factor (Spiegel et al., 2005). Another cellular signaling pathway affected is the activation of AP-1 by S and N (He et al., 2003; Chang et al., 2004). N protein activates nuclear factor (NF)-kB in Vero E6 cells but not Vero cells, HeLa cells, or lung epithelial and fibroblast cell lines (Chang et al., 2004; Liao et al., 2005b). Other viruses that activate NF-kB include HIV-1, human T-cell lymphotropic virus type 1, herpes viruses, hepatitis C virus, hepatitis B virus, and influenza viruses, among others (Santoro et al., 2003). The protean roles of NF-kB in inflammation, cell proliferation, cell survival, apoptosis, and as a central regulator of innate and adaptive immune responses, make it an ideal intracellular target for the virus.

The most important aspect of SARS-CoV evasion of the immune response occurs by abrogation of intracellular antiviral responses, aptly described as "intracellular warfare" (Krug et al., 2003), which also occurs in most viral infections (Samuel, 2001; Webby et al., 2004). Vero cells stably expressing MxA (Samuel, 2001), a broad-spectrum anti-RNA virus large GTPase protein induced by IFNs α and β (but not γ), continue to produce the virus, suggesting that SARS-CoV has countermeasures against this important defense mechanism (Spiegel et al., 2004). The adaptive immune system is itself a viral target; direct viral infection of CD4 + and CD8 + lymphocytes (Gu et al., 2005), induction of lymphocyte apoptosis (Chen et al., 2005a), and the multiple toxic viral molecules that can cause apoptosis, namely E protein (Yang et al., 2005b), U274 (Law et al., 2005b), U154 (Yuan et al., 2005), U122 (Tan et al., 2004a), and S (Chow et al., 2005). Harnessing the power of computational biology, scientists at the Beijing Genomics Institute are investigating viral virulence and evasion strategies by comparing SARS-CoV protein motifs with those of known human proteins and other viral proteins. Toxic motifs were found to be localized to various SARS-CoV proteins potentially relevant for therapy and vaccine design (Li et al., 2004b). For example, superantigen-like motifs in the S, E, N, and some accessory proteins are thought to cause lymphocyte apoptosis by activation in the absence of appropriate co-stimulatory signals. An enterotoxin motif in S could account for the diarrhea seen in many SARS victims.

More viral countermeasures may be identified in the future, perhaps including anti-RNA interference (RNAi). Progress is being made in the application of RNAi-based therapeutics against SARS-CoV (Zhang et al., 2003; Wang et al., 2004c; Li et al., 2005a; Shi et al., 2005; Tao et al., 2005; Wu et al., 2005a), in particular the recent advances in delivery of siRNAs, with the hope of specifically targeting the scattered and relatively inaccessible lymphocytes and dendritic cells to ameliorate the assault on the immune system by SARS-CoV (Song et al., 2005a).

Molecular evolution

Comparisons of the genomes of SARS-CoV and SARS-CoV-like animal corona-viruses from palm civets and a raccoon dog (Guan et al., 2003) revealed that human isolates of SARS-CoV all shared some deletions not seen in civet SARS-CoV. Additional polymorphisms were also identified, showing that humanized SARS-CoV had evolved from civet SARS-CoV (Chen et al., 2005b). These initial efforts also cataloged important genomic data for comparison with newly discovered SARS-CoV-like viruses, such as bat-SARS-CoV (Lau et al., 2005) and SL-CoV Rp3 (Li et al., 2005c). Both of these bat-SARS-CoVs contained the sequences deleted in humanized SARS-CoV, revealing their even closer kinship with civet SARS-CoV.

The Chinese SARS Molecular Epidemiology Consortium collected spatially and temporally diverse specimens from humans and animals to study SARS-CoV evolution (Chinese, 2004). Several major SARS-CoV genotypes and 299 single-nucleotide variations (SNVs) were discovered among 63 sequences studied. Certain SNVs, for example, the second and third nucleotides of codon 479 of S (22927 and 22928) created the so-called multiple substitution codons, which have a chance occurrence of zero, pointing toward their development by natural selection.

Another observation was the phenomenon of G + C enrichment (Song et al., 2005b), thought to be metabolically expensive for intracellular pathogens (Rocha and Danchin, 2002), but which also could be due to pressure from host sabotage akin to G → T editing by host APOBEC3 family proteins, again suggesting adaptive pressure rather than random mutations. Genotyping based on SNVs in 5 loci (17564, 21721, 22222, 23823, and 27827) defined civet SARS-CoV (GACGC), an early GACTC motif in human isolates of SARS-CoV, GGCTC, or GATTC motifs in the middle of the epidemic, and a late TGTTT motif that has corresponding non-synonymous changes in ORF1b, S and the non-coding X3 (ORF6 or ORF7) regions (Liu, 2005). Similar changes occurred in the evolution of the three most significantly variable proteins S, sars3a (U274), and nsp3 (PL2pro), as the virus adapted to humans (Kan et al., 2005; Song et al., 2005b). Sequence deletions were observed in the dominant human strain, including entire ORFs specifying group-specific accessory proteins, such as a 29-nucleotide deletion in the ORF8 of civet SARS-CoV, creating ORF8a and ORF8b. An uncommon strain with limited range isolated early in the epidemic had an 82-nucleotide deletion in ORF8a, similar to animal SARS-CoV isolated in farmed civets in Hubei province, China (Chinese, 2004). Yet another strain isolated late in the epidemic in Hong Kong in May 2003 lacked a 415-nucleotide sequence corresponding to the entire ORF8a and ORF8b (Poon et al., 2004a).

These and other data indicate that there was a rapid viral genomic adjustment to the human host early in the epidemic, particularly at specific mutational hotspots in the receptor-binding region. This slowed in the middle of the epidemic, with late changes producing strong purifying selection (Chinese, 2004; Yeh et al., 2004; Kan et al., 2005). These investigations also revealed that critical viral adaptations to humans went down the same evolutionary path in Beijing as earlier in Guangzhou, with a switch from the GGCTC to the TGTTT motif in patients belonging to the same cluster (Liu, 2005). Some of these molecular events occurred again in the late 2003 to early 2004 outbreak in Guangzhou (Kan et al., 2005; Song et al., 2005b). Throughout this period, civet SARS-CoV had been evolving and adapting to civet cats, producing a higher viral load, confirming that the civet is not its normal reservoir (Song et al., 2005b). However, given the opportunity, it appeared that SARS-CoV could establish a reservoir in farmed civets. These findings and the elucidation of the adaptation of S to hACE2 sharpen our perception of molecular emergence.

Because the human isolates of SARS-CoV are much more virulent and con-tagious than the animal strains, it is important for public health officials to quickly find out which strain(s) they are dealing with in the event of an outbreak. As such, the genotyping of SARS-CoV has acquired public health significance. Scientists at the Chinese University of Hong Kong have developed an allelic discrimination genotyping assay using 5′ nuclease probes that has been validated for discriminat-ing between human and animal strains of SARS-CoV, by comparison with direct sequencing (Chung et al., 2005).

Human disease

Transmission

It is thought that SARS-CoV spreads from person to person through mucosal surfaces with virus-laden body fluids, primarily respiratory secretions (Anon., 2003a). Tears (Loon et al., 2004; Tong and Lai, 2005) and sweat (Ding et al., 2004) have also been found to contain SARS-CoV RNA, although their role in disease transmission is unknown. Coughing as a means of airborne dissemination was difficult to prove (Seto et al., 2003; Tong, 2003), but was demonstrated experimentally (Booth et al., 2005). Large droplets emitted by coughing and sneezing and having a projection range of 1 m are believed to have contributed to airborne transmission (Fowler et al., 2004; Yu et al., 2004b, 2005; Booth et al., 2005; Li et al., 2005f,g; Tong, 2005a), possibly by superspreaders (Edwards et al., 2004); inadvertent aerosolization of other infected body materials or feces is also thought to be a possible means of transmission (Yu and Sung, 2004; Yu et al., 2004b). Fecal-to-oral transmission has not been documented, although viral nucleic acid has been found in sewage (Wang et al., 2005a). Nuclei acid testing by RT-PCR, if instituted, theoretically could prevent transfusion-associated transmission during future epidemics if SARS-Cov is shown to be present in blood from asymptomatic persons (Schmidt et al., 2004).

Clinical features of SARS

The clinical course has been divided into three phases (Peiris et al., 2003a). Phase 1 correlates with upper respiratory viral replication and viremia. Phases 2 and 3 correlate with lower respiratory tract viral replication, with phase 3 characterized by functionally critical pulmonary injury, due either to virus alone (Mazzulli et al., 2004) or in conjunction with immunological damage (Lin et al., 2005b; Matsuyama et al., 2005).

The incubation period of SARS ranges from 2 to 11 days after exposure, with a mean of 4.6 days (Leung et al., 2004), and occasionally was as long as 16 days (Booth et al., 2003; Lee et al., 2003b; Tsang et al., 2003a). The prodrome consists of flu-like symptoms such as malaise, myalgia, headache, fever, and rigors. Cough as an initial symptom is present in greater than half of the patients. Coryza and sore throat are present in a minority of cases. By day 5 (range, 3–7 days), up to 76% of patients develop exertional dyspnea; chest X-rays reveal opacities in the lungs of almost all patients, consistent with alveolar and interstitial exudation (Zhong et al., 2003b). This phase lasts for up to a week. Watery diarrhea developed in 20.4% of patients admitted to Princess Margaret Hospital, Hong Kong (Kwan et al., 2005a). A higher incidence of diarrhea was found in the cohort of patients from the Amoy Gardens (74%) and correlated with higher viral load in stool (Hung et al., 2004).

More than 20% of patients require intensive care, and 13% require ventilatory support (Tsui et al., 2003).

Asymptomatic cases were extremely rare during the epidemic (Lai et al., 2005b), being the rule in the early phase of the epidemic in China, before SARS-CoV had adapted to the human host (Guan et al., 2003; Lee et al., 2003a). Some elderly patients were not febrile (Christian et al., 2004); in some cases, the incubation period and convalescence was protracted. Up to 5.8% of 138 patients in Prince of Wales Hospital presented with diarrhea and fever without respiratory symptoms (Leung et al., 2003b).

Children were also infected, although their symptoms and clinical course were typically mild (Hon et al., 2003; Leung et al., 2003a; Kwan et al., 2004). Pregnancy did not alter the course of SARS in the mother and perinatal infection has not been reported (Shek et al., 2003). Children have also presented solely with diarrhea (Kwan et al., 2005b).

Recovery, if it will occur, begins between 14 and 18 days after disease onset (Christian et al., 2004). Convalescent patients no longer excrete the virus in stools (Wang et al., 2005b). In some patients, apparent recovery is followed by exacerbation (Peiris et al., 2003a), with arterial oxygen desaturation, and variable degrees of respiratory impairment or failure. At one year post-infection, one-third of patients continue to have pulmonary function impairment (Hui et al., 2005; Ong et al., 2005). Osteonecrosis occurs in a significant proportion of patients who receive systemic steroids; children can also experience this complication (Chan et al., 2004a; Griffith et al., 2005).

Clinical laboratory findings

Lymphopenia (Peiris et al., 2003b; He et al., 2005b) and thrombocytopenia are commonly present (Choi et al., 2003). Decrease of both CD4+ and CD8+ T-lymphocytes occurs early and adversely affects the prognosis (Wong et al., 2003a). Serum chemistry often reveals elevated lactate dehydrogenase (LDH), aminotransferase levels, and creatine phosphokinase levels, with LDH being an independent predictor of mortality (Choi et al., 2003). Initially elevated C-reactive protein levels were reported to be correlated with poor outcome (Wang et al., 2004a).

Pathology of SARS-CoV pneumonia

In humans, ACE2 is expressed in the lungs, intestines, testes, kidneys, endothelium, and heart, and in large part determined the tissue tropism (Donoghue et al., 2000; Tipnis et al., 2000; Harmer et al., 2002; Leung et al., 2003b; Hamming et al., 2004; Xu et al., 2005). In respiratory epithelium, ACE2 is expressed only in differentiated cells (Jia et al., 2005), in particular, ciliated cells (Sims et al., 2005), implying that bronchioalveolar stem cells (Kim et al., 2005) are poorly infected.

Abundant evidence points to viral infection of pneumocytes as the mechanism of lung injury (Nicholls et al., 2003; To et al., 2004; Chan et al., 2005b; Shieh et al., 2005). However, induction of an immune response by viral proteins is also implicated in the pathogenesis. For example, the N-terminal aa324–488 and the C-terminal aa609–688 of S activate AP-1 and MAPKs independent of NF-kB in lung epithelial cells, monocytes, and fibroblasts *in vitro* leading to induction of IL-8 (Chang et al., 2004), consistent with observations that IL-8 and IL-2 levels are elevated in patients with SARS (Lee et al., 2004). In turn, IL-8 recruits neutrophils to the lungs, thereby facilitating SARS-CoV entry into pneumocytes by elaboration of proteases (Chang et al., 2004; Wong et al., 2004a; Matsuyama et al., 2005; Tang et al., 2005).

Host factors appear also to contribute to diffuse alveolar damage. The peptide hormone angiotensin II, positively and negatively regulated by ACE (product of ACE1 gene) and ACE2, respectively, has been shown to participate in spike-induced diffuse alveolar damage in mice (Imai et al., 2005; Kuba et al., 2005; Nicholls and Peiris, 2005). This explains why SARS patients carrying the D allele (deletion involving intron 16) polymorphism of the ACE1 gene, which is associated with higher level of sACE, are more prone to hypoxemia (Itoyama et al., 2004). The D allele, by increasing sACE, results in higher angiotensin II levels and hence susceptibility to injury by SARS-CoV S. ACE2 is protective by inactivating angiotensin II (Imai et al., 2005; Nicholls and Peiris, 2005). Interrupting the renin–angiotensin system protected mice from exacerbation of lung injury aggravated by injection of S (Kuba et al., 2005). These studies showed how viral proteins can tip the balance in normal physiology and cause disease. The therapeutic implications for acute respiratory distress syndrome (ARDS), beyond the respiratory damage caused by SARS-CoV, was noted, but an explanation is needed for the generally mild infections of HCoV-NL63, which also utilizes ACE2 (Nicholls and Peiris, 2005). Perhaps the similarity is limited between human and murine pathophysiology in this infection.

These viral and host factors cannot account for cases showing apparent improvement followed later by deterioration (Peiris et al., 2003a). One school of thought incriminates the innate immune system. Peiris et al. investigated the alveolar macrophages, sentinels of the lower respiratory tract (Cheung et al., 2005). They found that cultured macrophages were infected (as evidenced by translated N protein) but not supportive of SARS-CoV replication. In addition, whereas macrophages infected by HCoV-229E and influenza A (H1N1) produce IFN-β, there is no evidence of induction of IFN-β in SARS-CoV-infected macrophages. Instead, there is elaboration of chemokines CXCL10/IFN-inducible protein 10 (IP-10) and CCL2/monocyte chemotactic protein 1 (MCP-1), possibly explaining aspects of the pathogenesis.

An autoimmune explanation akin to influenza virus-induced Goodpasture syndrome, and dengue hemorrhagic fever and dengue shock syndrome, has been suggested (Lin et al., 2003a). Anti-S2 antibodies were discovered in convalescent sera that cross-reacted with lung epithelial cells. These antibodies were reported to be cytotoxic to type-2 pneumocytes and were not found in non-SARS pneumonia patients (Lin et al., 2005b). Translating this into therapeutic terms, these studies suggest that steroids and plasmapheresis might be tried to correct these pathogenetic mechanisms.

Histologically, the lungs have evidence of patchy "diffuse" alveolar damage with a mixed inflammatory infiltrate, edema, microthrombi (Lang et al., 2003) and hyaline membrane formation (Ding et al., 2003; Franks et al., 2003; Ksiazek et al., 2003; Nicholls et al., 2003). SARS-CoV has been identified within fibrin, macrophages, and type-1 and type-2 pneumocytes by immunohistochemistry (Chan et al., 2005b), *in situ* hybridization (To et al., 2004; Chan et al., 2005b; Xu et al., 2005), and electron microscopy (Nicholls et al., 2003; Shieh et al., 2005). Desquamation of type-1 pneumocytes with proliferation of type-2 pneumocytes were consistently present (Franks et al., 2003; Griffiths et al., 2005). Multinucleated type-2 pneumocytes and macrophages similar to those observed in cell cultures were sometimes found (Franks et al., 2003).

SARS-CoV-infected cells displaying S on the surface fuse with adjacent cells expressing hACE2 (Petit et al., 2005), resulting in a little-appreciated route by which adjacent cells appear to become infected by accretion, even before the release of mature progeny virus. The nuclei may be enlarged and nucleoli prominent, but intranuclear inclusions have not been observed (Ksiazek et al., 2003), consistent with the fact that SARS-CoV replicates in the cytoplasm. When healing begins, it is accompanied by squamous metaplasia (Franks et al., 2003) and fibrosis in some patients. Pneumomediastinum has been reported in 10% of patients, unrelated to intubation or positive pressure ventilation (Peiris et al., 2003a; Chu et al., 2004b).

Extrapulmonary pathology

Although enteric infections by SARS-CoV were common in SARS patients and viral replication in the g.i. tract was documented, morphological changes there were minimal (Leung et al., 2003b; Chan et al., 2005b). In patients with lymphopenia, lymphoid depletion was observed in the splenic white pulp and in mucosa-associated lymphoid tissue of the g.i. tract (Ding et al., 2003; Zhong et al., 2003a; Tse et al., 2004; Gu et al., 2005). Striking hepatic mitotic activity was reported in two patients (Chau et al., 2004). Proof of SARS-CoV infection of the liver, however, has remained elusive (Chan et al., 2005b). Evidence of systemic vasculitis was reported in patients who died in a Chinese hospital (Ding et al., 2003). Recently, immune-mediated orchitis was described in men who died from SARS. Unlike mumps orchitis, which is usually (but not always) unilateral, the involvement was bilateral and appeared to target the germ cells, with the possibility of reduced fertility in men who recovered from the infection (Xu et al., 2005).

Immune response

The innate immune response to SARS-CoV infection included elaboration of acute-phase proteins, chemokines, inflammatory cytokines, and C-type lectins such as MBL. Ip et al. showed that MBL prevents SARS-CoV infection of FRhK-4 cells *in vitro*, in accordance with the non-specific role of this lectin that functions before the antibody response (Ip et al., 2005). They further investigated 569 SARS patients and demonstrated significantly lower serum levels of MBL and a significant prevalence of low-secretor genetic polymorphism than in 1188 controls. Similar conclusions were drawn in a genetic association study in northern China involving 352 SARS patients and 392 control subjects. Reduced expression of functional MBL was attributed to the codon 54 variant (Zhang et al., 2005b). Leikins et al. showed that the θ-defensin retrocyclin 2 inhibits influenza virus entry into cells by cross-linking surface glycoprotein and that the related MBL and human β-defensin 3 similarly inhibited the step that precedes viral entry (Leikina et al., 2005).

Evidence suggests that adaptive immunity in convalescent patients confers not only lasting protection against SARS-CoV, but also determines the outcome of infection (Zhang et al., 2005c). Convalescent patients develop IgG-class neutralizing antibodies against S protein (Traggiai et al., 2004; Lau and Peiris, 2005; Temperton et al., 2005). These antibodies prevent infection of permissive cell lines *in vitro*. At 7–8 months post-infection, the titer of neutralizing antibody to SARS-CoV remains stable (Traggiai et al., 2004; Chan et al., 2005a), suggesting the potential for lasting immunity and the possibility that developing an effective vaccine might be feasible.

Virologic diagnosis

The identification of SARS-CoV played a crucial role in the development of reliable diagnostic tests. These diagnostic tests were important because viral culture was only available in a few BSL3 laboratories. RT-PCR was developed as soon as SARS-CoV was identified (Drosten et al., 2003a; Ksiazek et al., 2003; Peiris et al., 2003b). At the same time, real-time quantitative reverse transcriptase-PCR (qRT-PCR) assays using intercalating dye, or in conjunction with single or, later, dual TaqMan probes, resulted in a significant increase in sensitivity and throughput compared to conventional RT-PCR (Drosten et al., 2003a; Poon et al., 2003; Jiang et al., 2004; Poon et al., 2004b; Yip et al., 2005). WHO network laboratories made available various primers and protocols for these tests (http://www.who.int/csr/sars/primers/en/index.html). Specimens from the upper respiratory tract, sputum, blood, stool, and urine have all yielded viral nucleic acid at various stages of the illness (Grant et al., 2003; Ng et al., 2003; Tong et al., 2003; Chan et al., 2004d; Hung et al., 2004; Ng et al., 2004). Viral load data generated from qRT-PCR were later shown to correlate with outcome (Chu et al., 2004c; Hung et al., 2004). For laboratories with fewer resources and those concerned about the shelf life of diagnostic kits, a highly sensitive gel-based RT-PCR protocol targeting the proteinase gene has been useful (Inoue et al., 2005).

Tests for antibodies to SARS-CoV, however, were plagued by concerns about sensitivity (only 60% positivity) (Chan et al., 2004b) and specificity. Peiris, Ksiazek, and Drosten used indirect fluorescence antibody (IFA) and cell culture extract-based ELISA assays to demonstrate seroconversion and a progressive increase in antibody titers in SARS (Drosten et al., 2003a; Ksiazek et al., 2003; Peiris et al., 2003b). IFA is specific (Chan et al., 2004c), but labor intensive and has an additional theoretical risk because virus-infected cells are used on the microscopic slides. ELISA assays using Vero cell extracts may yield false-positive results because of autoantibodies in patients with autoimmune disorders as well as in some normal subjects (Wang et al., 2004b). Recombinant N-based ELISA tests (Woo et al., 2004b) have cross-reacted with other HCoV. Protein immunoblotting against N and S could be used in conjunction with these other assays by identifying the false-positive results (Woo et al., 2004a). Recently, Chan et al. showed that SARS-CoV induces an anamnestic response to HCoV OC43, 229E, and NL63, demanding care in the interpretation of serological findings (Chan et al., 2005a).

Employing Pepscan analyses against convalescent patient sera and vaccine-induced laboratory animal antisera, He et al. identified regions in the M protein (M1-31 and M132-161) unique to SARS-CoV. Recombinant peptides from those regions have been exploited to overcome cross-reactivity in a recently developed ELISA test that correctly discriminated 40 SARS convalescent sera from 30 control sera (He et al., 2005a). Other advances led to the use of pseudotyped virus for the neutralization assay in lieu of SARS-CoV (Giroglou et al., 2004; Han et al., 2004; Yang et al., 2004b; Temperton et al., 2005).

Because of low sensitivity, none of the "rapid tests" can exclude SARS in a suspected case, and the testing of different types of specimens collected at different times is now recommended (Peiris et al., 2003c; Bermingham et al., 2004). The prolonged infectivity of respiratory and stool specimens demand careful handling of specimens (Lai et al., 2005a). Microarray and investigational plasma proteomic approaches to diagnosis [17, 82, 88] are under development. Issues in molecular diagnosis have been reviewed elsewhere (Poon et al., 2004a; Mahony and Richardson, 2005).

Drug therapy

The number of pharmacological agents with a significant selectivity index (CC_{50} divided by EC_{50}) against SARS-CoV has increased as knowledge of SARS-CoV biology has increased (Holmes, 2003). Thomas Lai has reviewed the therapeutic experience during the SARS epidemic (Lai, 2005).

Ribavirin

Ribavirin is a purine nucleoside analog that interacts with viral RNA polymerases as well as having other poorly characterized activities against viruses (Parker, 2005). In therapy of the hepatitis C virus, ribavirin is thought to act by inhibition of GTP synthesis by an effect on inosine monophosphate dehydrogenase, thereby limiting viral RNA synthesis, and by enhancement of Th1 responses, which may assist viral clearance (Thomas et al., 1999). For SARS-CoV, however, its *in vitro* activity is inconsistent (Morgenstern et al., 2005), and it has had no demonstrable clinical benefit in uncontrolled series of patients (Avendano et al., 2003; van Vonderen et al., 2003). In addition to the fact that it is a teratogen, it can cause a dose-dependent but reversible hemolytic anemia (Knowles et al., 2003). Its continued empirical use in SARS is not recommended (Knowles et al., 2003; van Vonderen et al., 2003).

Other antiviral therapies

Glycyrrhizin (Cinatl et al., 2003) and its derivatives (Wu et al., 2004; Hoever et al., 2005) have shown promising selective activity (selective activity index > 33) against SARS-CoV. Its antiviral activities may be related to its effects on cellular signaling pathways, transcription factors (AP-1, NF-kB), and its upregulation of inducible nitrous oxide synthase (Cinatl et al., 2003). Moreover, its effect on lowering plasma membrane fluidity and hence impeding viral entry, is consistent with its observed broad antiviral activity (Harada, 2005).

Chloroquine, discovered by the German chemist Hans Andersag in 1934 and used for the treatment of malaria, amebiasis, HIV, and autoimmune diseases, was recognized to have activity against SARS-CoV *in vitro*, with a selectivity index of 30 against SARS-CoV in Vero E6 cell culture (Savarino et al., 2003; Keyaerts et al., 2004; Vincent et al., 2005). Chloroquine elevates endosomal pH and interferes with terminal glycosylation of ACE2 (Vincent et al., 2005), thus having both non-specific and specific anti-SARS-CoV activities.

Drugs that target viral proteases

Inhibiting SARS-CoV 3CLpro prevents the assembly of a functional replication complex (Bacha et al., 2004; Lee et al., 2005a; Martina et al., 2005). Conservation among coronaviruses suggests that a wide-spectrum inhibitor against the main protease is feasible (Yang et al., 2005a), which may be useful against the several related strains of SARS-CoV-like viruses (Lau et al., 2005; Li et al., 2005c). Homology modeling has revealed remarkable conservation of substrate-binding sites among SARS-CoV, HCoV-229E, and PEDV (Anand et al., 2003). However, one such inhibitor of viral proteases, AG7088, did not show *in vitro* activity at the concentration of 10 μM (Wu et al., 2004).

During the epidemic in Guangzhou, clinicians observed that HIV-positive patients on highly active anti-retroviral therapy (HAART) appear to be protected against SARS (Chen et al., 2003; Chen and Cao, 2004). In Hong Kong, the utility of lopinavir–ritonavir combination therapy was investigated in a multicenter retrospective matched cohort study as initial and rescue therapy for SARS (Chan et al., 2003). Patients who received this therapy as initial treatment for SARS had better outcome (reduced death and intubation rate) compared with an uncontrolled group, with a lower rate of use of methylprednisolone at a lower mean dose. The results were similar in a subset of those patients reported separately (Chu et al., 2004a). These clinical trials are in agreement with structural studies that predicted the utility of lopinavir, ritonavir, niclosamide, and promazine against 3CL pro

(Zhang and Yap, 2004), with lopinavir and nelfinavir also showing *in vitro* activity (Chen et al., 2004a; Chu et al., 2004a; Yamamoto et al., 2004).

Therapy by blocking viral entry

The interactions between SARS-CoV and host cell involve binding, conformational change of S2, and membrane fusion, all of which are possible targets for therapy. Novel chimeric immunoglobulins such as CD4-IgG (Arthos et al., 2002), have shown benefit in treating HIV-1, and similarly, multivalent sACE2-immuno-globulin might be efficacious against SARS-CoV (Dimitrov, 2003), which can be improved by using residues 90–93 of civet ACE2 (Li et al., 2005e).

Because of the similar mechanism by which SARS-CoV S2 and HIV-1 gp41 mediate viral entry, S protein HR-derived peptides have been predicted to inhibit (Kliger and Levanon, 2003) and later shown to inhibit (Bosch et al., 2004) SARS-CoV infection of Vero cells. Recombinant proteins containing HR1 and HR2 were further shown to have potent inhibitory activities on entry of the HIV/SARS pseudoviruses into cells (Ni et al., 2005). These proteins are cheaper to produce than synthetic peptides and are more stable. Cathepsin L inhibitors could also be studied as entry inhibitors (Simmons et al., 2005).

Monoclonal antibody therapy

Monoclonal antibody with viral neutralizing activity has therapeutic potential against SARS and other viruses (Zhang et al., 2005d) and has been shown to be capable of preventing neonatal respiratory syncytial virus infection (Johnson et al., 1997). Monoclonal antibodies can protect ferrets against SARS-CoV infection (ter Meulen et al., 2004). Convalescent serum has been used in SARS patients, though its efficacy is unknown, and in experimentally infected mice, with possible activity against SARS-CoV infection in the latter (Wong et al., 2003b; Traggiai et al., 2004; Yeh et al., 2005).

An improved B-cell immortalization technique employing a CpG oligonucleotide (CpG 2006) as a polyclonal B-cell activator, was used with Epstein–Barr virus and irradiated allogeneic mononuclear cells to study the B-cell memory of a convalescent SARS patient. Neutralizing antibodies from one stable B-cell clone (S3.1) were found to protect mouse lungs from SARS-CoV challenge (Traggiai et al., 2004). Thirty-five neutralizing monoclonal antibodies were isolated in this study.

Eight recombinant human single-chain variable region fragments (scFvs) against the receptor-binding region of S protein were identified (Sui et al., 2004, 2005). One of these engineered monoclonal antibodies (80R IgG1) showed potent neutralization of SARS-CoV in *in vitro* and animal studies.

Interferons

The IFN signaling pathway is one of the targets of SARS-CoV (Cheung et al., 2005; Law et al., 2005a; Spiegel et al., 2005), suggesting that it may play an important role in host defense against SARS-CoV. Not unexpectedly, type-I IFN (α/β) but not type-II INF (γ) have shown potent inhibition of SARS-CoV infection and replication (Zheng et al., 2004a). Swedish scientists found that natural IFN-α and IFN-β have more potent *in vitro* activity than recombinant IFN-α (Chen et al., 2004b). A CpG oligodeoxynucleotide (BW001) strongly stimulated IFN-α secretion by dendritic cells and peripheral blood mononuclear cells; the supernatant fluid from these cells protected Vero cells from SARS-CoV infection (Bao et al., 2005). Macaques were protected by prophylactic use of pegylated IFN-α (Haagmans et al., 2004). Post-exposure prophylaxis of SARS by IFN yielded intermediate results. Uncontrolled clinical experience with IFN in the treatment of SARS has been reported. However, no randomized double-blind controlled trial has yet been conducted.

Vaccines

No effective vaccine has been developed so far. However, there is some evidence to suggest that successful vaccination may be possible. Molecular emergence studies have shown that SARS-CoV adapts to human ACE2, which presumably is not subject to much evolutionary pressure, and therefore it is likely that SARS-CoV making subsequent jumps to humans from animals will be covered by a vaccine developed against the 2003 human isolate (Lau et al., 2005; Li et al., 2005c; Zhi et al., 2005).

NIAID researchers engineered attenuated bovine-human parainfluenza virus (BHPIV3) to express various SARS-CoV structural proteins (Buchholz et al., 2004). They found that S, but not the other structural proteins (M, E, N), elicited neutralizing antibodies that protected the lungs of hamsters against SARS-CoV (Roberts et al., 2005). When a similar vaccine was given by the nasal route to African green monkeys (*Cercopithecus aethiops*), they shed no virus from the upper respiratory tract after challenge with SARS-CoV (Bukreyev et al., 2004).

Although the receptor-binding region of SARS-CoV is the most important target for neutralizing antibodies, the S2 "region" (Leu 803 to Ala 828), conserved across 45 viral isolates and containing a neutralizing antigenic determinant, was able to elicit neutralizing antibodies that protected some but not all small laboratory mammals against infection with SARS-CoV pseudovirus (Zhang et al., 2004). Over 100 potential cytotoxic T-lymphocyte (CTL) vaccine candidates that cover $>99\%$ of all individuals of all major human populations were identified within 6 months of the publication of the virus sequence (Sylvester-Hvid et al., 2004).

Antibody-enhanced viral pathogenicity is generally a concern with coronaviruses (Zhang et al., 2005a). With SARS-CoV infection, ferrets get a more severe hepatitis when first given a vaccinia-based recombinant SARS vaccine (Czub et al., 2005). More recently, NIAID scientists revealed that a pseudovirus expressing a *partially* humanized strain S (GD03T13) (GZ-03-01, Fig. 1 of Ref. (Song et al., 2005b) is markedly resistant to neutralization by immune IgG purified from mice vaccinated against S from strains derived from human isolates (Urbani strain) (Yang et al., 2005c). Antibodies raised against the human strain mediated enhanced entry of a lentiviral vector expressing civet S, but resistance to IgG enhancement of civet S is not limited to vaccinated mice; human monoclonal antibodies (S3.1, S111, S117) created from the immune repertoire of a convalescent patient (Traggiai et al., 2004) also exhibited these phenomena. Thus, a vaccine against humanized SARS-CoV might enhance the pathogenicity of a normally low-pathogenic animal SARS-CoV-like virus.

Another study showed that for SARS-CoV, which epitope *not* to employ in a vaccine is important. Interaction of antibody with conformational epitopes in the receptor-binding region was shown to be responsible for antibody-enhanced viral pathogenicity (Yang et al., 2005c). By deleting portions of S (truncated at aa1153), it was seen that the antibodies it induced did not promote enhancement. One monoclonal antibody (S110) was also found that did not mediate enhancement. This is consistent with other studies that have shown cross-reactivity between anti-S2 (aa927–937 and aa942–951) and lung cell antigens (Jiang et al., 2005a; Lin et al., 2005b).

Inactivated SARS-CoV can elicit neutralizing antibody (Takasuka et al., 2004; Tang et al., 2004) and cellular immunity. Mice vaccinated with inactivated SARS-CoV have been protected against challenge with intranasal SARS-CoV (Spruth et al., 2005).

Safety concerns about inactivated SARS-CoV vaccines are those of any inactivated vaccines, and they include the possibility that viral nucleic acid might remain infectious, as in the early days of the inactivated poliovirus vaccine (Katz, 2004; Offit, 2005). Another concern is the autoantibodies induced when Vero cells were used to cultivate SARS-CoV for experimental vaccines; the SARS-CoV neutralizing antibodies cross-reacted with an abundant human serum glycoprotein asialo-orosomucoid (ASOR) (Wang and Lu, 2004). An inactivated SARS-CoV vaccine using alum adjuvant has entered into a clinical trial in China, but the results are not yet available (Enserink, 2004).

The most attenuated SARS-CoV would be a genetically engineered version that could express proteins but that would not be transmissible from cell to cell (Holmes, 2003). Cross-reacting epitopes and toxic viral proteins (Chang et al., 2004; Imai et al., 2005; Kuba et al., 2005) would need to be excised or edited through genetic engineering techniques such as the construction and manipulation of full-length SARS-CoV cDNA (Yount et al., 2002, 2003).

Vectors for such an engineered vaccine could include a weakened version of the human parainfluenza virus 3, called BHPIV3. It is non-invasive (limited to the mucosa) and not known to recombine, unlike the coronaviruses. It replicates efficiently in children and with some engineering, might also replicate in non-naïve adults (Buchholz et al., 2004; Bukreyev et al., 2004), potentially yielding a vaccine with broad applications.

Other possible vectors such as adenovirus have been used to express SARS-CoV genes, and have been used to vaccinate macaque monkeys, eliciting neutralizing antibody and N-specific T-cell response (Gao et al., 2003). A highly attenuated vaccinia virus Ankara modified to express full-length S was given intranasally or intramuscularly to mice; it elicited cross-transferable (to other mice) humoral immunity that protected the upper as well as lower respiratory tracts against SARS-CoV (Bisht et al., 2004). Virus-like particles with no viral nucleic acid but containing S, M, and E proteins have been produced in Taiwan and the UK using insect cells infected by recombinant baculoviruses (Ho et al., 2004; Mortola and Roy, 2004), and might be suitable for study as vaccines.

DNA vaccines have been used to elicit protective humoral and cellular immunity against SARS-CoV in a mouse model (Yang et al., 2004b). A gene-based vaccine has also been tested, boosted by inactivated virus to broaden the immune response (Kong et al., 2005; Talaat and Stemke-Hale, 2005). A combination of nucleocapsid DNA vaccine against SARS-CoV with N protein has been shown to be required to generate antibody and a CD8+ response, and the presence of adjuvant determined whether humoral or cellular immunity is elicited (Azizi et al., 2005). Immunization with plasmid DNA carrying various S fragments have been shown by scientists at Hong Kong University to elicit antibodies in some mice, with the S1 fragment promoting a Th1-mediated antibody isotype switching. Both anti-S1 and anti-S2 antibodies were required for virus neutralization (Zeng et al., 2004a). One study of an experimental DNA vaccine against SARS-CoV showed that N alone was sufficient to induce antibody and CTL responses in mice (Zhu et al., 2004). In another study, N sequences linked to those specifying calreticulin (enhances antigen presentation to CD8+ T-cells) was efficacious in inducing N-specific humoral and cellular immune responses and in reducing the viral titer in mice challenged with N-expressing vaccinia virus (Kim et al., 2004). In mice immunized with plasmids, S, N, and M DNA vaccines were all able to elicit immune responses, with S and M eliciting more potent humoral and cellular immune responses, respectively (Wang et al., 2005c).

Most experience with DNA vaccines in other human viral diseases have been limited to various animal models (Gurunathan et al., 2000), although human studies have begun recently. With careful design, safety could be assured because integration into the genome appears to happen much less often than spontaneous mutations. Targeted delivery of nucleic acids will enable wider application of DNA vaccines (Song et al., 2005a). The ability of DNA vaccines to elicit both cellular and humoral immune responses, and their stability, simplicity, and versatility makes them attractive for immunization against intracellular pathogens such as SARS-CoV. Recent advances in this area have been reviewed (Taylor, 2005).

Implications for the future

A significant public health question is whether SARS-CoV will return. Many infectious diseases have reemerged in recent history (Fauci, 2005). SARS-CoV made a fleeting reemergence in the winter of 2003–2004 (Liang et al., 2004; Normile, 2004; Song et al., 2005b). With the discovery that the bat is the natural reservoir, it appears likely that SARS-CoV will eventually reemerge. However, the prospect of another large outbreak is low because an animal strain would have to adapt to humans before becoming epidemic, although it is not impossible that human isolate of SARS-CoV could have escaped back to the wild. Human strains of SARS-CoV bind efficiently to civet ACE2 (Li et al., 2005e). It might also bind bat ACE2 with avidity. The ease of species jumping as humans move into areas with SARS-CoV is suggested by the finding of SARS-CoV in rats, and the identification of serologically positive civets raised for the pet market in a farm in Shanwei, Guangdong. In the latter case, seed animals for that farm were bought at various markets in the province (Tu et al., 2004). Bats, civets, rodents, and other small mammals will need to be included in the surveillance for the presence of SARS-CoV.

Molecular emergence studies showed that most of the adaptations required for humanization of SARS-CoV took place within a short span early in the epidemic. This indicates a narrow window of opportunity for prevention of reemergence of SARS or the emergence of other viral infections. We missed the opportunity to prevent the emergence of SARS but managed to limit the damage. The conditions that can lead to reemergence are over-development and habitat destruction, excessive civet consumption, poor hygiene in markets and farms, etc.

Because poor market hygiene and management were major factors in the recent epidemic, major effort should be made to rectify the situation. Culinary culture needs to be modified in the interest of public health. Civets have been removed from the menu in Guandong and should remain so. Animals raised for food must be provided care and veterinary service, and wild animals should be left alone. Anthropocentric modification of the natural environment can lead to serious consequences (Dobson, 2005).

The careful design of hospitals (Li et al., 2005g), housing projects, and public places, with the unseen microbe in mind and with a view of providing clean breathing air will bring about the next quantum leap in public health (Tong and Liang, 2004; Tong, 2005a). Within health care facilities, awareness of infection control should be regularly refreshed so as to convert health care workers from "vectors" to infection controllers (Lloyd-Smith et al., 2003).

Amidst the exciting progress in vaccine development and drug discovery, we should be mindful that vaccines seldom achieve perfect immunity, and drug resistance is to be expected. However, the best time to face up to an emerging infectious disease is "now"—even before the outbreaks occur (Zhong et al., 2003b; Kuiken et al., 2005). Vaccines and drugs would be in the second line of defense, with public health measures being the first. Prevention of viral adaptation to the human receptor as a strategy against emerging viral diseases is the single most important translation from molecular emergence studies to public health management.

Last but not least, physicians must serve as sentinels for danger from this virus (Reilley et al., 2003). The lessons learned from this epidemic reinforced the need to strengthen surveillance and international cooperation, to maintain/upgrade time-honored infectious disease control practices, and to invest in rapid response capabilities such as the WHO. A paradigm shift to a better balance between defense (treatment) and preempting (prevention) is in order.

References

Anon., Cluster of severe acute respiratory syndrome cases among protected health-care workers—Toronto, Canada, April 2003. MMWR Morb Mortal Wkly Rep 2003a; 52: 433–436.

Anon., A multicentre collaboration to investigate the cause of severe acute respiratory syndrome. Lancet 2003b; 361: 1730–1733.

Anon., Prevalence of IgG antibody to SARS-associated coronavirus in animal traders—Guangdong Province, China, 2003. MMWR Morb Mortal Wkly Rep 2003c; 52: 986–987.

Anon., Update: outbreak of severe acute respiratory syndrome—worldwide, 2003. MMWR Morb Mortal Wkly Rep 2003d; 52: 269–272.

Anand K, Ziebuhr J, Wadhwani P, Mesters JR, Hilgenfeld R. Coronavirus main proteinase (3CLpro) structure: basis for design of anti-SARS drugs. Science 2003; 300: 1763–1767.

Anderson LJ. Infectious diseases: escaping an epidemic. Science 2005; 310: 444–445.

Arthos J, Cicala C, Steenbeke TD, Chun TW, Dela Cruz C, Hanback DB, Khazanie P, Nam D, Schuck P, Selig SM, Van Ryk D, Chaikin MA, Fauci AS. Biochemical and biological characterization of a dodecameric CD4-Ig fusion protein: implications for therapeutic and vaccine strategies. J Biol Chem 2002; 277: 11456–11464.

Avendano M, Derkach P, Swan S. Clinical course and management of SARS in health care workers in Toronto: a case series. CMAJ 2003; 168: 1649–1660.

Azizi A, Aucoin S, Ghorbani M, Soare C, Naas T, Tadesse H, Frost R, Diaz-Mitoma F. A combined nucleocapsid vaccine induces vigorous SARS-CD8+ T-cell immune responses. Genet Vaccines Ther 2005; 3: 7.

Bacha U, Barrila J, Velazquez-Campoy A, Leavitt SA, Freire E. Identification of novel inhibitors of the SARS coronavirus main protease 3CLpro. Biochemistry 2004; 43: 4906–4912.

Bao M, Zhang Y, Wan M, Dai L, Hu X, Wu X, Wang L, Deng P, Wang J, Chen J, Liu Y, Yu Y, Wang L. Anti-SARS-CoV immunity induced by a novel CpG oligodeoxynucleotide. Clin. Immunol. 2005; 118: 180–187.

Bergeron E, Vincent MJ, Wickham L, Hamelin J, Basak A, Nichol ST, Chretien M, Seidah NG. Implication of proprotein convertases in the processing and spread of severe acute respiratory syndrome coronavirus. Biochem Biophys Res Commun 2005; 326: 554–563.

Bermingham A, Heinen P, Iturriza-Gomara M, Gray J, Appleton H, Zambon MC. Laboratory diagnosis of SARS. Philos Trans R Soc Lond B Biol Sci 2004; 359: 1083–1089.

Bisht H, Roberts A, Vogel L, Bukreyev A, Collins PL, Murphy BR, Subbarao K, Moss B. Severe acute respiratory syndrome coronavirus spike protein expressed by attenuated vaccinia virus protectively immunizes mice. Proc Natl Acad Sci USA 2004; 101: 6641–6646.

Booth CM, Matukas LM, Tomlinson GA, Rachlis AR, Rose DB, Dwosh HA, Walmsley SL, Mazzulli T, Avendano M, Derkach P, Ephtimios IE, Kitai I, Mederski BD,

Shadowitz SB, Gold WL, Hawryluck LA, Rea E, Chenkin JS, Cescon DW, Poutanen SM, Detsky AS. Clinical features and short-term outcomes of 144 patients with SARS in the greater Toronto area. JAMA 2003; 289: 2801–2809.

Booth TF, Kournikakis B, Bastien N, Ho J, Kobasa D, Stadnyk L, Li Y, Spence M, Paton S, Henry B, Mederski B, White D, Low DE, McGeer A, Simor A, Vearncombe M, Downey J, Jamieson FB, Tang P, Plummer F. Detection of airborne severe acute respiratory syndrome (SARS) coronavirus and environmental contamination in SARS outbreak units. J Infect Dis 2005; 191: 1472–1477.

Bosch BJ, Martina BE, Van Der Zee R, Lepault J, Haijema BJ, Versluis C, Heck AJ, De Groot R, Osterhaus AD, Rottier PJ. Severe acute respiratory syndrome coronavirus (SARS-CoV) infection inhibition using spike protein heptad repeat-derived peptides. Proc Natl Acad Sci USA 2004; 101: 8455–8460.

Breslin JJ, Mork I, Smith MK, Vogel LK, Hemmila EM, Bonavia A, Talbot PJ, Sjostrom H, Noren O, Holmes KV. Human coronavirus 229E: receptor binding domain and neutralization by soluble receptor at 37 degrees C. J Virol 2003; 77: 4435–4438.

Buchholz UJ, Bukreyev A, Yang L, Lamirande EW, Murphy BR, Subbarao K, Collins PL. Contributions of the structural proteins of severe acute respiratory syndrome coronavirus to protective immunity. Proc Natl Acad Sci USA 2004; 101: 9804–9809.

Bukreyev A, Lamirande EW, Buchholz UJ, Vogel LN, Elkins WR, St Claire M, Murphy BR, Subbarao K, Collins PL. Mucosal immunisation of African green monkeys (*Cercopithecus aethiops*) with an attenuated parainfluenza virus expressing the SARS coronavirus spike protein for the prevention of SARS. Lancet 2004; 363: 2122–2127.

Cai CZ, Han LY, Chen X, Cao ZW, Chen YZ. Prediction of functional class of the SARS coronavirus proteins by a statistical learning method. J Proteome Res 2005; 4: 1855–1862.

Campanacci V, Egloff MP, Longhi S, Ferron F, Rancurel C, Salomoni A, Durousseau C, Tocque F, Bremond N, Dobbe JC, Snijder EJ, Canard B, Cambillau C. Structural genomics of the SARS coronavirus: cloning, expression, crystallization and preliminary crystallographic study of the Nsp9 protein. Acta Crystallogr D Biol Crystallogr 2003; 59: 1628–1631.

Cavanagh D. Nidovirales: a new order comprising *Coronaviridae* and *Arteriviridae*. Arch Virol 1997; 142: 629–633.

Chan CW, Chiu WK, Chan CC, Chow EY, Cheung HM, Ip PL. Osteonecrosis in children with severe acute respiratory syndrome. Pediatr Infect Dis J 2004a; 23: 888–890.

Chan KH, Cheng VCC, Woo PCY, Lau SKP, Poon LLM, Guan Y, Seto WH, Yuen KY, Peiris JSM. Serological responses in patients with severe acute respiratory syndrome coronavirus infection and cross-reactivity with human coronaviruses 229E, OC43, and NL63. Clin Diagn Lab Immunol 2005a; 12: 1317–1321.

Chan KH, Poon LL, Cheng VC, Guan Y, Hung IF, Kong J, Yam LY, Seto WH, Yuen KY, Peiris JS. Detection of SARS coronavirus in patients with suspected SARS. Emerg Infect Dis 2004b; 10: 294–299.

Chan KS, Lai ST, Chu CM, Tsui E, Tam CY, Wong MM, Tse MW, Que TL, Peiris JS, Sung J, Wong VC, Yuen KY. Treatment of severe acute respiratory syndrome with lopinavir/ritonavir: a multicentre retrospective matched cohort study. Hong Kong Med J 2003; 9: 399–406.

Chan PK, Ng KC, Chan RC, Lam RK, Chow VC, Hui M, Wu A, Lee N, Yap FH, Cheng FW, Sung JJ, Tam JS. Immunofluorescence assay for serologic diagnosis of SARS. Emerg Infect Dis 2004c; 10: 530–532.

Chan PK, To WK, Ng KC, Lam RK, Ng TK, Chan RC, Wu A, Yu WC, Lee N, Hui DS, Lai ST, Hon EK, Li CK, Sung JJ, Tam JS. Laboratory diagnosis of SARS. Emerg Infect Dis 2004d; 10: 825–831.

Chan WS, Wu C, Chow SC, Cheung T, To KF, Leung WK, Chan PK, Lee KC, Ng HK, Au DM, Lo AW. Coronaviral hypothetical and structural proteins were found in the intestinal surface enterocytes and pneumocytes of severe acute respiratory syndrome (SARS). Mod. Pathol. 2005; 18: 1432–1439.

Chandran K, Sullivan NJ, Felbor U, Whelan SP, Cunningham JM. Endosomal proteolysis of the Ebola virus glycoprotein is necessary for infection. Science 2005; 308: 1643–1645.

Chang CK, Sue SC, Yu TH, Hsieh CM, Tsai CK, Chiang YC, Lee SJ, Hsiao HH, Wu WJ, Chang WL, Lin CH, Huang TH. Modular organization of SARS coronavirus nucleocapsid protein. J. Biomed Sci. 2005; 13: 59–72.

Chang YJ, Liu CY, Chiang BL, Chao YC, Chen CC. Induction of IL-8 release in lung cells via activator protein-1 by recombinant baculovirus displaying severe acute respiratory syndrome-coronavirus spike proteins: identification of two functional regions. J Immunol 2004; 173: 7602–7614.

Chau TN, Lee KC, Yao H, Tsang TY, Chow TC, Yeung YC, Choi KW, Tso YK, Lau T, Lai ST, Lai CL. SARS-associated viral hepatitis caused by a novel coronavirus: report of three cases. Hepatology 2004; 39: 302–310.

Chen F, Chan KH, Jiang Y, Kao RY, Lu HT, Fan KW, Cheng VC, Tsui WH, Hung IF, Lee TS, Guan Y, Peiris JS, Yuen KY. *In vitro* susceptibility of 10 clinical isolates of SARS coronavirus to selected antiviral compounds. J Clin Virol 2004a; 31: 69–75.

Chen L, Liu P, Gao H, Sun B, Chao D, Wang F, Zhu Y, Hedenstierna G, Wang CG. Inhalation of nitric oxide in the treatment of severe acute respiratory syndrome: a rescue trial in Beijing. Clin Infect Dis 2004b; 39: 1531–1535.

Chen RF, Chang JC, Yeh WT, Lee CH, Liu JW, Eng HL, Yang KD. Role of vascular cell adhesion molecules and leukocyte apoptosis in the lymphopenia and thrombocytopenia of patients with severe acute respiratory syndrome (SARS). Microbes Infect. 2005; 8: 122–127.

Chen W, Yan M, Yang L, Ding B, He B, Wang Y, Liu X, Liu C, Zhu H, You B, Huang S, Zhang J, Mu F, Xiang Z, Feng X, Wen J, Fang J, Yu J, Yang H, Wang J. SARS-associated coronavirus transmitted from human to pig. Emerg Infect Dis 2005b; 11: 446–448.

Chen XP, Cao Y. Consideration of highly active antiretroviral therapy in the prevention and treatment of severe acute respiratory syndrome. Clin Infect Dis 2004; 38: 1030–1032.

Chen XP, Li GH, Tang XP, Xiong Y, Chen XJ, Cao Y. Lack of severe acute respiratory syndrome in 19 AIDS patients hospitalized together. J Acquir Immune Defic Syndr 2003; 34: 242–243.

Cheng PK, Wong DA, Tong LK, Ip SM, Lo AC, Lau CS, Yeung EY, Lim WW. Viral shedding patterns of coronavirus in patients with probable severe acute respiratory syndrome. Lancet 2004; 363: 1699–1700.

Cheung CY, Poon LL, Ng IH, Luk W, Sia SF, Wu MH, Chan KH, Yuen KY, Gordon S, Guan Y, Peiris JS. Cytokine responses in severe acute respiratory syndrome coronavirus-infected macrophages *in vitro*: possible relevance to pathogenesis. J Virol 2005; 79: 7819–7826.

Chinese SMEC. Molecular evolution of the SARS coronavirus during the course of the SARS epidemic in China. Science 2004; 303: 1666–1669.

Choi KW, Chau TN, Tsang O, Tso E, Chiu MC, Tong WL, Lee PO, Ng TK, Ng WF, Lee KC, Lam W, Yu WC, Lai JY, Lai ST. Outcomes and prognostic factors in 267 patients with severe acute respiratory syndrome in Hong Kong. Ann Intern Med 2003; 139: 715–723.

Chow KY, Yeung YS, Hon CC, Zeng F, Law KM, Leung FC. Adenovirus-mediated expression of the C-terminal domain of SARS-CoV spike protein is sufficient to induce apoptosis in Vero E6 cells. FEBS Lett. 2005; 579: 6699–6704.

Chowell G, Castillo-Chavez C, Fenimore PW, Kribs-Zaleta CM, Arriola L, Hyman JM. Model parameters and outbreak control for SARS. Emerg Infect Dis 2004; 10: 1258–1263.

Christian MD, Poutanen SM, Loutfy MR, Muller MP, Low DE. Severe acute respiratory syndrome. Clin Infect Dis 2004; 38: 1420–1427.

Chu CM, Cheng VC, Hung IF, Wong MM, Chan KH, Chan KS, Kao RY, Poon LL, Wong CL, Guan Y, Peiris JS, Yuen KY. Role of lopinavir/ritonavir in the treatment of SARS: initial virological and clinical findings. Thorax 2004a; 59: 252–256.

Chu CM, Leung YY, Hui JY, Hung IF, Chan VL, Leung WS, Law KI, Chan CS, Chan KS, Yuen KY. Spontaneous pneumomediastinum in patients with severe acute respiratory syndrome. Eur Respir J 2004b; 23: 802–804.

Chu CM, Poon LL, Cheng VC, Chan KS, Hung IF, Wong MM, Chan KH, Leung WS, Tang BS, Chan VL, Ng WL, Sim TC, Ng PW, Law KI, Tse DM, Peiris JS, Yuen KY. Initial viral load and the outcomes of SARS. CMAJ 2004c; 171: 1349–1352.

Chung GT, Chiu RW, Cheung JL, Jin Y, Chim SS, Chan PK, Lo YD. A simple and rapid approach for screening of SARS-coronavirus genotypes: an evaluation study. BMC Infect Dis 2005; 5: 87.

Cinatl J, Morgenstern B, Bauer G, Chandra P, Rabenau H, Doerr HW. Glycyrrhizin, an active component of liquorice roots, and replication of SARS-associated coronavirus. Lancet 2003; 361: 2045–2046.

Crotty S, Cameron CE, Andino R. RNA virus error catastrophe: direct molecular test by using ribavirin. Proc Natl Acad Sci USA 2001; 98: 6895–6900.

Czub M, Weingartl H, Czub S, He R, Cao J. Evaluation of modified vaccinia virus Ankara based recombinant SARS vaccine in ferrets. Vaccine 2005; 23: 2273–2279.

Dimitrov DS. The secret life of ACE2 as a receptor for the SARS virus. Cell 2003; 115: 652–653.

Ding Y, He L, Zhang Q, Huang Z, Che X, Hou J, Wang H, Shen H, Qiu L, Li Z, Geng J, Cai J, Han H, Li X, Kang W, Weng D, Liang P, Jiang S. Organ distribution of severe acute respiratory syndrome (SARS) associated coronavirus (SARS-CoV) in SARS patients: implications for pathogenesis and virus transmission pathways. J Pathol 2004; 203: 622–630.

Ding Y, Wang H, Shen H, Li Z, Geng J, Han H, Cai J, Li X, Kang W, Weng D, Lu Y, Wu D, He L, Yao K. The clinical pathology of severe acute respiratory syndrome (SARS): a report from China. J Pathol 2003; 200: 282–289.

Dobson AP. Virology: what links bats to emerging infectious diseases? Science 2005; 310: 628–629.

Donoghue M, HsiehF, Baronas E, Godbout K, Gosselin M, Stagliano N, Donovan M, Woolf B, Robison K, Jeyaseelan R, Breitbart RE, Acton S. A novel angiotensin-converting enzyme-related carboxypeptidase (ACE2) converts angiotensin I to angiotensin 1-9. Circ Res 2000; 87: E1–E9.

Drosten C, Gunther S, Preiser W, van der Werf S, Brodt HR, Becker S, Rabenau H, Panning M, Kolesnikova L, Fouchier RA, Berger A, Burguiere AM, Cinatl J, Eickmann M,

Escriou N, Grywna K, Kramme S, Manuguerra JC, Muller S, Rickerts V, Sturmer M, Vieth S, Klenk HD, Osterhaus AD, Schmitz H, Doerr HW. Identification of a novel coronavirus in patients with severe acute respiratory syndrome. N Engl J Med 2003a; 348: 1967–1976.

Drosten C, Preiser W, Gunther S, Schmitz H, Doerr HW. Severe acute respiratory syndrome: identification of the etiological agent. Trends Mol Med 2003b; 9: 325–327.

Edwards DA, Man JC, Brand P, Katstra JP, Sommerer K, Stone HA, Nardell E, Scheuch G. Inhaling to mitigate exhaled bioaerosols. Proc Natl Acad Sci USA 2004; 101: 17383–17388.

Egloff MP, Ferron F, Campanacci V, Longhi S, Rancurel C, Dutartre H, Snijder EJ, Gorbalenya AE, Cambillau C, Canard B. The severe acute respiratory syndrome-coronavirus replicative protein nsp9 is a single-stranded RNA-binding subunit unique in the RNA virus world. Proc Natl Acad Sci USA 2004; 101: 3792–3796.

Eigen M. New concepts for dealing with the evolution of nucleic acids. Cold Spring Harb Symp Quant Biol 1987; 52: 307–320.

Emeny JM, Morgan MJ. Regulation of the interferon system: evidence that Vero cells have a genetic defect in interferon production. J Gen Virol 1979; 43: 247–252.

Enserink M. Albert Osterhaus profile. The virus collector. Science 2003a; 300: 1228–1229.

Enserink M. Breakthrough of the year. SARS: a pandemic prevented. Science 2003b; 302: 2045.

Enserink M. SARS in China. The big question now: will it be back? Science 2003c; 301: 299.

Enserink M. Infectious diseases. One year after outbreak, SARS virus yields some secrets. Science 2004; 304: 1097.

Fang X, Ye L, Timani KA, Li S, Zen Y, Zhao M, Zheng H, Wu Z. Peptide domain involved in the interaction between membrane protein and nucleocapsid protein of SARS-associated coronavirus. J Biochem Mol Biol 2005; 38: 381–385.

Fauci AS. Emerging and reemerging infectious diseases: the perpetual challenge. Acad Med 2005; 80: 1079–1085.

Fouchier RA, Kuiken T, Schutten M, van Amerongen G, van Doornum GJ, van den Hoogen BG, Peiris M, Lim W, Stohr K, Osterhaus AD. Aetiology: Koch's postulates fulfilled for SARS virus. Nature 2003; 423: 240.

Fowler RA, Scales DC, Ilan R. Evidence of airborne transmission of SARS. N Engl J Med 2004; 351: 609–611.

Franks TJ, Chong PY, Chui P, Galvin JR, Lourens RM, Reid AH, Selbs E, McEvoy CP, Hayden CD, Fukuoka J, Taubenberger JK, Travis WD. Lung pathology of severe acute respiratory syndrome (SARS): a study of 8 autopsy cases from Singapore. Hum Pathol 2003; 34: 743–748.

Galvani AP, May RM. Epidemiology: dimensions of superspreading. Nature 2005; 438: 293–295.

Gao W, Tamin A, Soloff A, D'Aiuto L, Nwanegbo E, Robbins PD, Bellini WJ, Barratt-Boyes S, Gambotto A. Effects of a SARS-associated coronavirus vaccine in monkeys. Lancet 2003; 362: 1895–1896.

Giroglou T, Cinatl Jr. J, Rabenau H, Drosten C, Schwalbe H, Doerr HW, von Laer D. Retroviral vectors pseudotyped with severe acute respiratory syndrome coronavirus S protein. J Virol 2004; 78: 9007–9015.

Gorbalenya AE, Snijder EJ, Spaan WJ. Severe acute respiratory syndrome coronavirus phylogeny: toward consensus. J Virol 2004; 78: 7863–7866.

Graham RL, Sims AC, Brockway SM, Baric RS, Denison MR. The nsp2 replicase proteins of murine hepatitis virus and severe acute respiratory syndrome coronavirus are dispensable for viral replication. J Virol 2005; 79: 13399–13411.

Gramberg T, Hofmann H, Moller P, Lalor PF, Marzi A, Geier M, Krumbiegel M, Winkler T, Kirchhoff F, Adams DH, Becker S, Munch J, Pohlmann S. LSECtin interacts with filovirus glycoproteins and the spike protein of SARS coronavirus. Virology 2005; 340: 224–236.

Grant PR, Garson JA, Tedder RS, Chan PK, Tam JS, Sung JJ. Detection of SARS coronavirus in plasma by real-time RT-PCR. N Engl J Med 2003; 349: 2468–2469.

Griffith JF, Antonio GE, Kumta SM, Hui DS, Wong JK, Joynt GM, Wu AK, Cheung AY, Chiu KH, Chan KM, Leung PC, Ahuja AT. Osteonecrosis of hip and knee in patients with severe acute respiratory syndrome treated with steroids. Radiology 2005; 235: 168–175.

Griffiths MJ, Bonnet D, Janes SM. Stem cells of the alveolar epithelium. Lancet 2005; 366: 249–260.

Groneberg DA, Hilgenfeld R, Zabel P. Molecular mechanisms of severe acute respiratory syndrome (SARS). Respir Res 2005; 6: 8.

Gu J, Gong E, Zhang B, Zheng J, Gao Z, Zhong Y, Zou W, Zhan J, Wang S, Xie Z, Zhuang H, Wu B, Zhong H, Shao H, Fang W, Gao D, Pei F, Li X, He Z, Xu D, Shi X, Anderson VM, Leong ASY. Multiple organ infection and the pathogenesis of SARS. J Exp Med 2005; 202: 415–424.

Guan Y, Peiris JS, Zheng B, Poon LL, Chan KH, Zeng FY, Chan CW, Chan MN, Chen JD, Chow KY, Hon CC, Hui KH, Li J, Li VY, Wang Y, Leung SW, Yuen KY, Leung FC. Molecular epidemiology of the novel coronavirus that causes severe acute respiratory syndrome. Lancet 2004; 363: 99–104.

Guan Y, Zheng BJ, He YQ, Liu XL, Zhuang ZX, Cheung CL, Luo SW, Li PH, Zhang LJ, Guan YJ, Butt KM, Wong KL, Chan KW, Lim W, Shortridge KF, Yuen KY, Peiris JS, Poon LL. Isolation and characterization of viruses related to the SARS coronavirus from animals in southern China. Science 2003; 302: 276–278.

Guarino LA, Bhardwaj K, Dong W, Sun J, Holzenburg A, Kao C. Mutational analysis of the SARS virus Nsp15 endoribonuclease: identification of residues affecting hexamer formation. J Mol Biol. 2005; 353: 1106–1117.

Guillen J, Perez-Berna AJ, Moreno MR, Villalain J. Identification of the membrane-active regions of the severe acute respiratory syndrome coronavirus spike membrane glycoprotein using a 16/18-mer peptide scan: implications for the viral fusion mechanism. J Virol 2005; 79: 1743–1752.

Gurunathan S, Klinman DM, Seder RA. DNA vaccines: immunology, application, and optimization. Annu Rev Immunol 2000; 18: 927–974.

Gutierrez AL, Denova-Ocampo M, Racaniello VR, del Angel RM. Attenuating mutations in the poliovirus 5′ untranslated region alter its interaction with polypyrimidine tract-binding protein. J Virol 1997; 71: 3826–3833.

Haagmans BL, Kuiken T, Martina BE, Fouchier RA, Rimmelzwaan GF, van Amerongen G, van Riel D, de Jong T, Itamura S, Chan KH, Tashiro M, Osterhaus AD. Pegylated interferon-alpha protects type 1 pneumocytes against SARS coronavirus infection in macaques. Nat Med 2004; 10: 290–293.

Hamming I, Timens W, Bulthuis ML, Lely AT, Navis GJ, van Goor H. Tissue distribution of ACE2 protein, the functional receptor for SARS coronavirus. A first step in understanding SARS pathogenesis. J Pathol 2004; 203: 631–637.

Han DP, Kim HG, Kim YB, Poon LL, Cho MW. Development of a safe neutralization assay for SARS-CoV and characterization of S-glycoprotein. Virology 2004; 326: 140–149.

Harada S. Broad anti-viral agent glycyrrhizin directly modulates the fluidity of plasma membrane and HIV-1 envelope. Biochem J 2005; 392: 191–199.

Harmer D, Gilbert M, Borman R, Clark KL. Quantitative mRNA expression profiling of ACE 2, a novel homologue of angiotensin converting enzyme. FEBS Lett 2002; 532: 107–110.

He R, Leeson A, Andonov A, Li Y, Bastien N, Cao J, Osiowy C, Dobie F, Cutts T, Ballantine M, Li X. Activation of AP-1 signal transduction pathway by SARS coronavirus nucleocapsid protein. Biochem Biophys Res Commun 2003; 311: 870–876.

He R, Leeson A, Ballantine M, Andonov A, Baker L, Dobie F, Li Y, Bastien N, Feldmann H, Strocher U, Theriault S, Cutts T, Cao J, Booth TF, Plummer FA, Tyler S, Li X. Characterization of protein–protein interactions between the nucleocapsid protein and membrane protein of the SARS coronavirus. Virus Res 2004a; 105: 121–125.

He Y, Zhou Y, Siddiqui P, Jiang S. Inactivated SARS-CoV vaccine elicits high titers of spike protein-specific antibodies that block receptor binding and virus entry. Biochem Biophys Res Commun 2004b; 325: 445–452.

He Y, Zhou Y, Siddiqui P, Niu J, Jiang S. Identification of immunodominant epitopes on the membrane protein of the severe acute respiratory syndrome-associated coronavirus. J Clin Microbiol 2005a; 43: 3718–3726.

He Y, Zhou Y, Wu H, Luo B, Chen J, Li W, Jiang S. Identification of immunodominant sites on the spike protein of severe acute respiratory syndrome (SARS) coronavirus: implication for developing SARS diagnostics and vaccines. J Immunol 2004c; 173: 4050–4057.

He Z, Zhao C, Dong Q, Zhuang H, Song S, Peng G, Dwyer DE. Effects of acute severe acute respiratory syndrome (SARS) coronavirus infection on peripheral blood lymphocytes and their subsets. Int J Infect Dis. 2005; 9: 323–330.

Heymann D. David Heymann—WHO's public health guru. Interview by Haroon Ashraf. Lancet Infect Dis 2004; 4: 785–788.

Ho Y, Lin PH, Liu CY, Lee SP, Chao YC. Assembly of human severe acute respiratory syndrome coronavirus-like particles. Biochem Biophys Res Commun 2004; 318: 833–838.

Hoever G, Baltina L, Michaelis M, Kondratenko R, Baltina L, Tolstikov GA, Doerr HW, Cinatl Jr. J. Antiviral activity of glycyrrhizic acid derivatives against SARS-coronavirus. J Med Chem 2005; 48: 1256–1259.

Hofmann H, Geier M, Marzi A, Krumbiegel M, Peipp M, Fey GH, Gramberg T, Pohlmann S. Susceptibility to SARS coronavirus S protein-driven infection correlates with expression of angiotensin converting enzyme 2 and infection can be blocked by soluble receptor. Biochem Biophys Res Commun 2004; 319: 1216–1221.

Hofmann H, Pyrc K, van der Hoek L, Geier M, Berkhout B, Pohlmann S. Human coronavirus NL63 employs the severe acute respiratory syndrome coronavirus receptor for cellular entry. Proc Natl Acad Sci USA 2005; 102: 7988–7993.

Holmes EC, Rambaut A. Viral evolution and the emergence of SARS coronavirus. Philos Trans R Soc Lond B Biol Sci 2004; 359: 1059–1065.

Holmes KV. SARS coronavirus: a new challenge for prevention and therapy. J Clin Invest 2003; 111: 1605–1609.

Holmes KV. Structural biology. Adaptation of SARS coronavirus to humans. Science 2005; 309: 1822–1823.

Hon KL, Leung CW, Cheng WT, Chan PK, Chu WC, Kwan YW, Li AM, Fong NC, Ng PC, Chiu MC, Li CK, Tam JS, Fok TF. Clinical presentations and outcome of severe acute respiratory syndrome in children. Lancet 2003; 361: 1701–1703.

Horimoto T, Kawaoka Y. Influenza: lessons from past pandemics, warnings from current incidents. Nat Rev Microbiol 2005; 3: 591–600.

Hsieh P-K, Chang SC, Huang C-C, Lee T-T, Hsiao C-W, Kou Y-H, Chen IY, Chang C-K, Huang T-H, Chang M-F. Assembly of severe acute respiratory syndrome coronavirus RNA packaging signal into virus-like particles is nucleocapsid dependent. J Virol 2005; 79: 13848–13855.

Hui DS, Wong KT, Ko FW, Tam LS, Chan DP, Woo J, Sung JJY. The 1-year impact of severe acute respiratory syndrome on pulmonary function, exercise capacity, and quality of life in a cohort of survivors. Chest 2005; 128: 2247–2261.

Hung IF, Cheng VC, Wu AK, Tang BS, Chan KH, Chu CM, Wong MM, Hui WT, Poon LL, Tse DM, Chan KS, Woo PC, Lau SK, Peiris JS, Yuen KY. Viral loads in clinical specimens and SARS manifestations. Emerg Infect Dis 2004; 10: 1550–1557.

Imai Y, Kuba K, Rao S, Huan Y, Guo F, Guan B, Yang P, Sarao R, Wada T, Leong-Poi H, Crackower MA, Fukamizu A, Hui CC, Hein L, Uhlig S, Slutsky AS, Jiang C, Penninger JM. Angiotensin-converting enzyme 2 protects from severe acute lung failure. Nature 2005; 436: 112–116.

Inoue M, Barkham T, Keong LK, Gee LS, Wanjin H. Performance of single-step gel-based reverse transcription-PCR (RT-PCR) assays equivalent to that of real-time RT-PCR assays for detection of the severe acute respiratory syndrome-associated coronavirus. J Clin Microbiol 2005; 43: 4262–4265.

Ip WK, Chan KH, Law HK, Tso GH, Kong EK, Wong WH, To YF, Yung RW, Chow EY, Au KL, Chan EY, Lim W, Jensenius JC, Turner MW, Peiris JS, Lau YL. Mannose-binding lectin in severe acute respiratory syndrome coronavirus infection. J Infect Dis 2005; 191: 1697–1704.

Ito N, Mossel EC, Narayanan K, Popov VL, Huang C, Inoue T, Peters CJ, Makino S. Severe acute respiratory syndrome coronavirus 3a protein is a viral structural protein. J Virol 2005; 79: 3182–3186.

Itoyama S, Keicho N, Quy T, Phi NC, Long HT, Ha le D, Ban VV, Ohashi J, Hijikata M, Matsushita I, Kawana A, Yanai H, Kirikae T, Kuratsuji T, Sasazuki T. ACE1 polymorphism and progression of SARS. Biochem Biophys Res Commun 2004; 323: 1124–1129.

Jeffers SA, Tusell SM, Gillim-Ross L, Hemmila EM, Achenbach JE, Babcock GJ, Thomas Jr. WD, Thackray LB, Young MD, Mason RJ, Ambrosino DM, Wentworth DE, Demartini JC, Holmes KV. CD209L (L-SIGN) is a receptor for severe acute respiratory syndrome coronavirus. Proc Natl Acad Sci USA 2004; 101: 15748–15753.

Jia HP, Look DC, Shi L, Hickey M, Pewe L, Netland J, Farzan M, Wohlford-Lenane C, Perlman S, McCray Jr PB. ACE2 receptor expression and severe acute respiratory syndrome coronavirus infection depend on differentiation of human airway epithelia. J Virol 2005; 79: 14614–14621.

Jiang S, He Y, Liu S. SARS vaccine development. Emerg Infect Dis 2005a; 11: 1016–1020.

Jiang SS, Chen TC, Yang JY, Hsiung CA, Su IJ, Liu YL, Chen PC, Juang JL. Sensitive and quantitative detection of severe acute respiratory syndrome coronavirus infection by real-time nested polymerase chain reaction. Clin Infect Dis 2004; 38: 293–296.

Jiang XS, Tang LY, Dai J, Zhou H, Li SJ, Xia QC, Wu JR, Zeng R. Quantitative analysis of SARS-coronavirus infected cells using proteomic approaches: implications for cellular responses to virus infection. Mol Cell Proteomics 2005; 4: 902–913.

Johnson S, Oliver C, Prince GA, Hemming VG, Pfarr DS, Wang SC, Dormitzer M, O'Grady J, Koenig S, Tamura JK, Woods R, Bansal G, Couchenour D, Tsao E, Hall WC, Young JF. Development of a humanized monoclonal antibody (MEDI-493) with potent *in vitro* and *in vivo* activity against respiratory syncytial virus. J Infect Dis 1997; 176: 1215–1224.

Kan B, Wang M, Jing H, Xu H, Jiang X, Yan M, Liang W, Zheng H, Wan K, Liu Q, Cui B, Xu Y, Zhang E, Wang H, Ye J, Li G, Li M, Cui Z, Qi X, Chen K, Du L, Gao K, Zhao Y-t, Zou X-z, Feng Y-J, Gao Y-F, Hai R, Yu D, Guan Y, Xu J. Molecular evolution analysis and geographic investigation of severe acute respiratory syndrome coronavirus-like virus in palm civets at an animal market and on farms. J Virol 2005; 79: 11892–11900.

Kang X, Xu Y, Wu X, Liang Y, Wang C, Guo J, Wang Y, Chen M, Wu D, Wang Y, Bi S, Qiu Y, Lu P, Cheng J, Xiao B, Hu L, Gao X, Liu J, Wang Y, Song Y, Zhang L, Suo F, Chen T, Huang Z, Zhao Y, Lu H, Pan C, Tang H. Proteomic fingerprints for potential application to early diagnosis of severe acute respiratory syndrome. Clin Chem 2005; 51: 56–64.

Katz SL. From culture to vaccine—Salk and Sabin. N Engl J Med 2004; 351: 1485–1487.

Keyaerts E, Vijgen L, Maes P, Neyts J, Van Ranst M. *In vitro* inhibition of severe acute respiratory syndrome coronavirus by chloroquine. Biochem Biophys Res Commun 2004; 323: 264–268.

Kim CF, Jackson EL, Woolfenden AE, Lawrence S, Babar I, Vogel S, Crowley D, Bronson RT, Jacks T. Identification of bronchioalveolar stem cells in normal lung and lung cancer. Cell 2005; 121: 823–835.

Kim TW, Lee JH, Hung CF, Peng S, Roden R, Wang MC, Viscidi R, Tsai YC, He L, Chen PJ, Boyd DA, Wu TC. Generation and characterization of DNA vaccines targeting the nucleocapsid protein of severe acute respiratory syndrome coronavirus. J Virol 2004; 78: 4638–4645.

Kliger Y, Levanon EY. Cloaked similarity between HIV-1 and SARS-CoV suggests an anti-SARS strategy. BMC Microbiol 2003; 3: 20.

Knowles SR, Phillips EJ, Dresser L, Matukas L. Common adverse events associated with the use of ribavirin for severe acute respiratory syndrome in Canada. Clin Infect Dis 2003; 37: 1139–1142.

Kong W-p, Xu L, Stadler K, Ulmer JB, Abrignani S, Rappuoli R, Nabel GJ. Modulation of the immune response to the severe acute respiratory syndrome spike glycoprotein by gene-based and inactivated virus immunization. J Virol 2005; 79: 13915–13923.

Krug RM, Yuan W, Noah DL, Latham AG. Intracellular warfare between human influenza viruses and human cells: the roles of the viral NS1 protein. Virology 2003; 309: 181–189.

Ksiazek TG, Erdman D, Goldsmith CS, Zaki SR, Peret T, Emery S, Tong S, Urbani C, Comer JA, Lim W, Rollin PE, Dowell SF, Ling AE, Humphrey CD, Shieh WJ, Guarner J, Paddock CD, Rota P, Fields B, DeRisi J, Yang JY, Cox N, Hughes JM, LeDuc JW, Bellini WJ, Anderson LJ. A novel coronavirus associated with severe acute respiratory syndrome. N Engl J Med 2003; 348: 1953–1966.

Kuba K, Imai Y, Rao S, Gao H, Guo F, Guan B, Huan Y, Yang P, Zhang Y, Deng W, Bao L, Zhang B, Liu G, Wang Z, Chappell M, Liu Y, Zheng D, Leibbrandt A, Wada T, Slutsky AS, Liu D, Qin C, Jiang C, Penninger JM. A crucial role of angiotensin converting enzyme 2 (ACE2) in SARS coronavirus-induced lung injury. Nat Med 2005; 11: 875–879.

Kuiken T, Fouchier RA, Schutten M, Rimmelzwaan GF, van Amerongen G, van Riel D, Laman JD, de Jong T, van Doornum G, Lim W, Ling AE, Chan PK, Tam JS, Zambon MC, Gopal R, Drosten C, van der Werf S, Escriou N, Manuguerra JC, Stohr K, Peiris JS, Osterhaus AD. Newly discovered coronavirus as the primary cause of severe acute respiratory syndrome. Lancet 2003; 362: 263–270.

Kuiken T, Leighton FA, Fouchier RA, LeDuc JW, Peiris JS, Schudel A, Stohr K, Osterhaus AD. Public health. Pathogen surveillance in animals. Science 2005; 309: 1680–1681.

Kwan AC, Chau TN, Tong WL, Tsang OT, Tso EY, Chiu MC, Yu WC, Lai TS. Severe acute respiratory syndrome-related diarrhea. J Gastroenterol Hepatol 2005a; 20: 606–610.

Kwan MY, Chan WM, Ko PW, Leung CW, Chiu MC. Severe acute respiratory syndrome can be mild in children. Pediatr Infect Dis J 2004; 23: 1172–1174.

Kwan YW, Leung CW, Chiu MC. Diarrhoea as the presenting sign in an adolescent suffering from severe acute respiratory syndrome. Eur J Pediatr 2005b; 164: 227–230.

Lai MM, Cavanagh D. The molecular biology of coronaviruses. Adv Virus Res 1997; 48: 1–100.

Lai MYY, Cheng PKC, Lim WWL. Survival of severe acute respiratory syndrome coronavirus. Clin Infect Dis 2005a; 41: e67–e71.

Lai PC, Wong CM, Hedley AJ, Lo SV, Leung PY, Kong J, Leung GM. Understanding the spatial clustering of severe acute respiratory syndrome (SARS) in Hong Kong. Environ Health Perspect 2004; 112: 1550–1556.

Lai ST. Treatment of severe acute respiratory syndrome. Eur J Clin Microbiol Infect Dis 2005; 24: 583–591.

Lai TS, Keung Ng T, Seto WH, Yam L, Law KI, Chan J. Low prevalence of subclinical severe acute respiratory syndrome-associated coronavirus infection among hospital healthcare workers in Hong Kong. Scand J Infect Dis 2005b; 37: 500–503.

Lang ZW, Zhang LJ, Zhang SJ, Meng X, Li JQ, Song CZ, Sun L, Zhou YS, Dwyer DE. A clinicopathological study of three cases of severe acute respiratory syndrome (SARS). Pathology 2003; 35: 526–531.

Lau SKP, Woo PCY, Li KSM, Huang Y, Tsoi H-W, Wong BHL, Wong SSY, Leung S-Y, Chan K-H, Yuen K-Y. Severe acute respiratory syndrome coronavirus-like virus in Chinese horseshoe bats. Proc Natl Acad Sci USA 2005; 102: 14040–14045.

Lau YL, Peiris JM. Pathogenesis of severe acute respiratory syndrome. Curr Opin Immunol 2005; 17: 404–410.

Law HK, Cheung CY, Ng HY, Sia SF, Chan YO, Luk W, Nicholls JM, Peiris JS, Lau YL. Chemokine upregulation in SARS coronavirus infected human monocyte derived dendritic cells. Blood 2005a; 106: 2366–2374.

Law PT, Wong CH, Au TC, Chuck CP, Kong SK, Chan PK, To KF, Lo AW, Chan JY, Suen YK, Chan HY, Fung KP, Waye MM, Sung JJ, Lo YM, Tsui SK. The 3a protein of severe acute respiratory syndrome-associated coronavirus induces apoptosis in Vero E6 cells. J Gen Virol 2005b; 86: 1921–1930.

Lee CH, Chen RF, Liu JW, Yeh WT, Chang JC, Liu PM, Eng HL, Lin MC, Yang KD. Altered p38 mitogen-activated protein kinase expression in different leukocytes with increment of immunosuppressive mediators in patients with severe acute respiratory syndrome. J Immunol 2004; 172: 7841–7847.

Lee HK, Tso EY, Chau TN, Tsang OT, Choi KW, Lai TS. Asymptomatic severe acute respiratory syndrome-associated coronavirus infection. Emerg Infect Dis 2003a; 9: 1491–1492.

Lee N, Hui D, Wu A, Chan P, Cameron P, Joynt GM, Ahuja A, Yung MY, Leung CB, To KF, Lui SF, Szeto CC, Chung S, Sung JJ. A major outbreak of severe acute respiratory syndrome in Hong Kong. N Engl J Med 2003b; 348: 1986–1994.

Lee TW, Cherney MM, Huitema C, Liu J, James KE, Powers JC, Eltis LD, James MN. Crystal structures of the main peptidase from the SARS coronavirus inhibited by a substrate-like aza-peptide epoxide. J Mol Biol 2005; 353: 1137–1151.

Lee YS, Chen CH, Chao A, Chen ES, Wei ML, Chen LK, Yang KD, Lin MC, Wang YH, Liu JW, Eng HL, Chiang PC, Wu TS, Tsao KC, Huang CG, Tien YJ, Wang TH, Wang HS, Lee YS. Molecular signature of clinical severity in patients infected with severe acute respiratory syndrome coronavirus (SARS-CoV). BMC Genomics 2005b; 6: 132.

Leikina E, Delanoe-Ayari H, Melikov K, Cho M-S, Chen A, Waring AJ, Wang W, Xie Y, Loo JA, Lehrer RI, Chernomordik LV. Carbohydrate-binding molecules inhibit viral fusion and entry by crosslinking membrane glycoproteins. Nat Immunol 2005; 6: 995–1001.

Leroy EM, Kumulungui B, Pourrut X, Rouquet P, Hassanin A, Yaba P, Delicat A, Paweska JT, Gonzalez J-P, Swanepoel R. Fruit bats as reservoirs of Ebola virus. Nature 2005; 438: 575–576.

Leung FC. Hong Kong SARS sequence. Science 2003; 301: 309–310.

Leung GM, Hedley AJ, Ho LM, Chau P, Wong IO, Thach TQ, Ghani AC, Donnelly CA, Fraser C, Riley S, Ferguson NM, Anderson RM, Tsang T, Leung PY, Wong V, Chan JC, Tsui E, Lo SV, Lam TH. The epidemiology of severe acute respiratory syndrome in the 2003 Hong Kong epidemic: an analysis of all 1755 patients. Ann Intern Med 2004; 141: 662–673.

Leung TF, Wong GW, Hon KL, Fok TF. Severe acute respiratory syndrome (SARS) in children: epidemiology, presentation and management. Paediatr Respir Rev 2003a; 4: 334–339.

Leung WK, To KF, Chan PK, Chan HL, Wu AK, Lee N, Yuen KY, Sung JJ. Enteric involvement of severe acute respiratory syndrome-associated coronavirus infection. Gastroenterology 2003b; 125: 1011–1017.

Li B-j, Tang Q, Cheng D, Qin C, Xie FY, Wei Q, Xu J, Liu Y, Zheng B-j, Woodle MC, Zhong N, Lu PY. Using siRNA in prophylactic and therapeutic regimens against SARS coronavirus in rhesus macaque. Nat Med 2005a; 11: 944–951.

Li F, Li W, Farzan M, Harrison SC. Structure of SARS coronavirus spike receptor-binding domain complexed with receptor. Science 2005b; 309: 1864–1868.

Li W, Greenough TC, Moore MJ, Vasilieva N, Somasundaran M, Sullivan JL, Farzan M, Choe H. Efficient replication of severe acute respiratory syndrome coronavirus in mouse cells is limited by murine angiotensin-converting enzyme 2. J Virol 2004a; 78: 11429–11433.

Li W, Moore MJ, Vasilieva N, Sui J, Wong SK, Berne MA, Somasundaran M, Sullivan JL, Luzuriaga K, Greenough TC, Choe H, Farzan M. Angiotensin-converting enzyme 2 is a functional receptor for the SARS coronavirus. Nature 2003; 426: 450–454.

Li W, Shi Z, Yu M, Ren W, Smith C, Epstein JH, Wang H, Crameri G, Hu Z, Zhang H, Zhang J, McEachern J, Field H, Daszak P, Eaton BT, Zhang S, Wang L-F. Bats are natural reservoirs of SARS-like coronaviruses. Science 2005; 310: 676–679.

Li W, Shi Z, Yu M, Ren W, Smith C, Epstein JH, Wang H, Crameri G, Hu Z, Zhang H, Zhang J, McEachern J, Field H, Daszak P, Eaton BT, Zhang S, Wang L-F. Bats are natural reservoirs of SARS-like coronaviruses. Science 2005d; 310: 676–679.

Li W, Zhang C, Sui J, Kuhn JH, Moore MJ, Luo S, Wong SK, Huang IC, Xu K, Vasilieva N, Murakami A, He Y, Marasco WA, Guan Y, Choe H, Farzan M. Receptor and viral determinants of SARS-coronavirus adaptation to human ACE2. Embo J 2005e; 24: 1634–1643.

Li Y, Duan S, Yu IT, Wong TW. Multi-zone modeling of probable SARS virus transmission by airflow between flats in Block E, Amoy Gardens. Indoor Air 2005f; 15: 96–111.

Li Y, Huang X, Yu IT, Wong TW, Qian H. Role of air distribution in SARS transmission during the largest nosocomial outbreak in Hong Kong. Indoor Air 2005g; 15: 83–95.

Li Y, Luo C, Li W, Xu Z, Zeng C, Bi S, Yu J, Wu J, Yang H. Structure-based preliminary analysis of immunity and virulence of SARS coronavirus. Viral Immunol 2004b; 17: 528–534.

Liang G, Chen Q, Xu J, Liu Y, Lim W, Peiris JS, Anderson LJ, Ruan L, Li H, Kan B, Di B, Cheng P, Chan KH, Erdman DD, Gu S, Yan X, Liang W, Zhou D, Haynes L, Duan S, Zhang X, Zheng H, Gao Y, Tong S, Li D, Fang L, Qin P, Xu W. Laboratory diagnosis of four recent sporadic cases of community-acquired SARS, Guangdong Province, China. Emerg Infect Dis 2004; 10: 1774–1781.

Liao CM, Chang CF, Liang HM. A probabilistic transmission dynamic model to assess indoor airborne infection risks. Risk Anal 2005a; 25: 1097–1107.

Liao QJ, Ye LB, Timani KA, Zeng YC, She YL, Ye L, Wu ZH. Activation of NF-kappaB by the full-length nucleocapsid protein of the SARS coronavirus. Acta Biochim Biophys Sin (Shanghai) 2005b; 37: 607–612.

Lin CF, Lei HY, Shiau AL, Liu CC, Liu HS, Yeh TM, Chen SH, Lin YS. Antibodies from dengue patient sera cross-react with endothelial cells and induce damage. J Med Virol 2003a; 69: 82–90.

Lin M, Tseng HK, Trejaut JA, Lee HL, Loo JH, Chu CC, Chen PJ, Su YW, Lim KH, Tsai ZU, Lin RY, Lin RS, Huang CH. Association of HLA Class I with severe acute respiratory syndrome coronavirus infection. BMC Med Genet 2003b; 4: 9.

Lin S, Lee CK, Lee SY, Kao CL, Lin CW, Wang AB, Hsu SM, Huang LS. Surface ultrastructure of SARS coronavirus revealed by atomic force microscopy. Cell Microbiol 2005a; 7: 1763–1770.

Lin YS, Lin CF, Fang YT, Kuo YM, Liao PC, Yeh TM, Hwa KY, Shieh CC, Yen JH, Wang HJ, Su IJ, Lei HY. Antibody to severe acute respiratory syndrome (SARS)-associated coronavirus spike protein domain 2 cross-reacts with lung epithelial cells and causes cytotoxicity. Clin Exp Immunol 2005b; 141: 500–508.

Liu S, Xiao G, Chen Y, He Y, Niu J, Escalante CR, Xiong H, Farmar J, Debnath AK, Tien P, Jiang S. Interaction between heptad repeat 1 and 2 regions in spike protein of SARS-associated coronavirus: implications for virus fusogenic mechanism and identification of fusion inhibitors. Lancet 2004; 363: 938–947.

Liu W. Molecular epidemiology of SARS-associated coronavirus, Beijing. Emerg Infect Dis 2005; 11: 1420–1424.

Lloyd-Smith JO, Galvani AP, Getz WM. Curtailing transmission of severe acute respiratory syndrome within a community and its hospital. Proc Biol Sci 2003; 270: 1979–1989.

Lloyd-Smith JO, Schreiber SJ, Kopp PE, Getz WM. Superspreading and the effect of individual variation on disease emergence. Nature 2005; 438: 355–359.

Long WH, Xiao HS, Gu XM, Zhang QH, Yang HJ, Zhao GP, Liu JH. A universal microarray for detection of SARS coronavirus. J Virol Methods 2004; 121: 57–63.

Loon SC, Teoh SC, Oon LL, Se-Thoe SY, Ling AE, Leo YS, Leong HN. The severe acute respiratory syndrome coronavirus in tears. Br J Ophthalmol 2004; 88: 861–863.

Magiorkinis G, Magiorkinis E, Paraskevis D, Vandamme AM, Van Ranst M, Moulton V, Hatzakis A. Phylogenetic analysis of the full-length SARS-CoV sequences: evidence for phylogenetic discordance in three genomic regions. J Med Virol 2004; 74: 369–372.

Mahony JB, Richardson S. Molecular diagnosis of severe acute respiratory syndrome: the state of the art. J Mol Diagn 2005; 7: 551–559.

Marra MA, Jones SJ, Astell CR, Holt RA, Brooks-Wilson A, Butterfield YS, Khattra J, Asano JK, Barber SA, Chan SY, Cloutier A, Coughlin SM, Freeman D, Girn N, Griffith OL, Leach SR, Mayo M, McDonald H, Montgomery SB, Pandoh PK, Petrescu AS, Robertson AG, Schein JE, Siddiqui A, Smailus DE, Stott JM, Yang GS, Plummer F, Andonov A, Artsob H, Bastien N, Bernard K, Booth TF, Bowness D, Czub M, Drebot M, Fernando L, Flick R, Garbutt M, Gray M, Grolla A, Jones S, Feldmann H, Meyers A, Kabani A, Li Y, Normand S, Stroher U, Tipples GA, Tyler S, Vogrig R, Ward D, Watson B, Brunham RC, Krajden M, Petric M, Skowronski DM, Upton C, Roper RL. The genome sequence of the SARS-associated coronavirus. Science 2003; 300: 1399–1404.

Martina BE, Haagmans BL, Kuiken T, Fouchier RA, Rimmelzwaan GF, Van Amerongen G, Peiris JS, Lim W, Osterhaus AD. Virology: SARS virus infection of cats and ferrets. Nature 2003; 425: 915.

Martina E, Stiefl N, Degel B, Schulz F, Breuning A, Schiller M, Vicik R, Baumann K, Ziebuhr J, Schirmeister T. Screening of electrophilic compounds yields an aziridinyl peptide as new active-site directed SARS-CoV main protease inhibitor. Bioorg Med Chem Lett 2005; 15: 5365–5369.

Marzi A, Gramberg T, Simmons G, Moller P, Rennekamp AJ, Krumbiegel M, Geier M, Eisemann J, Turza N, Saunier B, Steinkasserer A, Becker S, Bates P, Hofmann H, Pohlmann S. DC-SIGN and DC-SIGNR interact with the glycoprotein of Marburg virus and the S protein of severe acute respiratory syndrome coronavirus. J Virol 2004; 78: 12090–12095.

Matsuyama S, Ujike M, Morikawa S, Tashiro M, Taguchi F. Protease-mediated enhancement of severe acute respiratory syndrome coronavirus infection. Proc Natl Acad Sci USA. 2005; 102: 12543–12547.

Mazzulli T, Farcas GA, Poutanen SM, Willey BM, Low DE, Butany J, Asa SL, Kain KC. Severe acute respiratory syndrome-associated coronavirus in lung tissue. Emerg Infect Dis 2004; 10: 20–24.

Meng B, Wang J, Liu J, Wu J, Zhong E. Understanding the spatial diffusion process of severe acute respiratory syndrome in Beijing. Public Health 2005; 119: 1080–1087.

Morgenstern B, Michaelis M, Baer PC, Doerr HW, Cinatl Jr. J. Ribavirin and interferon-beta synergistically inhibit SARS-associated coronavirus replication in animal and human cell lines. Biochem Biophys Res Commun 2005; 326: 905–908.

Mortola E, Roy P. Efficient assembly and release of SARS coronavirus-like particles by a heterologous expression system. FEBS Lett 2004; 576: 174–178.

Ng EK, Ng PC, Hon KL, Cheng WT, Hung EC, Chan KC, Chiu RW, Li AM, Poon LL, Hui DS, Tam JS, Fok TF, Lo YM. Serial analysis of the plasma concentration of SARS coronavirus RNA in pediatric patients with severe acute respiratory syndrome. Clin Chem 2003; 49: 2085–2088.

Ng LF, Wong M, Koh S, Ooi EE, Tang KF, Leong HN, Ling AE, Agathe LV, Tan J, Liu ET, Ren EC, Ng LC, Hibberd ML. Detection of severe acute respiratory syndrome coronavirus in blood of infected patients. J Clin Microbiol 2004; 42: 347–350.

Ni L, Zhu J, Zhang J, Yan M, Gao GF, Tien P. Design of recombinant protein-based SARS-CoV entry inhibitors targeting the heptad-repeat regions of the spike protein S2 domain. Biochem Biophys Res Commun 2005; 330: 39–45.

Nicholls J, Peiris M. Good ACE, bad ACE do battle in lung injury, SARS. Nat Med 2005; 11: 821–822.

Nicholls JM, Poon LL, Lee KC, Ng WF, Lai ST, Leung CY, Chu CM, Hui PK, Mak KL, Lim W, Yan KW, Chan KH, Tsang NC, Guan Y, Yuen KY, Peiris JS. Lung pathology of fatal severe acute respiratory syndrome. Lancet 2003; 361: 1773–1778.

Normile D. Infectious diseases. Viral DNA match spurs China's civet roundup. Science 2004; 303: 292.

Normile D. Virology: researchers tie deadly SARS virus to bats. Science 2005; 309: 2154–2155.

Normile D, Enserink M. SARS in China. Tracking the roots of a killer. Science 2003; 301: 297–299.

Offit PA. The Cutter incident, 50 years later. N Engl J Med 2005; 352: 1411–1412.

Olsen SJ, Chang HL, Cheung TY, Tang AF, Fisk TL, Ooi SP, Kuo HW, Jiang DD, Chen KT, Lando J, Hsu KH, Chen TJ, Dowell SF. Transmission of the severe acute respiratory syndrome on aircraft. N Engl J Med 2003; 349: 2416–2422.

Ong KC, Ng AW, Lee LS, Kaw G, Kwek SK, Leow MK, Earnest A. 1-year pulmonary function and health status in survivors of severe acute respiratory syndrome. Chest 2005; 128: 1393–1400.

Pager CT, Dutch RE. Cathepsin L is involved in proteolytic processing of the Hendra virus fusion protein. J Virol 2005; 79: 12714–12720.

Pariente N, Sierra S, Lowenstein PR, Domingo E. Efficient virus extinction by combinations of a mutagen and antiviral inhibitors. J Virol 2001; 75: 9723–9730.

Parker WB. Metabolism and antiviral activity of ribavirin. Virus Res 2005; 107: 165–171.

Peiris JM. Joseph Malik Peiris—on the trail of pneumonia in Hong Kong interviewed by Pam Das. Lancet Infect Dis 2003; 3: 309–311.

Peiris JS, Chu CM, Cheng VC, Chan KS, Hung IF, Poon LL, Law KI, Tang BS, Hon TY, Chan CS, Chan KH, Ng JS, Zheng BJ, Ng WL, Lai RW, Guan Y, Yuen KY. Clinical progression and viral load in a community outbreak of coronavirus-associated SARS pneumonia: a prospective study. Lancet 2003a; 361: 1767–1772.

Peiris JS, Lai ST, Poon LL, Guan Y, Yam LY, Lim W, Nicholls J, Yee WK, Yan WW, Cheung MT, Cheng VC, Chan KH, Tsang DN, Yung RW, Ng TK, Yuen KY. Coronavirus as a possible cause of severe acute respiratory syndrome. Lancet 2003b; 361: 1319–1325.

Peiris JS, Yuen KY, Osterhaus AD, Stohr K. The severe acute respiratory syndrome. N Engl J Med 2003c; 349: 2431–2441.

Petit CM, Melancon JM, Chouljenko VN, Colgrove R, Farzan M, Knipe DM, Kousoulas KG. Genetic analysis of the SARS-coronavirus spike glycoprotein functional domains involved in cell-surface expression and cell-to-cell fusion. Virology 2005; 341: 215–230.

Poon LL, Chan KH, Wong OK, Yam WC, Yuen KY, Guan Y, Lo YM, Peiris JS. Early diagnosis of SARS coronavirus infection by real time RT-PCR. J Clin Virol 2003; 28: 233–238.

Poon LL, Chu DK, Chan KH, Wong OK, Ellis TM, Leung YH, Lau SK, Woo PC, Suen KY, Yuen KY, Guan Y, Peiris JS. Identification of a novel coronavirus in bats. J Virol 2005; 79: 2001–2009.

Poon LL, Guan Y, Nicholls JM, Yuen KY, Peiris JS. The aetiology, origins, and diagnosis of severe acute respiratory syndrome. Lancet Infect Dis 2004a; 4: 663–671.

Poon LL, Wong BW, Chan KH, Leung CS, Yuen KY, Guan Y, Peiris JS. A one step quantitative RT-PCR for detection of SARS coronavirus with an internal control for PCR inhibitors. J Clin Virol 2004b; 30: 214–217.

Poon TC, Chan KC, Ng PC, Chiu RW, Ang IL, Tong YK, Ng EK, Cheng FW, Li AM, Hon EK, Fok TF, Lo YM. Serial analysis of plasma proteomic signatures in pediatric patients with severe acute respiratory syndrome and correlation with viral load. Clin Chem 2004c; 50: 1452–1455.

Prentice E, McAuliffe J, Lu X, Subbarao K, Denison MR. Identification and characterization of severe acute respiratory syndrome coronavirus replicase proteins. J Virol 2004; 78: 9977–9986.

Qin L, Xiong B, Luo C, Guo ZM, Hao P, Su J, Nan P, Feng Y, Shi YX, Yu XJ, Luo XM, Chen KX, Shen X, Shen JH, Zou JP, Zhao GP, Shi TL, He WZ, Zhong Y, Jiang HL, Li YX. Identification of probable genomic packaging signal sequence from SARS-CoV genome by bioinformatics analysis. Acta Pharmacol Sin 2003; 24: 489–496.

Reghunathan R, Jayapal M, Hsu LY, Chng HH, Tai D, Leung BP, Melendez AJ. Expression profile of immune response genes in patients with severe acute respiratory syndrome. BMC Immunol 2005; 6: 2.

Reilley B, Van Herp M, Sermand D, Dentico N. SARS and Carlo Urbani. N Engl J Med 2003; 348: 1951–1952.

Riley S, Fraser C, Donnelly CA, Ghani AC, Abu-Raddad LJ, Hedley AJ, Leung GM, Ho LM, Lam TH, Thach TQ, Chau P, Chan KP, Lo SV, Leung PY, Tsang T, Ho W, Lee KH, Lau EM, Ferguson NM, Anderson RM. Transmission dynamics of the etiological agent of SARS in Hong Kong: impact of public health interventions. Science 2003; 300: 1961–1966.

Roberts A, Vogel L, Guarner J, Hayes N, Murphy B, Zaki S, Subbarao K. Severe acute respiratory syndrome coronavirus infection of golden Syrian hamsters. J Virol 2005; 79: 503–511.

Rocha EP, Danchin A. Base composition bias might result from competition for metabolic resources. Trends Genet 2002; 18: 291–294.

Rota PA, Oberste MS, Monroe SS, Nix WA, Campagnoli R, Icenogle JP, Penaranda S, Bankamp B, Maher K, Chen MH, Tong S, Tamin A, Lowe L, Frace M, DeRisi JL, Chen Q, Wang D, Erdman DD, Peret TC, Burns C, Ksiazek TG, Rollin PE, Sanchez A, Liffick S, Holloway B, Limor J, McCaustland K, Olsen-Rasmussen M, Fouchier R, Gunther S, Osterhaus AD, Drosten C, Pallansch MA, Anderson LJ, Bellini WJ. Characterization of a novel coronavirus associated with severe acute respiratory syndrome. Science 2003; 300: 1394–1399.

Roy CJ, Milton DK. Airborne transmission of communicable infection—the elusive pathway. N Engl J Med 2004; 350: 1710–1712.

Ruan YJ, Wei CL, Ee AL, Vega VB, Thoreau H, Su ST, Chia JM, Ng P, Chiu KP, Lim L, Zhang T, Peng CK, Lin EO, Lee NM, Yee SL, Ng LF, Chee RE, Stanton LW, Long PM, Liu ET. Comparative full-length genome sequence analysis of 14 SARS coronavirus isolates and common mutations associated with putative origins of infection. Lancet 2003; 361: 1779–1785.

Sachdeva G, Kumar K, Jain P, Ramachandran S. SPAAN: a software program for prediction of adhesins and adhesin-like proteins using neural networks. Bioinformatics 2005; 21: 483–491.

Saikatendu KS, Joseph JS, Subramanian V, Clayton T, Griffith M, Moy K, Velasquez J, Neuman BW, Buchmeier MJ, Stevens RC, Kuhn P. Structural basis of severe acute respiratory syndrome coronavirus ADP-ribose-1''-phosphate dephosphorylation by a conserved domain of nsP3. Structure (Camb) 2005; 13: 1665–1675.

Samuel CE. Antiviral actions of interferons. Clin Microbiol Rev 2001; 14: 778–809.

Santoro MG, Rossi A, Amici C. New EMBO member's review: NF-{kappa}B and virus infection: who controls whom. EMBO J 2003; 22: 2552–2560.

Savarino A, Boelaert JR, Cassone A, Majori G, Cauda R. Effects of chloroquine on viral infections: an old drug against today's diseases? Lancet Infect Dis 2003; 3: 722–727.

Schmidt M, Brixner V, Ruster B, Hourfar MK, Drosten C, Preiser W, Seifried E, Roth WK. NAT screening of blood donors for severe acute respiratory syndrome coronavirus can potentially prevent transfusion associated transmissions. Transfusion 2004; 44: 470–475.

Seto WH, Tsang D, Yung RW, Ching TY, Ng TK, Ho M, Ho LM, Peiris JS. Effectiveness of precautions against droplets and contact in prevention of nosocomial transmission of severe acute respiratory syndrome (SARS). Lancet 2003; 361: 1519–1520.

Shek CC, Ng PC, Fung GP, Cheng FW, Chan PK, Peiris MJ, Lee KH, Wong SF, Cheung HM, Li AM, Hon EK, Yeung CK, Chow CB, Tam JS, Chiu MC, Fok TF. Infants born to mothers with severe acute respiratory syndrome. Pediatrics 2003; 112: e254.

Shen X, Xue JH, Yu CY, Luo HB, Qin L, Yu XJ, Chen J, Chen LL, Xiong B, Yue LD, Cai JH, Shen JH, Luo XM, Chen KX, Shi TL, Li YX, Hu GX, Jiang HL. Small envelope protein E of SARS: cloning, expression, purification, CD determination, and bioinformatics analysis. Acta Pharmacol Sin 2003; 24: 505–511.

Shen Z, Ning F, Zhou W, He X, Lin C, Chin DP, Zhu Z, Schuchat A. Superspreading SARS events, Beijing, 2003. Emerg Infect Dis 2004; 10: 256–260.

Shi Y, Yang de H, Xiong J, Jia J, Huang B, Jin YX. Inhibition of genes expression of SARS coronavirus by synthetic small interfering RNAs. Cell Res 2005; 15: 193–200.

Shieh WJ, Hsiao CH, Paddock CD, Guarner J, Goldsmith CS, Tatti K, Packard M, Mueller L, Wu MZ, Rollin P, Su IJ, Zaki SR. Immunohistochemical, *in situ* hybridization, and ultrastructural localization of SARS-associated coronavirus in lung of a fatal case of severe acute respiratory syndrome in Taiwan. Hum Pathol 2005; 36: 303–309.

Simmons G, Gosalia DN, Rennekamp AJ, Reeves JD, Diamond SL, Bates P. Inhibitors of cathepsin L prevent severe acute respiratory syndrome coronavirus entry. Proc Natl Acad Sci USA 2005; 102: 11876–11881.

Sims AC, Baric RS, Yount B, Burkett SE, Collins PL, Pickles RJ. Severe acute respiratory syndrome coronavirus infection of human ciliated airway epithelia: role of ciliated cells in viral spread in the conducting airways of the lungs. J Virol 2005; 79: 15511–15524.

Snijder EJ, Bredenbeek PJ, Dobbe JC, Thiel V, Ziebuhr J, Poon LL, Guan Y, Rozanov M, Spaan WJ, Gorbalenya AE. Unique and conserved features of genome and proteome of SARS-coronavirus, an early split-off from the coronavirus group 2 lineage. J Mol Biol 2003; 331: 991–1004.

Song E, Zhu P, Lee S-K, Chowdhury D, Kussman S, Dykxhoorn DM, Feng Y, Palliser D, Weiner DB, Shankar P, Marasco WA, Lieberman J. Antibody mediated *in vivo* delivery of small interfering RNAs via cell-surface receptors. Nat Biotech 2005a; 23: 709–717.

Song HD, Tu CC, Zhang GW, Wang SY, Zheng K, Lei LC, Chen QX, Gao YW, Zhou HQ, Xiang H, Zheng HJ, Chern SW, Cheng F, Pan CM, Xuan H, Chen SJ, Luo HM, Zhou DH, Liu YF, He JF, Qin PZ, Li LH, Ren YQ, Liang WJ, Yu YD, Anderson L, Wang M, Xu RH, Wu XW, Zheng HY, Chen JD, Liang G, Gao Y, Liao M, Fang L, Jiang LY, Li H, Chen F, Di B, He LJ, Lin JY, Tong S, Kong X, Du L, Hao P, Tang H, Bernini A, Yu XJ, Spiga O, Guo ZM, Pan HY, He WZ, Manuguerra JC, Fontanet A, Danchin A, Niccolai N, Li YX, Wu CI, Zhao GP. Cross-host evolution of severe acute respiratory syndrome coronavirus in palm civet and human. Proc Natl Acad Sci USA 2005b; 102: 2430–2435.

Spiegel M, Pichlmair A, Martinez-Sobrido L, Cros J, Garcia-Sastre A, Haller O, Weber F. Inhibition of beta interferon induction by severe acute respiratory syndrome coronavirus suggests a two-step model for activation of interferon regulatory factor 3. J Virol 2005; 79: 2079–2086.

Spiegel M, Pichlmair A, Muhlberger E, Haller O, Weber F. The antiviral effect of interferon-beta against SARS-coronavirus is not mediated by MxA protein. J Clin Virol 2004; 30: 211–213.

Spruth M, Kistner O, Savidis-Dacho H, Hitter E, Crowe B, Gerencer M, Bruhl P, Grillberger L, Reiter M, Tauer C, Mundt W, Barrett PN. A double-inactivated whole virus candidate SARS coronavirus vaccine stimulates neutralising and protective antibody responses. Vaccine 2005; 24: 652–661.

Stadler K, Masignani V, Eickmann M, Becker S, Abrignani S, Klenk HD, Rappuoli R. SARS—beginning to understand a new virus. Nat Rev Microbiol 2003; 1: 209–218.

Stafford N. Profile: Klaus Stohr: preparing for the next influenza pandemic. Lancet 2005; 365: 379.

Su MC, Chang CT, Chu CH, Tsai CH, Chang KY. An atypical RNA pseudoknot stimulator and an upstream attenuation signal for 1-ribosomal frameshifting of SARS coronavirus. Nucleic Acids Res 2005; 33: 4265–4275.

Sui J, Li W, Murakami A, Tamin A, Matthews LJ, Wong SK, Moore MJ, Tallarico AS, Olurinde M, Choe H, Anderson LJ, Bellini WJ, Farzan M, Marasco WA. Potent neutralization of severe acute respiratory syndrome (SARS) coronavirus by a human mAb to S1 protein that blocks receptor association. Proc Natl Acad Sci USA 2004; 101: 2536–2541.

Sui J, Li W, Roberts A, Matthews LJ, Murakami A, Vogel L, Wong SK, Subbarao K, Farzan M, Marasco WA. Evaluation of human monoclonal antibody 80R for immunoprophylaxis of severe acute respiratory syndrome by an animal study, epitope mapping, and analysis of spike variants. J Virol 2005; 79: 5900–5906.

Supekar VM, Bruckmann C, Ingallinella P, Bianchi E, Pessi A, Carfi A. Structure of a proteolytically resistant core from the severe acute respiratory syndrome coronavirus S2 fusion protein. Proc Natl Acad Sci USA 2004; 101: 17958–17963.

Surjit M, Kumar R, Mishra RN, Reddy MK, Chow VT, Lal SK. The severe acute respiratory syndrome coronavirus nucleocapsid protein is phosphorylated and localizes in the cytoplasm by 14-3-3-mediated translocation. J Virol 2005; 79: 11476–11486.

Sylvester-Hvid C, Nielsen M, Lamberth K, Roder G, Justesen S, Lundegaard C, Worning P, Thomadsen H, Lund O, Brunak S, Buus S. SARS CTL vaccine candidates; HLA supertype-, genome-wide scanning and biochemical validation. Tissue Antigens 2004; 63: 395–400.

Takasuka N, Fujii H, Takahashi Y, Kasai M, Morikawa S, Itamura S, Ishii K, Sakaguchi M, Ohnishi K, Ohshima M, Hashimoto S, Odagiri T, Tashiro M, Yoshikura H, Takemori T, Tsunetsugu-Yokota Y. A subcutaneously injected UV-inactivated SARS coronavirus vaccine elicits systemic humoral immunity in mice. Int Immunol 2004; 16: 1423–1430.

Talaat AM, Stemke-Hale K. Expression library immunization: a road map for discovery of vaccines against infectious diseases. Infect Immun 2005; 73: 7089–7098.

Tan YJ, Fielding BC, Goh PY, Shen S, Tan TH, Lim SG, Hong W. Overexpression of 7a, a protein specifically encoded by the severe acute respiratory syndrome coronavirus, induces apoptosis via a caspase-dependent pathway. J Virol 2004a; 78: 14043–14047.

Tan YJ, Teng E, Shen S, Tan TH, Goh PY, Fielding BC, Ooi EE, Tan HC, Lim SG, Hong W. A novel severe acute respiratory syndrome coronavirus protein, U274, is transported to the cell surface and undergoes endocytosis. J Virol 2004b; 78: 6723–6734.

Tang L, Zhu Q, Qin E, Yu M, Ding Z, Shi H, Cheng X, Wang C, Chang G, Zhu Q, Fang F, Chang H, Li S, Zhang X, Chen X, Yu J, Wang J, Chen Z. Inactivated SARS-CoV vaccine prepared from whole virus induces a high level of neutralizing antibodies in BALB/c mice. DNA Cell Biol 2004; 23: 391–394.

Tang NL, Chan PK, Wong CK, To KF, Wu AK, Sung YM, Hui DS, Sung JJ, Lam CW. Early enhanced expression of interferon-inducible protein-10 (CXCL-10) and other chemokines predicts adverse outcome in severe acute respiratory syndrome. Clin Chem 2005; 51: 2333–2340.

Tao P, Zhang J, Tang N, Zhang BQ, He TC, Huang AL. Potent and specific inhibition of SARS-CoV antigen expression by RNA interference. Chin Med J (Engl) 2005; 118: 714–719.

Taylor DR. Obstacles and advances in SARS vaccine development. Vaccine 2005; 24: 863–871.

Temperton NJ, Chan PK, Simmons G, Zambon MC, Tedder RS, Takeuchi Y, Weiss RA. Longitudinally profiling neutralizing antibody response to SARS coronavirus with pseudotypes. Emerg Infect Dis 2005; 11: 411–416.

ter Meulen J, Bakker AB, van den Brink EN, Weverling GJ, Martina BE, Haagmans BL, Kuiken T, de Kruif J, Preiser W, Spaan W, Gelderblom HR, Goudsmit J, Osterhaus AD. Human monoclonal antibody as prophylaxis for SARS coronavirus infection in ferrets. Lancet 2004; 363: 2139–2141.

Thiel V, Ivanov KA, Putics A, Hertzig T, Schelle B, Bayer S, Weissbrich B, Snijder EJ, Rabenau H, Doerr HW, Gorbalenya AE, Ziebuhr J. Mechanisms and enzymes involved in SARS coronavirus genome expression. J Gen Virol 2003; 84: 2305–2315.

Thomas HC, Torok ME, Forton DM, Taylor-Robinson SD. Possible mechanisms of action and reasons for failure of antiviral therapy in chronic hepatitis C. J Hepatol 1999; 31(Suppl 1): 152–159.

Tipnis SR, Hooper NM, Hyde R, Karran E, Christie G, Turner AJ. A human homolog of angiotensin-converting enzyme. Cloning and functional expression as a captopril-insensitive carboxypeptidase. J Biol Chem 2000; 275: 33238–33243.

To KF, Tong JH, Chan PK, Au FW, Chim SS, Chan KC, Cheung JL, Liu EY, Tse GM, Lo AW, Lo YM, Ng HK. Tissue and cellular tropism of the coronavirus associated with severe acute respiratory syndrome: an *in-situ* hybridization study of fatal cases. J Pathol 2004; 202: 157–163.

Tong T, Lai TS. The severe acute respiratory syndrome coronavirus in tears. Br J Ophthalmol 2005; 89: 392.

Tong TR. SARS infection control. Lancet 2003; 362: 76–77.

Tong TR. Airborne severe acute respiratory syndrome coronavirus and its implications. J Infect Dis 2005a; 191: 1401–1402.

Tong TR. SARS-CoV sampling from 3 portals. Emerg Infect Dis 2005b; 11: 167.

Tong TR, Lam BH, Ng TK, Lai ST, Tong MK, Chau TN. Conjunctiva-upper respiratory tract irrigation for early diagnosis of severe acute respiratory syndrome. J Clin Microbiol 2003; 41: 5352.

Tong TR, Liang C. Evidence of airborne transmission of SARS. N Engl J Med 2004; 351: 609–611.

Traggiai E, Becker S, Subbarao K, Kolesnikova L, Uematsu Y, Gismondo MR, Murphy BR, Rappuoli R, Lanzavecchia A. An efficient method to make human monoclonal antibodies from memory B cells: potent neutralization of SARS coronavirus. Nat Med 2004; 10: 871–875.

Tripet B, Howard MW, Jobling M, Holmes RK, Holmes KV, Hodges RS. Structural characterization of the SARS-coronavirus spike S fusion protein core. J Biol Chem 2004; 279: 20836–20849.

Tsang KW, Ho PL, Ooi GC, Yee WK, Wang T, Chan-Yeung M, Lam WK, Seto WH, Yam LY, Cheung TM, Wong PC, Lam B, Ip MS, Chan J, Yuen KY, Lai KN. A cluster of cases of severe acute respiratory syndrome in Hong Kong. N Engl J Med 2003a; 348: 1977–1985.

Tsang OT, Chau TN, Choi KW, Tso EY, Lim W, Chiu MC, Tong WL, Lee PO, Lam BH, Ng TK, Lai JY, Yu WC, Lai ST. Coronavirus-positive nasopharyngeal aspirate as predictor for severe acute respiratory syndrome mortality. Emerg Infect Dis 2003b; 9: 1381–1387.

Tse GM, To KF, Chan PK, Lo AW, Ng KC, Wu A, Lee N, Wong HC, Mak SM, Chan KF, Hui DS, Sung JJ, Ng HK. Pulmonary pathological features in coronavirus associated severe acute respiratory syndrome (SARS). J Clin Pathol 2004; 57: 260–265.

Tsui PT, Kwok ML, Yuen H, Lai ST. Severe acute respiratory syndrome: clinical outcome and prognostic correlates. Emerg Infect Dis 2003; 9: 1064–1069.

Tu C, Crameri G, Kong X, Chen J, Sun Y, Yu M, Xiang H, Xia X, Liu S, Ren T, Yu Y, Eaton BT, Xuan H, Wang LF. Antibodies to SARS coronavirus in civets. Emerg Infect Dis 2004; 10: 2244–2248.

van den Hoogen BG, de Jong JC, Groen J, Kuiken T, de Groot R, Fouchier RAM, Osterhaus ADME. A newly discovered human pneumovirus isolated from young children with respiratory tract disease. Nat Med 2001; 7: 719–724.

van Vonderen MG, Bos JC, Prins JM, Wertheim-van Dillen P, Speelman P. Ribavirin in the treatment of severe acute respiratory syndrome (SARS). Neth J Med 2003; 61: 238–241.

Vega VB, Ruan Y, Liu J, Lee WH, Wei CL, Se-Thoe SY, Tang KF, Zhang T, Kolatkar PR, Ooi EE, Ling AE, Stanton LW, Long PM, Liu ET. Mutational dynamics of the SARS coronavirus in cell culture and human populations isolated in 2003. BMC Infect Dis 2004; 4: 32.

Vincent MJ, Bergeron E, Benjannet S, Erickson BR, Rollin PE, Ksiazek TG, Seidah NG, Nichol ST. Chloroquine is a potent inhibitor of SARS coronavirus infection and spread. Virol J 2005; 2: 69.

von Grotthuss M, Wyrwicz LS, Rychlewski L. mRNA cap-1 methyltransferase in the SARS genome. Cell 2003; 113: 701–702.

Wang D, Lu J. Glycan arrays lead to the discovery of autoimmunogenic activity of SARS-CoV. Physiol Genomics 2004; 18: 245–248.

Wang D, Urisman A, Liu YT, Springer M, Ksiazek TG, Erdman DD, Mardis ER, Hickenbotham M, Magrini V, Eldred J, Latreille JP, Wilson RK, Ganem D, DeRisi JL. Viral discovery and sequence recovery using DNA microarrays. PLoS Biol 2003; 1: E2.

Wang JT, Sheng WH, Fang CT, Chen YC, Wang JL, Yu CJ, Chang SC, Yang PC. Clinical manifestations, laboratory findings, and treatment outcomes of SARS patients. Emerg Infect Dis 2004a; 10: 818–824.

Wang S, Browning KS, Miller WA. A viral sequence in the 3′-untranslated region mimics a 5′ cap in facilitating translation of uncapped mRNA. EMBO J 1997; 16: 4107–4116.

Wang XW, Li J, Guo T, Zhen B, Kong Q, Yi B, Li Z, Song N, Jin M, Xiao W, Zhu X, Gu C, Yin J, Wei W, Yao W, Liu C, Li J, Ou G, Wang M, Fang T, Wang G, Qiu Y, Wu H, Chao F, Li J. Concentration and detection of SARS coronavirus in sewage from Xiao Tang Shan Hospital and the 309th Hospital of the Chinese People's Liberation Army. Water Sci Technol 2005a; 52: 213–221.

Wang XW, Li JS, Guo TK, Zhen B, Kong QX, Yi B, Li Z, Song N, Jin M, Wu XM, Xiao WJ, Zhu XM, Gu CQ, Yin J, Wei W, Yao W, Liu C, Li JF, Ou GR, Wang MN, Fang TY, Wang GJ, Qiu YH, Wu HH, Chao FH, Li JW. Excretion and detection of SARS coronavirus and its nucleic acid from digestive system. World J Gastroenterol 2005b; 11: 4390–4395.

Wang YS, Sun SH, Shen H, Jiang LH, Zhang MX, Xiao DJ, Liu Y, Ma XL, Zhang Y, Guo NJ, Jia TH. Cross-reaction of SARS-CoV antigen with autoantibodies in autoimmune diseases. Cell Mol Immunol 2004b; 1: 304–307.

Wang Z, Ren L, Zhao X, Hung T, Meng A, Wang J, Chen YG. Inhibition of severe acute respiratory syndrome virus replication by small interfering RNAs in mammalian cells. J Virol 2004c; 78: 7523–7527.

Wang Z, Yuan Z, Matsumoto M, Hengge UR, Chang YF. Immune responses with DNA vaccines encoded different gene fragments of severe acute respiratory syndrome coronavirus in BALB/c mice. Biochem Biophys Res Commun 2005c; 327: 130–135.

Webby R, Hoffmann E, Webster R. Molecular constraints to interspecies transmission of viral pathogens. Nat Med 2004; 10: S77–S81.

Wentworth DE, Gillim-Ross L, Espina N, Bernard KA. Mice susceptible to SARS coronavirus. Emerg Infect Dis 2004; 10: 1293–1296.

Wong CK, Lam CW, Wu AK, Ip WK, Lee NL, Chan IH, Lit LC, Hui DS, Chan MH, Chung SS, Sung JJ. Plasma inflammatory cytokines and chemokines in severe acute respiratory syndrome. Clin Exp Immunol 2004a; 136: 95–103.

Wong RS, Wu A, To KF, Lee N, Lam CW, Wong CK, Chan PK, Ng MH, Yu LM, Hui DS, Tam JS, Cheng G, Sung JJ. Haematological manifestations in patients with severe acute respiratory syndrome: retrospective analysis. BMJ 2003a; 326: 1358–1362.

Wong SK, Li W, Moore MJ, Choe H, Farzan M. A 193-amino acid fragment of the SARS coronavirus S protein efficiently binds angiotensin-converting enzyme 2. J Biol Chem 2004b; 279: 3197–3201.

Wong VW, Dai D, Wu AK, Sung JJ. Treatment of severe acute respiratory syndrome with convalescent plasma. Hong Kong Med J 2003b; 9: 199–201.

Woo PC, Lau SK, Wong BH, Chan KH, Hui WT, Kwan GS, Peiris JS, Couch RB, Yuen KY. False-positive results in a recombinant severe acute respiratory syndrome-associated coronavirus (SARS-CoV) nucleocapsid enzyme-linked immunosorbent assay due to HCoV-OC43 and HCoV-229E rectified by Western blotting with recombinant SARS-CoV spike polypeptide. J Clin Microbiol 2004a; 42: 5885–5888.

Woo PC, Lau SK, Wong BH, Tsoi HW, Fung AM, Chan KH, Tam VK, Peiris JS, Yuen KY. Detection of specific antibodies to severe acute respiratory syndrome (SARS) coronavirus nucleocapsid protein for serodiagnosis of SARS coronavirus pneumonia. J Clin Microbiol 2004b; 42: 2306–2309.

Wu CJ, Huang HW, Liu CY, Hong CF, Chan YL. Inhibition of SARS-CoV replication by siRNA. Antiviral Res 2005a; 65: 45–48.

Wu CY, Jan JT, Ma SH, Kuo CJ, Juan HF, Cheng YS, Hsu HH, Huang HC, Wu D, Brik A, Liang FS, Liu RS, Fang JM, Chen ST, Liang PH, Wong CH. Small molecules targeting severe acute respiratory syndrome human coronavirus. Proc Natl Acad Sci USA 2004; 101: 10012–10017.

Wu D, Tu C, Xin C, Xuan H, Meng Q, Liu Y, Yu Y, Guan Y, Jiang Y, Yin X, Crameri G, Wang M, Li C, Liu S, Liao M, Feng L, Xiang H, Sun J, Chen J, Sun Y, Gu S, Liu N, Fu D, Eaton BT, Wang LF, Kong X. Civets are equally susceptible to experimental infection by two different severe acute respiratory syndrome coronavirus isolates. J Virol 2005b; 79: 2620–2625.

Xu D, Zhang Z, Chu F, Li Y, Jin L, Zhang L, Gao GF, Wang FS. Genetic variation of SARS coronavirus in Beijing Hospital. Emerg Infect Dis 2004a; 10: 789–794.

Xu D, Zhang Z, Wang FS. SARS-associated coronavirus quasispecies in individual patients. N Engl J Med 2004b; 350: 1366–1367.

Xu J, Qi L, Chi X, Yang J, Wei X, Gong E, Peh S, Gu J. Orchitis: a complication of severe acute respiratory syndrome (SARS). Biol Reprod 2006; 74: 410–416.

Xu RH, He JF, Evans MR, Peng GW, Field HE, Yu DW, Lee CK, Luo HM, Lin WS, Lin P, Li LH, Liang WJ, Lin JY, Schnur A. Epidemiologic clues to SARS origin in China. Emerg Infect Dis 2004c; 10: 1030–1037.

Xu Y, Liu Y, Lou Z, Qin L, Li X, Bai Z, Pang H, Tien P, Gao GF, Rao Z. Structural basis for coronavirus-mediated membrane fusion. Crystal structure of mouse hepatitis virus spike protein fusion core. J Biol Chem 2004d; 279: 30514–30522.

Xu Y, Lou Z, Liu Y, Pang H, Tien P, Gao GF, Rao Z. Crystal structure of severe acute respiratory syndrome coronavirus spike protein fusion core. J Biol Chem 2004e; 279: 49414–49419.

Yamamoto N, Yang R, Yoshinaka Y, Amari S, Nakano T, Cinatl J, Rabenau H, Doerr HW, Hunsmann G, Otaka A, Tamamura H, Fujii N, Yamamoto N. HIV protease inhibitor nelfinavir inhibits replication of SARS-associated coronavirus. Biochem Biophys Res Commun 2004; 318: 719–725.

Yamate M, Yamashita M, Goto T, Tsuji S, Li YG, Warachit J, Yunoki M, Ikuta K. Establishment of Vero E6 cell clones persistently infected with severe acute respiratory syndrome coronavirus. Microbes Infect 2005; 7: 1530–1540.

Yang H, Xie W, Xue X, Yang K, Ma J, Liang W, Zhao Q, Zhou Z, Pei D, Ziebuhr J, Hilgenfeld R, Yuen KY, Wong L, Gao G, Chen S, Chen Z, Ma D, Bartlam M, Rao Z. Design of wide-spectrum inhibitors targeting coronavirus main proteases. PLoS Biol 2005a; 3: e324.

Yang Y, Xiong Z, Zhang S, Yan Y, Nguyen J, Ng B, Lu H, Brendese J, Yang F, Wang H, Yang XF. Bcl-xL inhibits T cell apoptosis induced by expression of SARS coronavirus E protein in the absence of growth factors. Biochem J 2005; 392: 135–143.

Yang ZY, Huang Y, Ganesh L, Leung K, Kong WP, Schwartz O, Subbarao K, Nabel GJ. pH-dependent entry of severe acute respiratory syndrome coronavirus is mediated by the spike glycoprotein and enhanced by dendritic cell transfer through DC-SIGN. J Virol 2004a; 78: 5642–5650.

Yang ZY, Kong WP, Huang Y, Roberts A, Murphy BR, Subbarao K, Nabel GJ. A DNA vaccine induces SARS coronavirus neutralization and protective immunity in mice. Nature 2004b; 428: 561–564.

Yang ZY, Werner HC, Kong WP, Leung K, Traggiai E, Lanzavecchia A, Nabel GJ. Evasion of antibody neutralization in emerging severe acute respiratory syndrome coronaviruses. Proc Natl Acad Sci USA 2005c; 102: 797–801.

Yeh KM, Chiueh TS, Siu LK, Lin JC, Chan PK, Peng MY, Wan HL, Chen JH, Hu BS, Perng CL, Lu JJ, Chang FY. Experience of using convalescent plasma for severe acute respiratory syndrome among healthcare workers in a Taiwan hospital. J Antimicrob Chemother 2005; 56: 919–922.

Yeh SH, Wang HY, Tsai CY, Kao CL, Yang JY, Liu HW, Su IJ, Tsai SF, Chen DS, Chen PJ. Characterization of severe acute respiratory syndrome coronavirus genomes in Taiwan: molecular epidemiology and genome evolution. Proc Natl Acad Sci USA 2004; 101: 2542–2547.

Yi CE, Ba L, Zhang L, Ho DD, Chen Z. Single amino acid substitutions in the severe acute respiratory syndrome coronavirus spike glycoprotein determine viral entry and immunogenicity of a major neutralizing domain. J Virol 2005; 79: 11638–11646.

Yip SP, To SST, Leung PHM, Cheung TS, Cheng PKC, Lim WWL. Use of dual TaqMan probes to increase the sensitivity of 1-step quantitative reverse transcription-PCR: application to the detection of SARS coronavirus. Clin Chem 2005; 51: 1885–1888.

Yount B, Curtis KM, Fritz EA, Hensley LE, Jahrling PB, Prentice E, Denison MR, Geisbert TW, Baric RS. Reverse genetics with a full-length infectious cDNA of severe acute respiratory syndrome coronavirus. Proc Natl Acad Sci USA 2003; 100: 12995–13000.

Yount B, Denison MR, Weiss SR, Baric RS. Systematic assembly of a full-length infectious cDNA of mouse hepatitis virus strain A59. J Virol 2002; 76: 11065–11078.

Yount B, Roberts RS, Sims AC, Deming D, Frieman MB, Sparks J, Denison MR, Davis N, Baric RS. Severe acute respiratory syndrome coronavirus group-specific open reading frames encode nonessential functions for replication in cell cultures and mice. J Virol 2005; 79: 14909–14922.

Yu CJ, Chen YC, Hsiao CH, Kuo TC, Chang SC, Lu CY, Wei WC, Lee CH, Huang LM, Chang MF, Ho HN, Lee FJ. Identification of a novel protein 3a from severe acute respiratory syndrome coronavirus. FEBS Lett 2004a; 565: 111–116.

Yu IT, Li Y, Wong TW, Tam W, Chan AT, Lee JH, Leung DY, Ho T. Evidence of airborne transmission of the severe acute respiratory syndrome virus. N Engl J Med 2004b; 350: 1731–1739.

Yu IT, Sung JJ. The epidemiology of the outbreak of severe acute respiratory syndrome (SARS) in Hong Kong—what we do know and what we don't. Epidemiol Infect 2004; 132: 781–786.

Yu IT, Wong TW, Chiu YL, Lee N, Li Y. Temporal-spatial analysis of severe acute respiratory syndrome among hospital inpatients. Clin Infect Dis 2005; 40: 1237–1243.

Yuan XD, Shan Y, Zhao Z, Chen J, Cong Y. G0/G1 arrest and apoptosis induced by SARS-CoV 3b protein in transfected cells. Virol J 2005; 2: 66.

Zeng F, Chow KY, Hon CC, Law KM, Yip CW, Chan KH, Peiris JS, Leung FC. Characterization of humoral responses in mice immunized with plasmid DNAs encoding SARS-CoV spike gene fragments. Biochem Biophys Res Commun 2004a; 315: 1134–1139.

Zeng R, Ruan HQ, Jiang XS, Zhou H, Shi L, Zhang L, Sheng QH, Tu Q, Xia QC, Wu JR. Proteomic analysis of SARS associated coronavirus using two-dimensional liquid chromatography mass spectrometry and one-dimensional sodium dodecyl sulfate-polyacrylamide gel electrophoresis followed by mass spectrometric analysis. J Proteome Res 2004b; 3: 549–555.

Zhai Y, Sun F, Li X, Pang H, Xu X, Bartlam M, Rao Z. Insights into SARS-CoV transcription and replication from the structure of the nsp7–nsp8 hexadecamer. Nat Struct Mol Biol 2005; 12: 980–986.

Zhang DM, Wang GL, Lu JH. Severe acute respiratory syndrome: vaccine on the way. Chin Med J (Engl) 2005a; 118: 1468–1476.

Zhang H, Wang G, Li J, Nie Y, Shi X, Lian G, Wang W, Yin X, Zhao Y, Qu X, Ding M, Deng H. Identification of an antigenic determinant on the S2 domain of the severe acute respiratory syndrome coronavirus spike glycoprotein capable of inducing neutralizing antibodies. J Virol 2004; 78: 6938–6945.

Zhang H, Zhou G, Zhi L, Yang H, Zhai Y, Dong X, Zhang X, Gao X, Zhu Y, He F. Association between mannose-binding lectin gene polymorphisms and susceptibility to severe acute respiratory syndrome coronavirus infection. J Infect Dis 2005b; 192: 1355–1361.

Zhang L, Zhang F, Yu W, He T, Yu J, Yi CE, Ba L, Li W, Farzan M, Chen Z, Yuen KY, Ho D. Antibody responses against SARS coronavirus are correlated with disease outcome of infected individuals. J Med Virol 2005c; 78: 1–8.

Zhang MY, Choudhry V, Xiao X, Dimitrov DS. Human monoclonal antibodies to the S glycoprotein and related proteins as potential therapeutics for SARS. Curr Opin Mol Ther 2005d; 7: 151–156.

Zhang R, Guo Z, Lu J, Meng J, Zhou C, Zhan X, Huang B, Yu X, Huang M, Pan X, Ling W, Chen X, Wan Z, Zheng H, Yan X, Wang Y, Ran Y, Liu X, Ma J, Wang C, Zhang B. Inhibiting severe acute respiratory syndrome-associated coronavirus by small interfering RNA. Chin Med J (Engl) 2003; 116: 1262–1264.

Zhang XW, Yap YL. Old drugs as lead compounds for a new disease? Binding analysis of SARS coronavirus main proteinase with HIV, psychotic and parasite drugs. Bioorg Med Chem 2004; 12: 2517–2521.

Zheng B, He ML, Wong KL, Lum CT, Poon LL, Peng Y, Guan Y, Lin MC, Kung HF. Potent inhibition of SARS-associated coronavirus (SCOV) infection and replication by type I interferons (IFN-alpha/beta) but not by type II interferon (IFN-gamma). J Interferon Cytokine Res 2004a; 24: 388–390.

Zheng BJ, Wong KH, Zhou J, Wong KL, Young BW, Lu LW, Lee SS. SARS-related virus predating SARS outbreak, Hong Kong. Emerg Infect Dis 2004b; 10: 176–178.

Zhi Y, Wilson JM, Shen H. SARS vaccine: progress and challenge. Cell Mol Immunol 2005; 2: 101–105.

Zhong N, Ding Y, Mao Y, Wang Q, Wang G, Wang D, Cong Y, Li Q, Liu Y, Ruan L, Chen B, Du X, Yang Y, Zhang Z, Zhang X, Lin J, Zheng J, Zhu Q, Ni D, Xi X, Zeng G, Ma D, Wang C, Wang W, Wang B, Wang J, Liu D, Li X, Liu X, Chen J, Chen R, Min F, Yang P, Zhang Y, Luo H, Lang Z, Hu Y, Ni A, Cao W, Lei J, Wang S, Wang Y, Tong X, Liu W, Zhu M, Zhang Y, Zhang Z, Zhang X, Li X, Chen W, Xhen X, Lin L, Luo Y, Zhong J, Weng W, Peng S, Pan Z, Wang Y, Wang R, Zuo J, Liu B, Zhang N, Zhang J, Zhang B, Zhang Z, Wang W, Chen L, Zhou P, Luo Y, Jiang L, Chao E, Guo L, Tan X, Pan J. Consensus for the management of severe acute respiratory syndrome. Chin Med J (Engl) 2003a; 116: 1603–1635.

Zhong NS, Zheng BJ, Li YM, Poon, Xie ZH, Chan KH, Li PH, Tan SY, Chang Q, Xie JP, Liu XQ, Xu J, Li DX, Yuen KY, Peiris, Guan Y. Epidemiology and cause of severe acute respiratory syndrome (SARS) in Guangdong, People's Republic of China, in February, 2003. Lancet 2003b; 362: 1353–1358.

Zhu MS, Pan Y, Chen HQ, Shen Y, Wang XC, Sun YJ, Tao KH. Induction of SARS-nucleoprotein-specific immune response by use of DNA vaccine. Immunol Lett 2004; 92: 237–243.

Ziegler T, Matikainen S, Ronkko E, Osterlund P, Sillanpaa M, Siren J, Fagerlund R, Immonen M, Melen K, Julkunen I. Severe acute respiratory syndrome coronavirus fails to activate cytokine-mediated innate immune responses in cultured human monocyte-derived dendritic cells. J Virol 2005; 79: 13800–13805.

Emerging Viruses in Human Populations
Edward Tabor (Editor)
DOI 10.1016/S0168-7069(06)16005-X

The Pandemic Threat of Avian Influenza Viruses

Amorsolo L. Suguitan, Jr., Kanta Subbarao

Laboratory of Infectious Diseases, NIAID, NIH, Bethesda, MD 20892, USA

Introduction

Influenza viruses remain a significant cause of morbidity and mortality in both developing countries and developed countries (Simonsen, 1999). In temperate climates, influenza epidemics are common during winter months, while a biannual pattern has been reported in the tropics (Shek and Lee, 2003).

Influenza is transmitted by inhalation of microdroplets of respiratory secretions, often expelled by coughing or sneezing, that contain the virus or from fomites. The incubation period ranges from 1 to 5 days. Symptoms typically include fever, headache, malaise, myalgia, cough, nasal discharge, and sore throat (Cox and Subbarao, 1999). In severe cases of influenza, the cause of death is usually a secondary bacterial pneumonia.

Although most infections by influenza virus are self-limited, as many as 36,000 excess deaths in the United States every year are attributed to influenza, mostly in the elderly and in individuals with underlying pulmonary conditions (Thompson et al., 2003). It has been estimated that the total annual burden of influenza in the United States alone can range from US$1 to 3 billion in direct medical costs. Indirect costs, including lost earnings due to illness, hospitalizations, substantial reduction in productivity, and lost future earnings due to death, can range from US$10 to 15 billion a year (Szucs, 1999).

Of greater concern, however, is the ability of certain influenza viruses with novel antigenic properties to enter and spread in an immunologically naïve human population, with the potential to initiate a pandemic characterized by rapid global spread, morbidity, and mortality. Influenza pandemics were recorded as early as 412 B.C. by Hippocrates (Kuszewski and Brydak, 2000). The consequences of such pandemics can be devastating, as in the "Spanish" influenza pandemic that occurred in 1918 and resulted in the deaths of at least 40 million people worldwide

(Johnson and Mueller, 2002), making it one of the deadliest infectious diseases in mankind's history. In the absence of effective intervention, it is estimated that a pandemic today could cause 700,000 hospitalizations and 89,000–207,700 deaths in the United States alone, and 18–42 million individuals would require out-patient based care, and the economic impact would be between US$71.3 and 166.5 billion, excluding the cost of disruptions to commerce and society (Meltzer et al., 1999).

The recent outbreak in poultry of highly pathogenic avian influenza (HPAI) infections caused by H5N1 viruses began in 2003 in Southeast Asia. It has been unprecedented in magnitude, as it has spread to South and Central Asia, Europe, and Africa, resulting in the massive culling of poultry. More important, these outbreaks of HPAI in poultry have been associated with the transmission of the H5N1 virus to a small number of humans. As of this writing (April 2006), there have been more than 200 laboratory-confirmed cases of avian influenza H5N1 infections in humans reported in nine countries, more than 100 of which resulted in death (WHO, 2006b). These events have highlighted the potential for another influenza pandemic.

What causes a pandemic and how does it arise? What can be done to limit the devastating effects a pandemic usually brings and how prepared are we to meet such challenges? An examination of the biology of the avian influenza viruses and their relationship with their animal hosts may shed light on these questions.

Virology

Classification

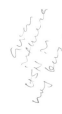

Influenza viruses are enveloped viruses with a segmented genome. They are in the virus family *Orthomyxoviridae*. Three types of influenza virus have been described, designated as influenza A, B, and C, based on the antigenicity of two of their internal proteins, the nucleoprotein (NP) and matrix (M) protein (Lamb and Krug, 2001). Influenza B and C viruses mainly infect humans, while influenza A viruses infect a wide variety of avian and mammalian species, including humans, pigs, sea mammals, and horses.

Influenza viral proteins

Influenza A and B viruses possess eight single-stranded negative-sense RNA segments that encode structural and nonstructural proteins. Hemagglutinin (HA), a surface glycoprotein that mediates viral entry by binding to sialic acid residues on host cells, is the main target of the protective humoral immune responses in the human host. Neuraminidase (NA) is the other major surface glycoprotein, whose enzymatic function allows the release of newly formed virions, permits the spread of infectious virus from cell to cell, and keeps newly budding virions from aggregating at the host cell surface. This catalytic function of the NA protein is the target of the anti-influenza virus drugs oseltamivir and zanamivir; although these compounds do not directly prevent infection of healthy cells, they limit the release of infectious progeny viruses thus curtailing their spread and shortening the duration of illness. These NA inhibitors are effective against all NA subtypes among the influenza A viruses and may be the primary antiviral drugs in the event of a future pandemic (Moscona, 2004). Antibodies to the NA protein do not neutralize infectivity but are protective (Murphy et al., 1972).

Three proteins comprise the viral polymerase of the influenza viruses: two basic proteins (PB1 and PB2) and an acidic protein (PA). Together with NP (mentioned above), these polymerase proteins associate with the RNA segments to form ribonucleoprotein (RNP) complexes. Two viral RNA segments encode at least two proteins each by alternative splicing. Gene segment 7 codes for two proteins: matrix protein M1, which is involved in maintaining the structural integrity of the virion, and M2, an integral membrane (surface) protein that acts as an ion channel and facilitates virus uncoating. The drugs amantadine and rimantadine bind to the influenza A M2 protein and interfere with its ability to transport hydrogen ions into the virion, preventing virus uncoating. Amantadine is only effective against influenza A viruses. Passively transferred antibodies to M2 can protect animals against influenza viruses, but such M2-specific antibodies are not consistently detected in human convalescent sera (Black et al., 1993), suggesting that this type of immunity may play a minor role in the clearance of influenza virus in humans. Gene segment 8 is responsible for the synthesis of the nonstructural protein NS1 and nuclear export protein (NEP, formerly called NS2). NS1 is involved in modulating the host's interferon response (Garcia-Sastre et al., 1998), while NEP plays a role in the export of RNP from the nucleus to the cytoplasm (O'Neill et al., 1998). Recently, an unusual 87-amino acid peptide arising from an alternative reading frame of the PB1 RNA segment has been described (Chen et al., 2001). This mitochondrial protein, PB1-F2, is believed to function in the induction of apoptosis as a means of down-regulating the host immune response to influenza infection (Zamarin et al., 2005).

Influenza A viral antigens and wild aquatic waterfowl as natural hosts

The HA and NA proteins of influenza A viruses display a greater degree of amino acid sequence variation than their counterparts in influenza B viruses and they are further divided into subtypes (Lamb, 2001). Sixteen serologically distinguishable HA (H1–H16) and 9 different NA (N1–N9) proteins have been identified to date (Lamb, 2001; Fouchier et al., 2005), all of which can be found in different combinations in waterfowl including mallards, ducks, shorebirds, and gulls (Ito, 1998; Hatchette et al., 2004) where they replicate mainly in the gastrointestinal tract and are shed in the feces (Webster et al., 1978). Wild aquatic birds rarely display symptoms of influenza disease, even though they may shed high titers of virus. This indicates that influenza A viruses have achieved an optimal level of adaptation to aquatic waterfowl as natural reservoirs, where they are believed to exist in relative evolutionary stasis (Webster et al., 1992).

Sources of variation: antigenic drift and antigenic shift

The extensive antigenic variation exhibited by the HA and NA proteins of human influenza viruses contributes to their evolutionary success as they undergo genetic change to elude the host's immune responses. These variations are brought about by two fundamental mechanisms: antigenic drift and antigenic shift. Antigenic drift results from the accumulation of point mutations in the HA and NA of influenza viruses that arise from a combination of the inherently low fidelity of the viral RNA-dependent polymerase complex (lacking proofreading ability) and from positive selection driven by the antibody response of the host (Steinhauer and Holland, 1987; Bush et al., 1999). Antigenic drift is an ongoing process of evolution that permits epidemic influenza A and B viruses to evade neutralization by antibodies elicited by prior infection or immunization. Influenza vaccines are updated annually to keep pace with antigenic drift so that the virus included in the vaccine formulation will closely match that of the current year's epidemic circulating strain.

While antigenic drift is a continuous process of change, antigenic shift arises less frequently, results in greater antigenic change, and is only seen with influenza A viruses. It occurs as a result of the introduction into the human population of a novel HA and/or NA protein that is immunologically distinct from the influenza A viruses circulating in recent years (Cox and Subbarao, 1999). The segmented nature of the influenza genome permits the possible exchange of gene segments (in a process referred to as genetic reassortment) when two different influenza A viruses infect the same cell. The isolation of viruses in nature with different combinations of HA and NA suggests that such genetic reassortments occur freely and frequently (Sharp et al., 1997).

Because wild waterfowl and migratory birds act as natural hosts of all known influenza A viruses, they are believed to be the original source of the influenza A viruses circulating in other animal species. Some avian influenza viruses cross the species barrier and are transferred from their natural host to another avian or mammalian host where they may cause disease outbreaks and may lead to endemicity through adaptation or genetic reassortment.

HA receptor specificity and host-range restriction

The affinity of HA for sialic-acid-containing molecules on target cells is a determinant of host-range restriction among influenza A viruses. The type of glycosidic linkage that exists between the sialic acid and the penultimate galactose residue in cell-surface oligosaccharides is associated with preferential binding of human (SAα2,6Gal linkage) and avian (SAα2,3Gal linkage) influenza viruses (Rogers and D'Souza, 1989; Ito et al., 1997a; Matrosovich et al., 2000). In support of this hypothesis, the human tracheal epithelium predominantly contains sugars of the SAα2,6Gal moiety (Couceiro et al., 1993) while there is an abundance of the SAα2,3Gal variety in the gastrointestinal tract of ducks (Ito, 1998). It has been proposed that as a virus adapts to its new host, it is under selective pressure toward the utilization of receptors available in its immediate environment, thus restricting the type of sialic acid linkage that is recognized (Gambaryan et al., 1999; Matrosovich et al., 2000). Amino acid residues in the HA protein, particularly in the receptor-binding domain, are believed to play a role in determining host-range specificity (Rogers et al., 1983; Connor et al., 1994; Vines et al., 1998). Human influenza A viruses with SAα2,6Gal specificity that are repeatedly passaged in the allantoic membrane of embryonated eggs develop HA with preference for SAα2,3Gal receptors. A single amino acid change (L226Q) has been shown to be sufficient to alter the receptor-binding preference of HA from SAα2,6Gal to SAα2,3Gal (Rogers et al., 1983; Ito et al., 1997b). In a recent study, Stevens and colleagues evaluated the receptor-binding preferences of several human and avian H1 and H3 viruses in a customized glycan microarray that contained 200 carbohydrates and glycoproteins (Stevens et al., 2006). By analyzing the amino acid sequence and receptor-binding specificity of two variants of the HA of the 1918 H1N1 virus, it was found that an amino acid at position 190 was crucial in recognizing either SAα2,6Gal (Asp190) or SAα2,3Gal receptors (Glu190). Taken together, these results demonstrate that even small changes in the HA receptor-binding site can broaden the host range of an influenza virus and potentially allow the infection to spread to different animal species.

When an H5N1 avian influenza virus directly infected several humans during an outbreak in Hong Kong in 1997, the virus retained its preference for SAα2,3Gal (Matrosovich et al., 1999), indicating that severe infection can occur in humans by avian viruses with HAs specific to SAα2,3Gal. Recent findings by two groups of investigators provide a possible explanation for this observation (Shinya et al., 2006; van Riel et al., 2006). Shinya and colleagues report that the human nasal mucosa, trachea, pharynx, and bronchus are abundant in SAα2,6Gal, while both SAα2,3Gal and SAα2,6Gal are detected in the respiratory bronchioles and alveoli (Shinya et al., 2006). Riel and colleagues observed H5N1 virus attachment to type II pneumocytes, alveolar macrophages, and nonciliated cuboidal epithelial cells in the terminal bronchioles of humans (van Riel et al., 2006). Thus, there are some SAα2,3Gal receptors expressed by cells in the lower respiratory tract of humans to which the H5N1 avian influenza virus can bind and infect. It should be noted, however, that even though receptor preference influences the host-range of influenza virus, this is not an absolute determinant of host-range. The infectivity and transmissibility in humans of avian influenza viruses with SAα2,3Gal or SAα2,6Gal specificity remains undefined and will require further study to understand fully the role of these receptors in host-range restriction.

Overcoming the species barrier

Avian influenza viruses shed by aquatic birds can occasionally infect terrestrial birds and a variety of mammalian species (Webster et al., 1992), but they seldom become endemic in these new hosts (Suarez and Schultz-Cherry, 2000). The infections are often transient; the new hosts may only be capable of infection by a limited number of influenza subtypes. Only three subtypes have widely circulated in humans during the past century (H1N1, H2N2, H3N2) and only a few subtypes have been repeatedly isolated from pigs (H1N1, H3N2, and H1N2) and horses (H7N7 and H3N8) (Webby and Webster, 2001). Attempts to infect humans or nonhuman primates experimentally with avian influenza viruses, and attempts to infect ducks with human influenza viruses (Kida et al., 1980), were not very successful, leading to the conclusions that avian influenza viruses replicate poorly in humans (Beare and Webster, 1991) and other primates (Murphy et al., 1982) and that human influenza viruses replicate poorly in waterfowl (Hinshaw et al., 1983). In order for viruses to establish themselves in a new host, they must establish interactions between viral proteins and host-cell machinery, subvert the host's innate and adaptive immune responses, and exploit host factors to permit transmission from one host to another (Parrish and Kawaoka, 2005). All of these adaptive changes necessitate viral alterations at the genetic level, and it is believed that the selection, accumulation, and maintenance of these mutations could occur during the passage of the virus in an intermediate host.

Possible involvement of an intermediate host

Although precursors of pandemic viruses have not actually been isolated from putative intermediate hosts, it was believed that pandemic influenza viruses arose by reassortment between an avain and a human influenza virus in an intermediate host. Pigs have long been suspected of being the intermediate host in which avian and human influenza viruses could reassort to form a virus with pandemic potential (Scholtissek, 1990), in a sense acting as "mixing vessels," because pigs are susceptible to infection with many influenza subtypes (Kida et al., 1994) and they express both the SAα2,3Gal and SAα2,6Gal moieties in their tracheas (Ito et al., 1998). For example, a reassortant influenza virus that surface protein genes of avian origin and gene segments from a human influenza virus that conferred the property of efficient replication and transmissibility in humans, could have pandemic potential. Alternatively, avian influenza viruses could gradually acquire the ability to recognize and bind to human virus receptors after replication in an intermediate host like the pig (Ito et al., 1998). It is also possible that adaptations of avian influenza viruses in domestic poultry or terrestrial birds could enhance their potential to infect humans (Banks and Plowright, 2003; Perez et al., 2003). Humans could also serve as a host in whom avian and human viruses could reassort. These findings suggest that there is a need to maintain virologic surveillance both in animals and in humans to monitor the emergence of new strains of influenza virus.

Pandemic influenza

Several influenza subtypes have infected humans. Based on historical accounts, an average of three influenza pandemics have occurred each century, at intervals ranging from 10 to 50 years (WHO, 2005). Three influenza pandemics occurred in the last century: the "Spanish" influenza pandemic of 1918 (H1N1 subtype), the 1957 "Asian flu" (H2N2), and the 1968 "Hong Kong flu" (H3N2). These pandemics resulted in high morbidity, loss of life, and considerable social and economic disruption. They provide health authorities information on which to base preparations for a future pandemic.

Asia has been referred to as an influenza epicenter (Shortridge and Stuart-Harris, 1982) because the two most recent pandemics originated there, and because it is a region where cultural and agricultural practices place very large numbers of people and domestic livestock in close proximity with each other. Pandemics have a propensity to unfold in waves, with subsequent waves tending to be more severe than the last (Reid et al., 2001). Containing the spread of the virus during the initial wave of a pandemic has been cited as a critical measure to mitigate the impact of a pandemic (WHO, 2005). Intensive influenza surveillance in humans, waterfowl, and poultry has been put in place by the World Health Organization and the World Organization for Animal Health (OIE) to provide prompt information about the emergence of a novel influenza virus.

1918 Spanish influenza pandemic

In addition to being one of the most devastating epidemics in history, the 1918 influenza pandemic had several additional interesting aspects. Although it had the same clinical manifestations as previous influenza outbreaks, with pathology largely confined to the respiratory tract, a higher percentage of cases in 1918 developed severe, fatal pneumonia (Reid and Taubenberger, 2003). Moreover, the 1918 H1N1 virus more frequently caused severe disease and mortality in young healthy adults between 20 and 40 years of age (Glezen, 1996; Luk et al., 2001; Langford, 2002). Typical age-specific epidemic curves follow a U-shape pattern, with peaks in mortality among infants and the elderly, age-specific mortality during the 1918 pandemic displayed a W-shaped curve that reflected an additional peak of mortality among young adults (Luk et al., 2001); this age group constituted almost half of the influenza-associated deaths during the pandemic (Reid and Taubenberger, 2003). The cause of this distribution remains a mystery.

Taubenberger and colleagues amplified viral RNA from formalin-fixed, paraffin-embedded lung tissue infected during the 1918 H1N1 pandemic from autopsy samples from two American soldiers, and from the frozen lung tissue of an Inuit woman who had died in the epidemic and was buried in the Alaskan permafrost (Reid et al., 1999). The generation of complete gene sequence information allowed detailed studies of each of the gene segments of the virus and led to the eventual reconstruction of the entire virus (Tumpey et al., 2005). Using techniques to generate infectious viruses from cloned complementary DNA, reassortant viruses possessing different combinations of the 1918 HA and NA genes in a background of different human influenza viruses were generated to determine the contribution of each gene to pathogenicity (Kobasa et al., 2004; Tumpey et al., 2005). It was found that the 1918 HA protein, but not NA, enhanced the virulence of influenza A viruses in mice and that the polymerase genes contributed to the virulence of the 1918 virus (Tumpey et al., 2005). In addition, a separate study on the receptor-binding specificity of the HA of two different strains of the 1918 virus showed that a single amino acid substitution (D190E) in the HA protein could restrict the ability of the HA from recognizing and binding both SAα2,6Gal and SAα2,3Gal to binding only the SAα2,6Gal (Glaser et al., 2005), an evolutionary step that may have facilitated its transmission in humans.

Phylogenetic analyses of the entire genome of the 1918 H1N1 virus suggest that it most likely originated from an avian source (Taubenberger et al., 2005). This indicates that, in the future, another avian influenza virus could acquire mutations that would alter its host range and cause a pandemic in humans (Russell and Webster, 2005). A survey of the amino acid changes between the 1918 virus and available avian influenza virus consensus sequences identified 10 differences in the polymerase genes that consistently distinguished the 1918 virus from its avian counterparts, changes that may have contributed to its adaptation to humans (Taubenberger et al., 2005). The predictive value of such analyses depends on the breadth of the database of available avian and human influenza virus gene sequences and will be enhanced by expansion of the database. Monitoring changes in key residues among circulating avian influenza viruses might provide an early warning that these viruses are gradually adapting to humans.

The H1N1 virus that appeared in the human population in 1918 circulated in a less virulent form until 1957, when it was replaced by the H2N2 pandemic virus during the Asian influenza pandemic in 1957. H1N1 viruses reappeared in 1977 in China (Kung et al., 1978) and Russia (Zakstelskaja et al., 1978; Zhdanov et al., 1978) and spread throughout the world, infecting mainly children and young adults, individuals in an age group that did not have prior natural immunity against the virus. Individuals who were born before 1957 were not as often infected, presumably because of the previous exposure of many of them to a similar strain (Nakajima et al., 1978; Scholtissek et al., 1978b; Zakstelskaja et al., 1978; Zhdanov et al., 1978).

The 1957 Asian and the 1968 Hong Kong influenza pandemics

Phylogenetic analyses of the viruses that caused the 1957 and 1968 pandemics revealed that these strains were reassortants between avian influenza viruses and previously circulating human influenza viruses (Scholtissek et al., 1978a; Kawaoka et al., 1989). The 1957 H2N2 pandemic virus derived its H2 HA, N2 NA, and PB1 genes from an avian virus, with remaining gene segments derived from the circulating H1N1 human influenza virus. The 1957 pandemic resulted in the death of about 1 million individuals worldwide (Kawaoka et al., 1989), with excess mortality largely confined to infants and the elderly.

In 1968, the H2N2 subtype was replaced by an H3N2 subtype reassortant virus that derived its H3 HA and PB1 genes from an avian influenza virus and remaining gene segments from the previously circulating H2N2 strain (Scholtissek et al.,

1978a). The 1968 pandemic resulted in milder clinical symptoms and led to few excess deaths except in the United States (Glezen, 1996). The relative mildness of this pandemic has been attributed to the genetic similarity of the H3N2 virus to the previously circulating viruses, particularly the conservation of the N2 NA from the 1957 H2N2 strain, which might have conferred partial protection to some individuals (Lipatov et al., 2004). Of interest, the PB1 genes for both pandemic viruses were derived from an avian source, suggesting a high degree of compatibility between avian PB1 protein and the other polymerase subunits of human influenza A viruses.

Today, influenza A H1N1 and H3N2 continue to co-circulate in humans (Subbarao et al., 2006b) along with influenza B viruses. Co-circulation of two subtypes of influenza A and two lineages of influenza B viruses in humans eventually led to the generation of reassortant virus strains, an influenza A H1N2 reassortant (Gregory et al., 2002; Xu et al., 2002) and an influenza B virus reassortant that acquired its HA from the B/Victoria lineage and its NA from the B/Yamagata lineage (Rota et al., 1990; Shaw et al., 2002).

Avian influenza

Avian influenza virus infections in poultry can cause a wide spectrum of clinical symptoms ranging from asymptomatic infections, decreased egg-laying capacity, depression, mild-to-severe respiratory disease, and high mortality.

These viruses are classified based on their lethality in chickens, as determined by a standard intravenous pathogenicity test (USAHA, 1994). In this procedure, eight 4–6-week-old specific pathogen-free (SPF) chickens are inoculated intravenously with a 1:10 dilution of the test virus and are observed for 10 days. Viruses are categorized as highly pathogenic if they result in the death of six or more inoculated chickens ($\geq 75\%$ mortality), mildly pathogenic if one to five chickens die, and nonpathogenic if all chickens survive. HPAI viruses are confined to the H5 and H7 subtypes, although not all viruses of these subtypes cause HPAI.

Determinants of pathogenicity

Studies of reassortant viruses have shown that virulence is a multi-genic trait that is not solely determined by the gene segments that have been substituted, but also by the resulting gene constellation (Rott et al., 1979; Scholtissek et al., 1979). The genes that have been identified as virulence determinants in naturally occurring and laboratory-adapted influenza viruses are summarized in Table 1.

Transmission of avian influenza viruses to humans

The three prerequisites for an influenza virus pandemic are the emergence of a novel viral subtype to which the general population has little or no immunity, a virus that can replicate in humans and cause serious illness, and efficient human-to-human

Table 1

Some virulence determinants of influenza viruses

Virus protein	Virulence factor	Comments	References
HA	Multiple basic amino acids at the HA cleavage site	• Known virulence motif in poultry • Contribution to virulence in mammals is unknown	Bosch et al. (1981), Bosch et al. (1979), Senne et al. (1996), Steinhauer (1999)
	Loss of carbohydrate side chain in the HA stalk region	• HA cleavage site becomes more accessible to host proteases, enhancing HA activation	Kawaoka et al. (1984)
	Glycosylation near the receptor-binding site	• Carbohydrate side chain enhances viral attachment to cells, resulting in higher rate of productive infection	Perdue et al. (1994), Perdue et al. (1995), Perdue and Suarez (2000)
NA	Presence of carboxy-terminal lysine and loss of glycosylation at amino acid 146	• NA gains ability to bind and sequester plasminogen, resulting in increased cleavage of HA • Has only been demonstrated with A/WSN/33 (H1N1)	Goto and Kawaoka (1998)
	Deletion in the stalk region	• Associated with decreased ability of viral release from cells and viral attenuation in mice • Correlation between stalk length and better viral replication in eggs • Influence on avian influenza infection in humans is unknown	Castrucci and Kawaoka (1993), Matrosovich et al. (1999)
	H274Y and E119V mutations	• Associated with resistance to oseltamivir	Gubareva et al. (2001), Molla et al. (2002)
PB2	E627K mutation	• Virulence appears to be limited to mice where it enhances viral replication that tends to overwhelm host immune responses	Hatta et al. (2001), Subbarao et al. (1993)

Table 1 (*continued*)

Virus protein	Virulence factor	Comments	References
NS1	Deletions in the C-terminal region	• Associated with decreased ability to prevent type I IFN synthesis in pigs, resulting in viral attenuation	Solorzano et al. (2005)
	D92E mutation	• Associated with resistance to the antiviral effects of type I IFN and TNF-α, resulting in disease exacerbation in pigs	Seo et al. (2002)

transmission of the virus (WHO, 2005). In the past few years, several novel influenza subtypes (H5, H7, and H9) have been reported to infect humans. These infections have generally occurred in people who were exposed to diseased poultry and the viruses isolated from human cases were genetically identical to the viruses isolated from infected poultry, demonstrating that direct transmission of influenza viruses from avian species to humans can occur in the absence of reassortment. These laboratory-confirmed cases of avian-to-human transmission have raised fears that one of these viruses may become transmissible and thus, acquire pandemic potential that have fulfilled the first two criteria for a pandemic virus.

H5 subtype viruses

In May 1997, an avian influenza A H5N1 virus (A/Hong Kong/156/97) was isolated from a 3-year-old child in Hong Kong who subsequently died due to severe pneumonia complicated by acute respiratory distress syndrome (ARDS), renal failure, and Reye's syndrome (Subbarao et al., 1998). Although no clear link was established between the child and infected birds, there were reports of outbreaks of fatal H5N1 avian influenza in poultry on farms in the northwestern part of Hong Kong that occurred around the time of the child's infection (Subbarao et al., 1998). Six months later, 17 additional cases of human H5N1 infections were identified in Hong Kong, five of which were fatal (Yuen et al., 1998). These cases occurred concomitantly with an outbreak of H5N1 influenza virus infections among chickens in poultry markets and on farms in Hong Kong. Sequence analysis of all gene segments from the human and avian H5N1 isolates revealed >99% homology, consistent with transmission from chickens to humans (Claas et al., 1998; Suarez et al., 1998; Subbarao et al., 1998). The cases in humans and the discovery that several species of birds in the live bird markets were infected with the H5N1 virus prompted intensified surveillance for avian influenza virus in poultry, the strict regulation of the importation of live poultry from mainland China, and the mass culling of about 1.5 million chickens in Hong Kong (Shortridge, 1999; Chan, 2002). These strategies successfully ended the outbreak of human infection and may have averted a pandemic.

Molecular and genetic characterization of the human H5N1 virus isolates confirmed that the viruses were of avian origin, with no evidence of genetic reassortment with circulating human influenza A viruses (Claas et al., 1998; Subbarao et al., 1998). By phylogenetic analysis, the virus source of the HA gene of the 1997 H5N1 virus was identified to be A/goose/Guangdong/1/96 (H5N1) (Xu et al., 1999), a virus that continued to circulate in geese in southeastern China (Webster et al., 2002), while the NA and the remaining internal protein gene segments were derived from either A/teal/Hong Kong/W312/97 (H6N1) or A/quail/Hong Kong/G1/97 (H9N2) (Guan et al., 1999; Lin et al., 2000). As a result of the killing of poultry in Hong Kong for the purpose of influenza control, the 1997 H5N1 virus was eradicated but the precursor viruses continued to circulate in the region (Guan et al., 2000), giving rise to different genotypes that had high pathogenicity in chickens (Guan et al., 2002). In 2002, some of these viruses acquired dramatic new pathogenicity for ducks and other aquatic birds (Sturm-Ramirez et al., 2004), a trait that is unusual for HPAI viruses. In 2003, three humans in a family of five developed severe respiratory illness and two succumbed to their illness (Peiris et al., 2004). The H5N1 virus that was isolated from two family members was genetically and antigenically different from the H5N1 viruses isolated during the 1997 outbreak in Hong Kong (Guan et al., 2004).

The outbreak of HPAI in poultry in several Asian countries that started in late 2003 is unprecedented in magnitude. Outbreaks caused by antigenically related viruses were reported in Vietnam, Japan, Thailand, Cambodia, Laos, Indonesia, China, and Malaysia, and HPAI H5N1 infections were eventually detected in more than 40 countries in Asia, Europe, and Africa (OIE, 2006). While some countries were able to efficiently contain the epidemic and have been declared virus-free, the H5N1 virus is currently endemic in poultry in several countries (de Jong and Hien, 2006; Chen et al., 2006a).

Migratory birds appear to play a significant role in the spread of the H5N1 virus over great distances (Sturm-Ramirez et al., 2004); antigenic drift variants of the earlier H5N1 strains that were isolated in 2002 in aquatic birds in Hong Kong (Lipatov et al., 2004) were isolated in migrating geese in western China (Chen et al., 2005). H5N1 viruses replicate in the intestinal tract and respiratory tract of ducks, with higher viral titers isolated in the trachea than in the cloaca (Sturm-Ramirez et al., 2005), and ducks shed virus for up to 17 days post-infection (Hulse-Post et al., 2005).

Studies indicate that H5N1 viruses are gaining virulence and expanding their host range. Increased virulence of H5N1 viruses has been noted in laboratory animals including ferrets and mice, with some viruses disseminating to extrapulmonary sites, including the brain (Gao et al., 1999; Lu et al., 1999; Lipatov et al., 2003; Govorkova et al., 2005; Maines et al., 2005). Lethal H5N1 infections have been reported in unconventional hosts such as felids (tigers, leopards), and domestic cats have been experimentally infected with H5N1 viruses (Keawcharoen et al., 2004; Kuiken et al., 2004).

While the majority of the HPAI H5N1 outbreaks are confined to poultry, reports of human H5N1 infections are rising. As of this writing (April 2006), there have been more than 200 laboratory-confirmed cases of H5N1 infections reported in humans and more than 100 have been fatal (WHO, 2006b). This figure is likely to be an underestimate because it represents only laboratory-confirmed cases. Other cases may have been missed due to lack of active surveillance and clinical awareness (Hien et al., 2004). Laboratory confirmation usually consists of detection of influenza A H5N1 viral RNA by polymerase chain reaction (PCR), recognition of influenza A H5N1 viral antigen by immunofluorescence or antigen-capture enzyme-linked immunosorbent assay (ELISA) (using monoclonal antibodies specific to H5), virus isolation, or various serological methods (WHO, 2004).

A summary of the clinical characteristics of humans infected with the H5N1 virus is shown in Table 2. Most reported H5N1 infections have occurred in otherwise healthy children or adults who had been exposed to infected poultry (Beigel et al., 2005; Chotpitayasunondh et al., 2005). The median age of eight patients hospitalized during the 1997 H5N1 outbreak in Hong Kong was 9.5 years (range 1–60) (Yuen et al., 1998; Chan, 2002).

Initial signs and symptoms of patients infected with avian influenza H5N1 virus in Hong Kong were typical of severe human influenza, including fever ($>38°C$), cough, dyspnea, and pneumonia (Yuen et al., 1998; Beigel et al., 2005). Gastrointestinal symptoms, including vomiting, abdominal pain, and diarrhea, were prominent in almost half of the patients. Abnormal liver function tests and pancytopenia were also noted in some cases (Yuen et al., 1998), and X-rays in some showed diffuse alveolar damage due to ARDS. Despite supportive therapy and intensive care support, several patients died with multiple organ failure. Amantadine was administered in a few cases, but its benefits could not be analyzed due to the small number of patients in which it was used. Risk factors associated with severe disease included delay in hospitalization, pneumonia, leukopenia, and lymphopenia (Yuen et al., 1998).

The clinical illness in 10 patients in Vietnam (mean age 13.7 years, range 5–24 years) and in 12 cases in Thailand (median age 12 years, range 2–58 years) with H5N1 infection in 2004 were similar to those in the 1997 H5N1 outbreak in Hong Kong (Tran et al., 2004; Chotpitayasunondh et al., 2005). Many of the patients reported close contact with poultry during the week before the onset of illness, suggesting an incubation period of 2–4 days. H5N1 infection in these patients was confirmed by virus culture or reverse transcription-PCR (RT-PCR) using H5 HA-specific primers. All patients presented with fever, dyspnea, and cough. Chest X-rays of patients in Vietnam were abnormal on admission, displaying extensive bilateral infiltrates, lobar collapse, and focal consolidation (Tran et al., 2004).

Table 2

Clinical characteristics of confirmed avian influenza A (H5N1) cases in humans

Variable	Hong Kong, 1997 ($n = 18$)	Thailand, 2004 ($n = 12$)	Vietnam, 2004 ($n = 10$)
Male sex—no. (%)	8 (44)	8 (67)	6 (60)
Age (year)			
Median	9.5	12	13.7 (mean)
Range	1–60	2–58	5–24
No. (%) exposed to ill poultry	11/16 (70)	7/12 (58)	8/9 (89)
Clinical symptoms [no. (%)]			
Fever	17/18 (94)	12/12 (100)	10/10 (100)
Cough	12/18 (67)	12/12 (100)	10/10 (100)
Dyspnea	11/18 (61)	12/12 (100)	10/10 (100)
Myalgia	2/18 (11)	5/12 (42)	0/10 (0)
Diarrhea	3/18 (17)	5/12 (42)	7/10 (70)
Conjunctivitis	NR[a]	0/12 (0)	0/10 (0)
Abdominal pain	3/18 (17)	2/12 (17)	NR
Rhinorrhea	7/12 (58)	4/12 (33)	0/10 (0)
Lymphopenia			
Laboratory findings [no. (%)]	11/18 (61)	7/12 (58)	10/10 (100)
Elevated serum aminotransferase levels	11/18 (61)	8/12 (67)	5/6 (83)
Outcome [no. (%)]			
Mortality	6/18 (33)	8/12 (67)	8/10 (80)

Note: Hong Kong, 1997: (Chan, 2002; Yuen et al., 1998), Thailand, 2004: (Beigel et al., 2005; Chotpitayasunondh et al., 2005), Vietnam, 2004: (Tran et al., 2004)
[a]NR—not reported.

A large proportion (70%) of patients also had diarrhea (Tran et al., 2004). Lymphopenia and thrombocytopenia were commonly observed among patients in both Vietnam and Thailand and were recognized as major risk factors for ARDS and death (Tran et al., 2004; Chotpitayasunondh et al., 2005). Six of the seven patients in Vietnam and six of the eight patients in Thailand who were treated with corticosteroids died, suggesting that corticosteroids may not be beneficial. The administration of oseltamivir has been reported, but its use at different stages of illness makes it difficult to assess its efficacy, although there appeared to be an association between early administration of oseltamivir and survival in some patients in Thailand (Chotpitayasunondh et al., 2005).

Elevated levels of pro-inflammatory cytokines (interleukin-6 and interferon-γ) and chemokines (interferon-inducible protein-10 [IP-10] and monocyte chemoattractant protein-1 [MCP-1]) have been detected in the sera of several H5N1-infected patients (To et al., 2001; Peiris et al., 2004). This suggests that an aggressive cytokine response against the H5N1 virus might exacerbate virus-mediated pathology.

Although several deaths have occurred as a result of H5N1 infection, few autopsies have been conducted to investigate the pathology caused by H5N1 viruses. Post-mortem examination of two fatal cases caused by the 1997 H5N1 virus identified hemophagocytosis as the most prominent feature, along with diffuse alveolar damage with interstitial fibrosis, extensive hepatic central lobular necrosis, acute renal tubular necrosis, and lymphoid depletion (To et al., 2001). An autopsy conducted on an H5N1 virus-infected 6-year-old boy who died during an outbreak in Thailand found viral RNA by RT-PCR in the lung, intestine, and spleen tissues, but found viral replication only in the lung and intestine (Uiprasertkul et al., 2005). The presence of the H5N1 virus in the intestine may explain the diarrhea seen among patients upon admission. There is one report of H5N1 virus dissemination to the central nervous system in a 4-year-old boy who presented with severe diarrhea and acute encephalitis but without respiratory symptoms typically associated with influenza; H5N1 virus was isolated from his cerebrospinal fluid, fecal, throat, and blood specimens (de Jong et al., 2005). This case suggests that disease surveillance of H5N1 influenza may need to focus on clusters of death of unknown etiology or with other symptoms than those of classical influenza (de Jong et al., 2005a).

A minority of H5N1 infections have resulted in milder symptoms and a few individuals with no history of clinical illness have been found to have antibodies to the H5N1 virus. A seroepidemiological survey of 1525 poultry workers who participated in the poultry culling during the 1997 H5N1 outbreak in Hong Kong revealed that approximately 10% had anti-H5 antibody; there were no documented cases of H5-related illness in this group (Bridges et al., 2002). While the vast majority of H5N1 infections have occurred as a result of poultry-to-human transmission, human-to-human transmission has been documented on a few occasions but is inefficient (Table 3). Human-to-human transmission of the H5N1 virus was suspected in a family cluster in Thailand, in which the child's aunt as well as the child's mother who provided unprotected nursing care to her infected daughter, apparently developed pneumonia (Ungchusak et al., 2005). However, related seroprevalence studies of health care workers in Vietnam and Thailand in 2004 did not detect any antibodies to H5 viruses (Apisarnthanarak et al., 2005; Liem and Lim, 2005).

H9 subtype viruses

Surveillance for influenza viruses in live bird markets during the H5N1 outbreak in November and December 1997 in Hong Kong identified the presence of other influenza subtypes in addition to H5N1, with H9N2 being one of the most common (Guan et al., 1999). However, infection of chickens with H9N2 viruses was not associated with severe morbidity or mortality (Lin et al., 2000). H9N2 viruses have been sporadically isolated in humans since 1999, including five patients with

Table 3

Serologic studies of H5N1 avian influenza infection among patient contacts

Year	Country	Group	Detection method	No. tested	No. positive or percent	Remarks	Reference
1997	Hong Kong, China	Poultry workers	Microneutralization assay, Western blot	1525	~10%	Mostly asymptomatic infections	Bridges et al. (2002)
1997	Hong Kong, China	Household contacts	Microneutralization assay, ELISA, Western blot	51	6 (12%)	5 of 6 individuals also had exposure to poultry	Katz et al. (1999)
1997	Hong Kong, China	Health care workers	Microneutralization assay, Western blot	217	8 (4%)	Exposed to H5N1-infected patients; 2 cases of seroconversion	Buxton Bridges et al. (2000)
2004	Vietnam	Health care workers	Microneutralization assay	83	0	No anti-H5 detected	Liem and Lim (2005)
2004	Thailand	Health care workers	Clinical presentation	25	0	Index case had an atypical presentation of influenza virus infection	Apisarnthanarak et al. (2005)

influenza-like illness in Guangdong province, China, in 1999 (Guo et al., 1999), two girls with mild influenza symptoms in Hong Kong in March 1999 (Peiris et al., 1999), and a child with influenza-like illness in Hong Kong in 2003 (Butt et al., 2005). Thus, it appears that this subtype can infect humans. There are multiple co-circulating genotypes of the H9N2 influenza viruses (Li et al., 2003). The H5N1 viruses isolated from humans and poultry during the outbreak in Hong Kong in 1997 were reassortants that obtained their internal gene segments from an avian H9N2 virus (A/quail/Hong Kong/G1/97) or an H6N1 virus (A/teal/Hong Kong/W312/97) (Guan et al., 1999; Guan et al., 2000; Lin et al., 2000). Some H9N2 viruses isolated in pigs in southern China displayed affinity for the SAα2,6Gal moiety found abundantly in human epithelial cells (Matrosovich et al., 2001; Peiris et al., 2001). No new human cases of H9N2 infections have been reported since 2003, and all the reported illnesses associated with these viruses were mild and self-limited.

H7 subtype viruses

Isolated human infections with H7 viruses, acquired from birds and seals, resulted in asymptomatic infections, conjunctivitis, and/or influenza-like illnesses (Webster et al., 1981; Kurtz et al., 1996; Fouchier et al., 2004; Koopmans et al., 2004; Tweed et al., 2004; Puzelli et al., 2005). There have been several large-scale outbreaks of H7 infections in poultry in Italy (H7N1, H7N3), the Netherlands (H7N7), and Canada (H7N3). Agricultural workers and veterinarians were exposed to large numbers of infected birds during these outbreaks and careful study of them has led to the identification of several H7 infections. Seven of 185 (3.8%) poultry workers in Italy were found to have H7 antibodies during an H7N3 low-pathogenic avian influenza outbreak in 2002–2003; one worker developed conjunctivitis while the rest were asymptomatic (Puzelli et al., 2005). An H7N7 outbreak in poultry in the Netherlands resulted in extensive transmission of the virus to individuals involved in farming or culling of infected fowl (Koopmans et al., 2004); 83 of 89 cases had conjunctivitis while the remaining six patients had influenza-like illnesses. A veterinarian developed pneumonia and later died of ARDS (Fouchier et al., 2004; Koopmans et al., 2004); this patient initially complained of fever and headache 4 days after visiting a poultry farm and initially had no signs of respiratory disease or conjunctivitis. Throat and eye swabs collected 7 days after exposure were negative by RT-PCR. However, he was admitted to the hospital 2 days later where interstitial opacities were seen in the right lower lobe of the lung on X-ray. He developed bilateral pneumonia and died of respiratory insufficiency 6 days after admission (Fouchier et al., 2004). H7 RNA was detected by real-time PCR in a broncho-alveolar lavage specimen collected 11 days after exposure and the H7 virus [A/Netherlands/219/03 (H7N7)] was isolated from post-mortem specimens of the right and left lung. Significant lesions were not observed by gross or histologic examination in organs outside the respiratory tract (Fouchier et al., 2004).

There was some evidence of human-to-human transmission of the H7 virus during the outbreak in the Netherlands. Serological survey among family members of infected poultry workers detected that 59% had H7 antibodies (Du Ry van Beest Holle et al., 2005). In 2004, an H7N3 virus outbreak in poultry in British Columbia, Canada, resulted in the infection of two poultry workers who presented with conjunctivitis and mild respiratory symptoms (Tweed et al., 2004).

These reports indicate that conjunctivitis is an important feature of H7 influenza virus infection in humans, unlike infections with H5N1 viruses. It is possible that the conjunctiva may be a significant portal of entry for H7 viruses.

Other subtypes

Influenza A viruses of the H6 subtype have been consistently isolated from poultry in live bird markets in the United States (Panigrahy et al., 2002; Webby et al., 2003). The internal protein genes of H6N1 viruses isolated in Hong Kong in 1997 are genetically identical to those of 1997 H5N1 and H9N2 viruses (Hoffmann et al., 2000; Chin et al., 2002). As stated above, H5N1 viruses isolated from humans and poultry in Hong Kong in 1997 were reassortants that obtained their internal gene segments in some cases from an H6N1 virus (A/teal/Hong Kong/W312/97) (Guan et al., 1999, 2000; Lin et al., 2000). If the ability to infect humans lies in one or more of these internal protein genes, H6N1 viruses could also cross the species barrier and infect humans.

The H10 subtype has been associated with a severe avian influenza outbreak in turkeys (H10N7) (Karunakaran et al., 1983) and can be pathogenic to minks (H10N4) (Englund and Hard af Segerstad, 1998). There are reports of H10N7 virus transmission to two human infants in Egypt in 2004 (Anonymous, 2004).

The H2 subtype responsible for the 1957 pandemic continues to circulate in wild ducks (Makarova et al., 1999). This virus has clearly demonstrated the ability to infect humans. Should it reemerge, individuals born after 1968 will lack immunity against this subtype because they were born after H2N2 viruses ceased to circulate in humans.

Prevention and treatment of influenza

Antiviral prevention and treatment of influenza virus infections

Two classes of antiviral drugs are licensed for the prevention and treatment of influenza in humans. These are the M2 ion channel inhibitors, amantadine and rimantadine, and the NA inhibitors, oseltamivir and zanamivir. The discussion in this section refers mainly to recommendations for use of antivirals in prevention and treatment of human influenza virus infections. The limited experience in treating avian influenza virus infections in humans is also addressed.

In a typical influenza epidemic, treatment with antiviral drugs can offer a significant benefit to individuals such as the elderly and those with chronic underlying diseases, who are at risk for developing severe illness or complications of influenza (Stiver, 2003). Epidemiological modeling suggests that in the event of a pandemic, the early use of antivirals for prophylaxis could have a marked impact in limiting its spread (Longini et al., 2004).

Effective antiviral treatment for pandemic influenza should have efficacy against avian strains, limited development of resistance, ability to be stockpiled in large quantities, and ability to be used to treat patients with severe influenza symptoms (Kandel and Hartshorn, 2005). Based on these features, the NA inhibitors are preferred over the adamantanes.

However, M2 ion channel inhibitors are effective for prophylaxis of influenza. In a recent comprehensive review of the efficacy of antiviral drugs in preventing influenza in healthy adults, Jefferson and colleagues determined that amantadine significantly prevented 61% of influenza A cases and 25% cases of influenza-like illnesses (Jefferson et al., 2006). Amantadine and rimantadine are also useful in treatment, as they significantly shorten the duration of fever, although neither drug has any effect on nasal viral shedding or persistence of influenza A viruses in the upper respiratory tract (Jefferson et al., 2006).

A major concern regarding the use of the M2 ion channel inhibitors is the rapid development of resistance against these drugs. Resistance can occur in up to 30% of individuals within 5 days of treatment (Belshe et al., 1988; Hayden and Hay, 1992; Stiver, 2003) and drug-resistant strains can be transmitted to contacts (Hayden et al., 1989). Furthermore, some H5N1 viruses isolated from birds and human patients have displayed resistance to amantadine due to a fixed mutation in their M2 gene (Li et al., 2004; Puthavathana et al., 2005). M2 ion channel inhibitors can also have unpleasant side effects, including CNS stimulation characterized by jitteriness, confusion, anxiety, nightmares, and hallucinations (Keyser et al., 2000).

On the other hand, administration of the NA inhibitors zanamivir or oseltamivir once daily for 4–6 weeks is effective and well tolerated in preventing influenza infection in healthy adults (Hayden et al., 1999; Monto et al., 1999). NA inhibitors can reduce viral shedding and shorten the duration of symptoms when administered within 48 h of disease onset (Hayden et al., 1997; Englund, 2002). Early treatment of human influenza virus infection with oseltamivir provides clinical benefit, but there is no evidence of benefit when treatment is initiated more than 48 h after the onset of symptoms (Chotpitayasunondh et al., 2005; Wong and Yuen, 2006). Both oseltamivir and zanamivir are effective in preventing death following infection with H5N1 viruses in animal models (Gubareva et al., 1998; Leneva et al., 2001), although more recently isolated H5N1 strains tend to require higher doses of oseltamivir and prolonged administration to achieve similar efficacy (Yen et al., 2005; Wong and Yuen, 2006). During the H7N7 avian influenza outbreak in the Netherlands in 2003, immediate treatment with oseltamivir was recommended for individuals with recent onset of conjunctivitis and for all personnel in bird culling operations (a daily prophylactic regimen of oseltamivir [75 mg/day] to be continued 2 days after the last exposure) (Koopmans et al., 2004).

Currently, the WHO recommendation for influenza prophylaxis is that adults with household exposure to H5N1 influenza infections be given 75 mg of oseltamivir/day for 7–10 days from the last day of a potentially infective exposure. Continuous treatment may be required for individuals with repeated or prolonged exposure such as health care workers and poultry workers involved in bird culling operations (WHO, 2006a).

The optimum dosage of oseltamivir for treating H5N1 virus-infected patients is unknown; ill patients might benefit from a longer duration of therapy (up to 10 days) or higher doses (~300 mg/day), but clinical studies of these have not been conducted (WHO, 2006a). Some NA inhibitor-resistant strains of H5N1 have been reported (Le et al., 2005; de Jong et al., 2005b), but they are still uncommon. NA inhibitors have few side effects; these include mild nausea and vomiting with oseltamivir (Treanor et al., 2000) and possible exacerbation of bronchospasm among individuals with asthma after using zanamivir (which is inhaled) (Moscona, 2005).

Vaccines

Immunization is the cornerstone of influenza prophylaxis and is considered to be the most cost-effective strategy of preventing its spread in the community. The two types of licensed vaccines against human influenza viruses are formalin-inactivated (whole or split) virus vaccines and live-attenuated influenza virus vaccines. Both types of vaccines are trivalent and contain influenza A/H1N1, A/H3N2 and B components to protect against circulating strains of human influenza viruses. Unlike vaccines for other infectious pathogens, vaccines for influenza need to be reformulated annually to keep up with antigenic drift of influenza A and B viruses. New variants with epidemic potential are identified through the global surveillance conducted by the WHO network of laboratories (Cox et al., 1994; Subbarao and Katz, 2004). The antigenicity of these viruses' HA proteins are evaluated and the nucleotide sequences are of the genes also determined.

Inactivated virus vaccines

Inactivated virus vaccines are generated by propagation of the virus in embryonated hen's eggs and are manufactured as whole virion vaccines, split-product vaccines, and subunit vaccines. Split-product vaccines are whole virus particles that have been treated with detergents to remove the virus' lipid component. Subunit vaccines contain highly purified HA and NA proteins.

Live-attenuated influenza vaccines

Attenuated, cold-adapted (ca) vaccine viruses have HA and NA proteins from a wild-type virus, while the six internal gene segments from an attenuated master strain whose genes confer the temperature-sensitive (ts), ca, and attenuation phenotypes. Influenza A (A/Ann Arbor/6/60) and B (B/Ann Arbor/1/66) master donor ca strains are used to generate live-attenuated influenza virus vaccines in the United States. Comparison of the nucleotide sequence of cloned ca donor strains with those of the wild-type viruses have led to the identification of mutations in several gene segments that are associated with the ca, ts, and attenuation phenotypes (Herlocher et al., 1996; Jin et al., 2003; Chen et al., 2006b) and this polygenic nature of attenuation may be responsible for the high degree of stability exhibited by ca reassortant vaccine strains (Murphy and Coelingh, 2002).

Advantages of live, attenuated influenza virus vaccine over the inactivated vaccine include the ability of the live-attenuated vaccine to induce a mucosal IgA antibody response and to stimulate $CD8^+$ T-cell-mediated immune responses that play a role in viral clearance and recovery (Murphy and Clements, 1989). Live-attenuated influenza virus vaccine is delivered intranasally using a syringe-like spraying device that delivers a 0.25-ml volume of a large particle aerosol into each nostril (Belshe et al., 2004); the attenuated vaccine virus replicates to a limited extent in the upper respiratory tract, inducing both a secretory and a systemic immune response that closely resemble the response induced by natural infection (Subbarao and Katz, 2004).

Live-attenuated influenza virus vaccine is well-tolerated, although it is associated with runny nose or sore throat in some individuals (Mendelman et al., 2001). Perhaps one of the greatest advantages of the live-attenuated vaccine is its ability to induce broader cross-protection against antigenically drifted strains, in addition to eliciting protection against homologous influenza strains (Belshe et al., 2000; Mendelman et al., 2004).

Pandemic vaccines

The development of vaccines against a newly emerged pandemic influenza strain is hampered by the considerable lag time that is required before an appropriate vaccine can be generated after the infections with the new strain begin, estimated to be at least 6 months (Kandel and Hartshorn, 2005). Reliance on the use of embryonated eggs for vaccine virus production is also a concern. In addition to the challenge of a limited egg supply, most of the virulent H5 and H7 subtypes are highly pathogenic in chickens and are thus lethal for chick embryos as well, so they often cannot be propagated efficiently in eggs. Due to their high pathogenicity, handling of the wild-type viruses requires a biosafety level-3 containment that also impacts the pace of vaccine development.

Several strategies have been explored in attempts to overcome these obstacles, mostly applied to the development of vaccines against the H5N1 virus. These include the use of a nonpathogenic isolate that is antigenically related to circulating strains (Nicholson et al., 2001), the use of baculovirus-expressed recombinant HA protein (Treanor et al., 2001), and the production of attenuated seed viruses with an H5 HA modified by means of reverse genetics (Subbarao et al., 2003; Webby et al., 2004). Most of the studies employing inactivated vaccines against H9N2 and H5 subtypes of avian influenza virus have found that these vaccines are poorly immunogenic and that two doses of vaccine will be required to immunize a naïve population. The use of adjuvants may enhance the immunogenicity of the vaccine (Nicholson et al., 2001; Treanor et al., 2001; Hehme et al., 2002; Stephenson et al., 2003a,b, 2005). It should be noted that natural or experimental infections with the H5N1 virus yield a poor hemagglutination inhibition antibody response, and the immunogenicity of the vaccines are evaluated using neutralization tests for H5-specific antibodies (Katz et al., 1999).

These observations highlight critical gaps in our current knowledge about avian influenza viruses. Further structural studies of the H5 HA protein need to be undertaken to help understand the biological basis for its poor immunogenicity. There is also a pressing need to identify the correlates of protection in avian influenza infections.

Live-attenuated vaccines against potential pandemic strains of influenza are also being actively developed, with the goal of determining whether vaccines that possess the HA and the NA gene segments of the wild-type (potentially pandemic) virus, placed in the A/Ann Arbor/6/60 ca backbone, will be safe and immunogenic in humans (Luke and Subbarao, 2006). The experience gained from this research can be used to direct vaccine development efforts in case that seed virus happens to be antigenically mismatched with the actual pandemic virus (Luke and Subbarao, 2006).

If the behavior of the 1918 pandemic is any indication, it will be difficult to predict which segment of the population will be most vulnerable to the next pandemic strain, making planning to target certain groups for vaccination a challenge (Luke and Subbarao, 2006). With a limited supply of vaccine generated during the early phase of a pandemic, one of the primary goals will center on stimulating a protective immune response in the target population using the least amount of antigen (Monto, 2006). To this end, alternative ways of improving the immunogenicity of vaccines should be explored such as varying the routes of vaccine administration, determining the efficacy of known and novel adjuvants, and evaluating the feasibility of pre-emptive vaccination with a vaccine of the same subtype even if it does not match the strain that eventually emerges as pandemic strain to prime the population for an antibody response to a novel HA (Subbarao et al., 2006a). The pandemic vaccine must be able to prevent mortality and severe morbidity, which will require the development of vaccines that elicit sufficient titers of systemic antibodies to limit virus replication in the lower respiratory tract and thereby to prevent pneumonia and its complications (Subbarao et al., 2006a).

To circumvent some of the difficulties associated with traditional vaccine production, alternative technologies are being investigated. One of these is to use adenovirus-based vaccines that do not need to be grown on embryonated eggs and can replicate to high titers in standard cell lines. Vaccines containing the full-length H5 HA of either A/HK/156/1997 (Hoelscher et al., 2006) or A/Vietnam/1203/2004 viruses (Gao et al., 2006), expressed in a replication-defective, recombinant human adenovirus vector, have been reported to be immunogenic in mice and protected mice from lethal challenge against homologous and heterologous H5N1 viruses.

These studies demonstrated that the vaccines induced broad cross-protection even in the absence of adjuvants.

Control of avian influenza in poultry

Methods to limit H5N1 virus infections in poultry, thereby minimizing the risk of transmission to humans, have included increased viral and disease surveillance, strict quarantine measures, and restriction of movement of animals and equipment used to care for them (Swayne, 2003). In developed countries, the disease is often controlled by killing potentially infected flocks, although the severe economic impact of this strategy precludes its use in developing countries may discourage. In many instances, vaccination of poultry is also included as a control measure; however, vaccination can result in restrictions on the marketing and importation of poultry and related products because it is difficult to differentiate vaccinated poultry from infected poultry (Capua et al., 2003). Methods are being developed to distinguish infected from vaccinated poultry, and this is making veterinary vaccination an attractive option (Halvorson, 2002).

A number of methods for differentiation of infected from vaccinated animals (DIVA) have been employed, with varying degrees of success (Suarez, 2005). These include the introduction of unvaccinated sentinels in vaccinated flocks to detect exposure to avian influenza; the use of recombinant virus-vectored subunit HA vaccines, after which vaccinated poultry will only have antibodies to HA and infected poultry will have antibodies to other viral proteins as well; the administration of an HA vaccine with a different NA subtype, so antibodies to NA will reveal whether a bird was infected or vaccinated (but protective antibodies directed against the HA will still be elicited by the vaccine), or the use of tests to detect anti-NS1 antibodies (which should only be detected in infected poultry).

Ideally, a vaccine for controlling HPAI in poultry must be able to reduce or prevent clinical disease, reduce or eliminate virus shedding to prevent its spread to uninfected poultry, and create sufficient immunity to raise the threshold of viral load required for infectivity (Suarez, 2005). The resulting reduction in the prevalence of influenza virus in the environment may also lower the likelihood of an epidemic arising from low pathogenic avian influenza H5 and H7 viruses (Capua et al., 2004). Inactivated oil emulsion vaccines and recombinant fowlpox virus vaccines expressing the H7 and H5 HAs have been widely used to control these infections in poultry. It appears that vaccination of poultry reduces infectiousness of infected chickens as well as the susceptibility of uninfected chickens (van der Goot et al., 2005). The efficacy of veterinary vaccination and its average cost of $0.025–0.05 prohibitively expansive for a poultry vaccine, suggest it may be a cost-effective alternative to the large-scale killing of poultry and will ultimately reduce human exposure to the virus as well. Concerns about the possible antigenic drift in avian influenza viruses driven by vaccination (Lee et al., 2004) can be monitored by intensified viral surveillance and periodic updating of the vaccine composition. Preparation for pandemic influenza will require a multi-pronged approach and vaccination of poultry against avian influenza appears to be an important component of such a program.

Acknowledgment

This work was supported in part by the Intramural Research Program of the NIH, NIAID.

References

Anonymous. Avian influenza virus A (H10N7) circulating among humans in Egypt. EID Wkly Updates: Emerging and Reemerging infections Diseases, Region of the Americas. 2004; 2 (18). http://www.paho.org/English/AD/DPC/CD/eid-eer-07-may-2004.htm#birdflu.

Apisarnthanarak A, Erb S, Stephenson I, Katz JM, Chittaganpitch M, Sangkitporn S, Kitphati R, Thawatsupha P, Waicharoen S, Pinitchai U, Apisarnthanarak P, Fraser VJ, Mundy LM. Seroprevalence of anti-H5 antibody among Thai health care workers after exposure to avian influenza (H5N1) in a tertiary care center. Clin Infect Dis 2005; 40: e16–e18.

Banks J, Plowright L. Additional glycosylation at the receptor binding site of the hemagglutinin (HA) for H5 and H7 viruses may be an adaptation to poultry hosts, but does it influence pathogenicity? Avian Dis 2003; 47: 942–950.

Beare AS, Webster RG. Replication of avian influenza viruses in humans. Arch Virol 1991; 119: 37–42.

Beigel JH, Farrar J, Han AM, Hayden FG, Hyer R, de Jong MD, Lochindarat S, Nguyen TK, Nguyen TH, Tran TH, Nicoll A, Touch S, Yuen KY. Avian influenza A (H5N1) infection in humans. N Engl J Med 2005; 353: 1374–1385.

Belshe RB, Gruber WC, Mendelman PM, Cho I, Reisinger K, Block SL, Wittes J, Iacuzio D, Piedra P, Treanor J, King J, Kotloff K, Bernstein DI, Hayden FG, Zangwill K, Yan L, Wolff M. Efficacy of vaccination with live attenuated, cold-adapted, trivalent, intranasal influenza virus vaccine against a variant (A/Sydney) not contained in the vaccine. J Pediatr 2000; 136: 168–175.

Belshe RB, Nichol KL, Black SB, Shinefield H, Cordova J, Walker R, Hessel C, Cho I, Mendelman PM. Safety, efficacy, and effectiveness of live, attenuated, cold-adapted influenza vaccine in an indicated population aged 5–49 years. Clin Infect Dis 2004; 39: 920–927.

Belshe RB, Smith MH, Hall CB, Betts R, Hay AJ. Genetic basis of resistance to rimantadine emerging during treatment of influenza virus infection. J Virol 1988; 62: 1508–1512.

Black RA, Rota PA, Gorodkova N, Klenk HD, Kendal AP. Antibody response to the M2 protein of influenza A virus expressed in insect cells. J Gen Virol 1993; 74(Pt 1): 143–146.

Bosch FX, Garten W, Klenk HD, Rott R. Proteolytic cleavage of influenza virus hemagglutinins: primary structure of the connecting peptide between HA1 and HA2 determines proteolytic cleavability and pathogenicity of avian influenza viruses. Virology 1981; 113: 725–735.

Bosch FX, Orlich M, Klenk HD, Rott R. The structure of the hemagglutinin, a determinant for the pathogenicity of influenza viruses. Virology 1979; 95: 197–207.

Bridges CB, Lim W, Hu-Primmer J, Sims L, Fukuda K, Mak KH, Rowe T, Thompson WW, Conn L, Lu X, Cox NJ, Katz JM. Risk of influenza A (H5N1) infection among poultry workers, Hong Kong, 1997–1998. J Infect Dis 2002; 185: 1005–1010.

Bush RM, Bender CA, Subbarao K, Cox NJ, Fitch WM. Predicting the evolution of human influenza A. Science 1999; 286: 1921–1925.

Butt KM, Smith GJ, Chen H, Zhang LJ, Leung YH, Xu KM, Lim W, Webster RG, Yuen KY, Peiris JS, Guan Y. Human infection with an avian H9N2 influenza A virus in Hong Kong in 2003. J Clin Microbiol 2005; 43: 5760–5767.

Buxton Bridges C, Katz JM, Seto WH, Chan PK, Tsang D, Ho W, Mak KH, Lim W, Tam JS, Clarke M, Williams SG, Mounts AW, Bresee JS, Conn LA, Rowe T, Hu-Primmer J, Abernathy RA, Lu X, Cox NJ, Fukuda K. Risk of influenza A (H5N1) infection among health care workers exposed to patients with influenza A (H5N1), Hong Kong. J Infect Dis 2000; 181: 344–348.

Capua I, Cattoli G, Marangon S. DIVA—a vaccination strategy enabling the detection of field exposure to avian influenza. Dev Biol (Basel) 2004; 119: 229–233.

Capua I, Terregino C, Cattoli G, Mutinelli F, Rodriguez JF. Development of a DIVA (differentiating infected from vaccinated animals) strategy using a vaccine containing a heterologous neuraminidase for the control of avian influenza. Avian Pathol 2003; 32: 47–55.

Castrucci MR, Kawaoka Y. Biologic importance of neuraminidase stalk length in influenza A virus. J Virol 1993; 67: 759–764.

Chan PK. Outbreak of avian influenza A (H5N1) virus infection in Hong Kong in 1997. Clin Infect Dis 2002; 34(Suppl 2): S58–S64.

Chen H, Smith GJ, Li KS, Wang J, Fan XH, Rayner JM, Vijaykrishna D, Zhang JX, Zhang LJ, Guo CT, Cheung CL, Xu KM, Duan L, Huang K, Qin K, Leung YH, Wu WL, Lu HR, Chen Y, Xia NS, Naipospos TS, Yuen KY, Hassan SS, Bahri S, Nguyen TD, Webster RG, Peiris JS, Guan Y. Establishment of multiple sublineages of H5N1 influenza virus in Asia: implications for pandemic control. Proc Natl Acad Sci USA 2006a; 103: 2845–2850.

Chen H, Smith GJ, Zhang SY, Qin K, Wang J, Li KS, Webster RG, Peiris JS, Guan Y. Avian flu: H5N1 virus outbreak in migratory waterfowl. Nature 2005; 436: 191–192.

Chen W, Calvo PA, Malide D, Gibbs J, Schubert U, Bacik I, Basta S, O'Neill R, Schickli J, Palese P, Henklein P, Bennink JR, Yewdell JW. A novel influenza A virus mitochondrial protein that induces cell death. Nat Med 2001; 7: 1306–1312.

Chen Z, Aspelund A, Kemble G, Jin H. Genetic mapping of the cold-adapted phenotype of B/Ann Arbor/1/66, the master donor virus for live attenuated influenza vaccines (FluMist). Virology 2006b; 345: 416–423.

Chin PS, Hoffmann E, Webby R, Webster RG, Guan Y, Peiris M, Shortridge KF. Molecular evolution of H6 influenza viruses from poultry in southeastern China: prevalence of H6N1 influenza viruses possessing seven A/Hong Kong/156/97 (H5N1)-like genes in poultry. J Virol 2002; 76: 507–516.

Chotpitayasunondh T, Ungchusak K, Hanshaoworakul W, Chunsuthiwat S, Sawanpanyalert P, Kijphati R, Lochindarat S, Srisan P, Suwan P, Osotthanakorn Y, Anantasetagoon T, Kanjanawasri S, Tanupattarachai S, Weerakul J, Chaiwirattana R, Maneerattanaporn M, Poolsavathitikool R, Chokephaibulkit K, Apisarnthanarak A, Dowell SF. Human disease from influenza A (H5N1), Thailand, 2004. Emerg Infect Dis 2005; 11: 201–209.

Claas EC, Osterhaus AD, van Beek R, De Jong JC, Rimmelzwaan GF, Senne DA, Krauss S, Shortridge KF, Webster RG. Human influenza A H5N1 virus related to a highly pathogenic avian influenza virus. Lancet 1998; 351: 472–477.

Connor RJ, Kawaoka Y, Webster RG, Paulson JC. Receptor specificity in human, avian, and equine H2 and H3 influenza virus isolates. Virology 1994; 205: 17–23.

Couceiro JN, Paulson JC, Baum LG. Influenza virus strains selectively recognize sialyloligosaccharides on human respiratory epithelium; the role of the host cell in selection of hemagglutinin receptor specificity. Virus Res 1993; 29: 155–165.

Cox NJ, Brammer TL, Regnery HL. Influenza: global surveillance for epidemic and pandemic variants. Eur J Epidemiol 1994; 10: 467–470.

Cox NJ, Subbarao K. Influenza. Lancet 1999; 354: 1277–1282.

de Jong MD, Bach VC, Phan TQ, Vo MH, Tran TT, Nguyen BH, Beld M, Le TP, Truong HK, Nguyen VV, Tran TH, Do QH, Farrar J. Fatal avian influenza A (H5N1) in a child presenting with diarrhea followed by coma. N Engl J Med 2005; 352: 686–691.

De Jong MD, Tran TT, Truong HK, Vo MH, Smith GJ, Nguyen VC, Bach VC, Phan TQ, Do QH, Guan Y, Peireis JS, Tran TH, Farrar J. Oseltamivir resistance during treatment of influenza A (H5N1) infection. N Engl J Med 2005; 353: 2667–2672.

de Jong MD, Hien TT. Avian influenza A (H5N1). J Clin Virol 2006; 35: 2–13.

Du Ry van Beest Hoell M, Meijer A, Koopmans M, de Jager C. Human-to-human transmission of avain influenza A/H7N7. The Netherlands, 2003. Euro Survie l 2005; 10: 264–268.

Englund JA. Antiviral therapy of influenza. Semin Pediatr Infect Dis 2002; 13: 120–128.

Englund L, Hard af Segerstad C. Two avian H10 influenza A virus strains with different pathogenicity for mink (Mustela vison). Arch Virol 1998; 143: 653–666.

Fouchier RA, Munster V, Wallensten A, Bestebroer TM, Herfst S, Smith D, Rimmelzwaan GF, Olsen B, Osterhaus AD. Characterization of a novel influenza A virus hemagglutinin subtype (H16) obtained from black-headed gulls. J Virol 2005; 79: 2814–2822.

Fouchier RA, Schneeberger PM, Rozendaal FW, Broekman JM, Kemink SA, Munster V, Kuiken T, Rimmelzwaan GF, Schutten M, Van Doornum GJ, Koch G, Bosman A, Koopmans M, Osterhaus AD. Avian influenza A virus (H7N7) associated with human conjunctivitis and a fatal case of acute respiratory distress syndrome. Proc Natl Acad Sci USA 2004; 101: 1356–1361.

Gambaryan AS, Robertson JS, Matrosovich MN. Effects of egg-adaptation on the receptor-binding properties of human influenza A and B viruses. Virology 1999; 258: 232–239.

Gao P, Watanabe S, Ito T, Goto H, Wells K, McGregor M, Cooley AJ, Kawaoka Y. Biological heterogeneity, including systemic replication in mice, of H5N1 influenza A virus isolates from humans in Hong Kong. J Virol 1999; 73: 3184–3189.

Gao W, Soloff AC, Lu X, Montecalvo A, Nguyen DC, Matsuoka Y, Robbins PD, Swayne DE, Donis RO, Katz JM, Barratt-Boyes SM, Gambotto A. Protection of mice and poultry from lethal H5N1 avian influenza virus through adenovirus-based immunization. J Virol 2006; 80: 1959–1964.

Garcia-Sastre A, Egorov A, Matassov D, Brandt S, Levy DE, Durbin JE, Palese P, Muster T. Influenza A virus lacking the NS1 gene replicates in interferon-deficient systems. Virology 1998; 252: 324–330.

Glaser L, Stevens J, Zamarin D, Wilson IA, Garcia-Sastre A, Tumpey TM, Basler CF, Taubenberger JK, Palese P. A single amino acid substitution in 1918 influenza virus hemagglutinin changes receptor binding specificity. J Virol 2005; 79: 11533–11536.

Glezen WP. Emerging infections: pandemic influenza. Epidemiol Rev 1996; 18: 64–76.

Goto H, Kawaoka Y. A novel mechanism for the acquisition of virulence by a human influenza A virus. Proc Natl Acad Sci USA 1998; 95: 10224–10228.

Govorkova EA, Rehg JE, Krauss S, Yen HL, Guan Y, Peiris M, Nguyen TD, Hanh TH, Puthavathana P, Long HT, Buranathai C, Lim W, Webster RG, Hoffmann E. Lethality to ferrets of H5N1 influenza viruses isolated from humans and poultry in 2004. J Virol 2005; 79: 2191–2198.

Gregory V, Bennett M, Orkhan MH, Al Hajjar S, Varsano N, Mendelson E, Zambon M, Ellis J, Hay A, Lin YP. Emergence of influenza A H1N2 reassortant viruses in the human population during 2001. Virology 2002; 300: 1–7.

Guan Y, Peiris JS, Lipatov AS, Ellis TM, Dyrting KC, Krauss S, Zhang LJ, Webster RG, Shortridge KF. Emergence of multiple genotypes of H5N1 avian influenza viruses in Hong Kong SAR. Proc Natl Acad Sci USA 2002; 99: 8950–8955.

Guan Y, Poon LL, Cheung CY, Ellis TM, Lim W, Lipatov AS, Chan KH, Sturm-Ramirez KM, Cheung CL, Leung YH, Yuen KY, Webster RG, Peiris JS. H5N1 influenza: a protean pandemic threat. Proc Natl Acad Sci USA 2004; 101: 8156–8161.

Guan Y, Shortridge KF, Krauss S, Chin PS, Dyrting KC, Ellis TM, Webster RG, Peiris M. H9N2 influenza viruses possessing H5N1-like internal genomes continue to circulate in poultry in southeastern China. J Virol 2000; 74: 9372–9380.

Guan Y, Shortridge KF, Krauss S, Webster RG. Molecular characterization of H9N2 influenza viruses: were they the donors of the "internal" genes of H5N1 viruses in Hong Kong? Proc Natl Acad Sci USA 1999; 96: 9363–9367.

Gubareva LV, Kaiser L, Matrosovich MN, Soo-Hoo Y, Hayden FG. Selection of influenza virus mutants in experimentally infected volunteers treated with oseltamivir. J Infect Dis 2001; 183: 523–531.

Gubareva LV, McCullers JA, Bethell RC, Webster RG. Characterization of influenza A/HongKong/156/97 (H5N1) virus in a mouse model and protective effect of zanamivir on H5N1 infection in mice. J Infect Dis 1998; 178: 1592–1596.

Guo Y, Li J, Cheng X. [Discovery of men infected by avian influenza A (H9N2) virus]. Zhonghua Shi Yan He Lin Chuang Bing Du Xue Za Zhi 1999; 13: 105–108.

Halvorson DA. The control of H5 or H7 mildly pathogenic avian influenza: a role for inactivated vaccine. Avian Pathol 2002; 31: 5–12.

Hatchette TF, Walker D, Johnson C, Baker A, Pryor SP, Webster RG. Influenza A viruses in feral Canadian ducks: extensive reassortment in nature. J Gen Virol 2004; 85: 2327–2337.

Hatta M, Gao P, Halfmann P, Kawaoka Y. Molecular basis for high virulence of Hong Kong H5N1 influenza A viruses. Science 2001; 293: 1840–1842.

Hayden FG, Atmar RL, Schilling M, Johnson C, Poretz D, Paar D, Huson L, Ward P, Mills RG. Use of the selective oral neuraminidase inhibitor oseltamivir to prevent influenza. N Engl J Med 1999; 341: 1336–1343.

Hayden FG, Belshe RB, Clover RD, Hay AJ, Oakes MG, Soo W. Emergence and apparent transmission of rimantadine-resistant influenza A virus in families. N Engl J Med 1989; 321: 1696–1702.

Hayden FG, Hay AJ. Emergence and transmission of influenza A viruses resistant to amantadine and rimantadine. Curr Top Microbiol Immunol 1992; 176: 119–130.

Hayden FG, Osterhaus AD, Treanor JJ, Fleming DM, Aoki FY, Nicholson KG, Bohnen AM, Hirst HM, Keene O, Wightman K. Efficacy and safety of the neuraminidase inhibitor zanamivir in the treatment of influenza virus infections. GG167 Influenza Study Group. N Engl J Med 1997; 337: 874–880.

Hehme N, Engelmann H, Kunzel W, Neumeier E, Sanger R. Pandemic preparedness: lessons learnt from H2N2 and H9N2 candidate vaccines. Med Microbiol Immunol (Berl) 2002; 191: 203–208.

Herlocher ML, Clavo AC, Maassab HF. Sequence comparisons of A/AA/6/60 influenza viruses: mutations which may contribute to attenuation. Virus Res 1996; 42: 11–25.

Hien TT, de Jong M, Farrar J. Avian influenza—a challenge to global health care structures. N Engl J Med 2004; 351: 2363–2365.

Hinshaw VS, Webster RG, Naeve CW, Murphy BR. Altered tissue tropism of human-avian reassortant influenza viruses. Virology 1983; 128: 260–263.

Hoelscher MA, Garg S, Bangari DS, Belser JA, Lu X, Stephenson I, Bright RA, Katz JM, Mittal SK, Sambhara S. Development of adenoviral-vector-based pandemic influenza vaccine against antigenically distinct human H5N1 strains in mice. Lancet 2006; 367: 475–481.

Hoffmann E, Stech J, Leneva I, Krauss S, Scholtissek C, Chin PS, Peiris M, Shortridge KF, Webster RG. Characterization of the influenza A virus gene pool in avian species in southern China: was H6N1 a derivative or a precursor of H5N1? J Virol 2000; 74: 6309–6315.

Hulse-Post DJ, Sturm-Ramirez KM, Humberd J, Seiler P, Govorkova EA, Krauss S, Scholtissek C, Puthavathana P, Buranathai C, Nguyen TD, Long HT, Naipospos TS, Chen H, Ellis TM, Guan Y, Peiris JS, Webster RG. Role of domestic ducks in the propagation and biological evolution of highly pathogenic H5N1 influenza viruses in Asia. Proc Natl Acad Sci USA 2005; 102: 10682–10687.

Ito T, Couceiro JN, Kelm S, Baum LG, Krauss S, Castrucci MR, Donatelli I, Kida H, Paulson JC, Webster RG, Kawaoka Y. Molecular basis for the generation in pigs of influenza A viruses with pandemic potential. J Virol 1998; 72: 7367–7373.

Ito T, Suzuki Y, Mitnaul L, Vines A, Kida H, Kawaoka Y. Receptor specificity of influenza A viruses correlates with the agglutination of erythrocytes from different animal species. Virology 1997a; 227: 493–499.

Ito T, Suzuki Y, Takada A, Kawamoto A, Otsuki K, Masuda H, Yamada M, Suzuki T, Kida H, Kawaoka Y. Differences in sialic acid-galactose linkages in the chicken egg amnion and allantois influence human influenza virus receptor specificity and variant selection. J Virol 1997b; 71: 3357–3362.

Ito T, Kawaoka Y. Avian influenza. In: Textbook of Influenza (Nicholson KG, Webster RG, Hay RG, editors). Oxford, UK: Blackwell Science; 1998; pp. 126–136.

Jefferson T, Demicheli V, Rivetti D, Jones M, Di Pietrantonj C, Rivetti A. Antivirals for influenza in healthy adults: systematic review. Lancet 2006; 367: 303–313.

Jin H, Lu B, Zhou H, Ma C, Zhao J, Yang CF, Kemble G, Greenberg H. Multiple amino acid residues confer temperature sensitivity to human influenza virus vaccine strains (FluMist) derived from cold-adapted A/Ann Arbor/6/60. Virology 2003; 306: 18–24.

Johnson NP, Mueller J. Updating the accounts: global mortality of the 1918–1920 "Spanish" influenza pandemic. Bull Hist Med 2002; 76: 105–115.

Kandel R, Hartshorn KL. Novel strategies for prevention and treatment of influenza. Expert Opin Ther Targets 2005; 9: 1–22.

Karunakaran D, Hinshaw V, Poss P, Newman J, Halvorson D. Influenza A outbreaks in Minnesota turkeys due to subtype H10N7 and possible transmission by waterfowl. Avian Dis 1983; 27: 357–366.

Katz JM, Lim W, Bridges CB, Rowe T, Hu-Primmer J, Lu X, Abernathy RA, Clarke M, Conn L, Kwong H, Lee M, Au G, Ho YY, Mak KH, Cox NJ, Fukuda K. Antibody response in individuals infected with avian influenza A (H5N1) viruses and detection of anti-H5 antibody among household and social contacts. J Infect Dis 1999; 180: 1763–1770.

Kawaoka Y, Krauss S, Webster RG. Avian-to-human transmission of the PB1 gene of influenza A viruses in the 1957 and 1968 pandemics. J Virol 1989; 63: 4603–4608.

Kawaoka Y, Naeve CW, Webster RG. Is virulence of H5N2 influenza viruses in chickens associated with loss of carbohydrate from the hemagglutinin? Virology 1984; 139: 303–316.

Keawcharoen J, Oraveerakul K, Kuiken T, Fouchier RA, Amonsin A, Payungporn S, Noppornpanth S, Wattanodorn S, Theambooniers A, Tantilertcharoen R, Pattanarangsan R, Arya N, Ratanakorn P, Osterhaus DM, Poovorawan Y. Avian influenza H5N1 in tigers and leopards. Emerg Infect Dis 2004; 10: 2189–2191.

Keyser LA, Karl M, Nafziger AN, Bertino Jr. JS. Comparison of central nervous system adverse effects of amantadine and rimantadine used as sequential prophylaxis of influenza A in elderly nursing home patients. Arch Intern Med 2000; 160: 1485–1488.

Kida H, Ito T, Yasuda J, Shimizu Y, Itakura C, Shortridge KF, Kawaoka Y, Webster RG. Potential for transmission of avian influenza viruses to pigs. J Gen Virol 1994; 75(Pt 9): 2183–2188.

Kida H, Yanagawa R, Matsuoka Y. Duck influenza lacking evidence of disease signs and immune response. Infect Immun 1980; 30: 547–553.

Kobasa D, Takada A, Shinya K, Hatta M, Halfmann P, Theriault S, Suzuki H, Nishimura H, Mitamura K, Sugaya N, Usui T, Murata T, Maeda Y, Watanabe S, Suresh M, Suzuki T, Suzuki Y, Feldmann H, Kawaoka Y. Enhanced virulence of influenza A viruses with the haemagglutinin of the 1918 pandemic virus. Nature 2004; 431: 703–707.

Koopmans M, Wilbrink B, Conyn M, Natrop G, van der Nat H, Vennema H, Meijer A, van Steenbergen J, Fouchier R, Osterhaus A, Bosman A. Transmission of H7N7 avian influenza A virus to human beings during a large outbreak in commercial poultry farms in the Netherlands. Lancet 2004; 363: 587–593.

Kuiken T, Rimmelzwaan G, van Riel D, van Amerongen G, Baars M, Fouchier R, Osterhaus A. Avian H5N1 influenza in cats. Science 2004; 306: 241.

Kung HC, Jen KF, Yuan WC, Tien SF, Chu CM. Influenza in China in 1977: recurrence of influenza virus A subtype H1N1. Bull World Health Organ 1978; 56: 913–918.

Kurtz J, Manvell RJ, Banks J. Avian influenza virus isolated from a woman with conjunctivitis. Lancet 1996; 348: 901–902.

Kuszewski K, Brydak L. The epidemiology and history of influenza. Biomed Pharmacother 2000; 54: 188–195.

Lamb RA, Krug RM. *Orthomyxoviridae*: The Viruses and Their Replication. In: Fields Virology, 4th edition (Knipe DM, Howley PM, Griffin DT, Lamb RA, Martin MA, Roizman B, Straus SE, editors). Philadelphia, PA: Lippincott, Williams & Wilkins; 2001; pp. 1487–1531.

Langford C. The age pattern of mortality in the 1918–19 influenza pandemic: an attempted explanation based on data for England and Wales. Med Hist 2002; 46: 1–20.

Le QM, Kiso M, Someya K, Sakai YT, Nguyen KH, Pham ND, Nguyen HH, Yamada S, Muramoto Y, Horimoto T, Takada A, Goto H. Avian flu: isolation of drug-resistant H5N1 virus. Nature 2005; 437: 1108.

Lee CW, Senne DA, Suarez DL. Effect of vaccine use in the evolution of Mexican lineage H5N2 avian influenza virus. J Virol 2004; 78: 8372–8381.

Leneva IA, Goloubeva O, Fenton RJ, Tisdale M, Webster RG. Efficacy of zanamivir against avian influenza A viruses that possess genes encoding H5N1 internal proteins and are pathogenic in mammals. Antimicrob Agents Chemother 2001; 45: 1216–1224.

Li KS, Guan Y, Wang J, Smith GJ, Xu KM, Duan L, Rahardjo AP, Puthavathana P, Buranathai C, Nguyen TD, Estoepangestie AT, Chaisingh A, Auewarakul P, Long HT, Hanh NT, Webby RJ, Poon LL, Chen H, Shortridge KF, Yuen KY, Webster RG, Peiris JS. Genesis of a highly pathogenic and potentially pandemic H5N1 influenza virus in eastern Asia. Nature 2004; 430: 209–213.

Li KS, Xu KM, Peiris JS, Poon LL, Yu KZ, Yuen KY, Shortridge KF, Webster RG, Guan Y. Characterization of H9 subtype influenza viruses from the ducks of southern China: a candidate for the next influenza pandemic in humans? J Virol 2003; 77: 6988–6994.

Liem NT, Lim W. Lack of H5N1 avian influenza transmission to hospital employees, Hanoi, 2004. Emerg Infect Dis 2005; 11: 210–215.

Lin YP, Shaw M, Gregory V, Cameron K, Lim W, Klimov A, Subbarao K, Guan Y, Krauss S, Shortridge K, Webster R, Cox N, Hay A. Avian-to-human transmission of H9N2 subtype influenza A viruses: relationship between H9N2 and H5N1 human isolates. Proc Natl Acad Sci USA 2000; 97: 9654–9658.

Lipatov AS, Govorkova EA, Webby RJ, Ozaki H, Peiris M, Guan Y, Poon L, Webster RG. Influenza: emergence and control. J Virol 2004; 78: 8951–8959.

Lipatov AS, Krauss S, Guan Y, Peiris M, Rehg JE, Perez DR, Webster RG. Neurovirulence in mice of H5N1 influenza virus genotypes isolated from Hong Kong poultry in 2001. J Virol 2003; 77: 3816–3823.

Longini Jr. IM, Halloran ME, Nizam A, Yang Y. Containing pandemic influenza with antiviral agents. Am J Epidemiol 2004; 159: 623–633.

Lu X, Tumpey TM, Morken T, Zaki SR, Cox NJ, Katz JM. A mouse model for the evaluation of pathogenesis and immunity to influenza A (H5N1) viruses isolated from humans. J Virol 1999; 73: 5903–5911.

Luk J, Gross P, Thompson WW. Observations on mortality during the 1918 influenza pandemic. Clin Infect Dis 2001; 33: 1375–1378.

Luke CJ, Subbarao K. Vaccines for pandemic influenza. Emerg Infect Dis 2006; 12: 66–72.

Maines TR, Lu XH, Erb SM, Edwards L, Guarner J, Greer PW, Nguyen DC, Szretter KJ, Chen LM, Thawatsupha P, Chittaganpitch M, Waicharoen S, Nguyen DT, Nguyen T, Nguyen HH, Kim JH, Hoang LT, Kang C, Phuong LS, Lim W, Zaki S, Donis RO, Cox NJ, Katz JM, Tumpey TM. Avian influenza (H5N1) viruses isolated from humans in Asia in 2004 exhibit increased virulence in mammals. J Virol 2005; 79: 11788–11800.

Makarova NV, Kaverin NV, Krauss S, Senne D, Webster RG. Transmission of Eurasian avian H2 influenza virus to shorebirds in North America. J Gen Virol 1999; 80(Pt 12): 3167–3171.

Matrosovich M, Tuzikov A, Bovin N, Gambaryan A, Klimov A, Castrucci MR, Donatelli I, Kawaoka Y. Early alterations of the receptor-binding properties of H1, H2, and H3 avian influenza virus hemagglutinins after their introduction into mammals. J Virol 2000; 74: 8502–8512.

Matrosovich M, Zhou N, Kawaoka Y, Webster R. The surface glycoproteins of H5 influenza viruses isolated from humans, chickens, and wild aquatic birds have distinguishable properties. J Virol 1999; 73: 1146–1155.

Matrosovich MN, Krauss S, Webster RG. H9N2 influenza A viruses from poultry in Asia have human virus-like receptor specificity. Virology 2001; 281: 156–162.

Meltzer MI, Cox NJ, Fukuda K. The economic impact of pandemic influenza in the United States: priorities for intervention. Emerg Infect Dis 1999; 5: 659–671.

Mendelman PM, Cordova J, Cho I. Safety, efficacy and effectiveness of the influenza virus vaccine, trivalent, types A and B, live, cold-adapted (CAIV-T) in healthy children and healthy adults. Vaccine 2001; 19: 2221–2226.

Mendelman PM, Rappaport R, Cho I, Block S, Gruber W, August M, Dawson D, Cordova J, Kemble G, Mahmood K, Palladino G, Lee MS, Razmpour A, Stoddard J, Forrest BD. Live attenuated influenza vaccine induces cross-reactive antibody responses in children against an a/Fujian/411/2002-like H3N2 antigenic variant strain. Pediatr Infect Dis J 2004; 23: 1053–1055.

Molla A, Kati W, Carrick R, Steffy K, Shi Y, Montgomery D, Gusick N, Stoll VS, Stewart KD, Ng TI, Maring C, Kempf DJ, Kohlbrenner W. *In vitro* selection and characterization of influenza A (A/N9) virus variants resistant to a novel neuraminidase inhibitor, A-315675. J Virol 2002; 76: 5380–5386.

Monto AS. Vaccines and antiviral drugs in pandemic preparedness. Emerg Infect Dis 2006; 12: 55–60.

Monto AS, Robinson DP, Herlocher ML, Hinson Jr. JM, Elliott MJ, Crisp A. Zanamivir in the prevention of influenza among healthy adults: a randomized controlled trial. JAMA 1999; 282: 31–35.

Moscona A. Oseltamivir-resistant influenza? Lancet 2004; 364: 733–734.

Moscona A. Neuraminidase inhibitors for influenza. N Engl J Med 2005; 353: 1363–1373.

Murphy BR, Clements ML. The systemic and mucosal immune response of humans to influenza A virus. Curr Top Microbiol Immunol 1989; 146: 107–116.

Murphy BR, Coelingh K. Principles underlying the development and use of live attenuated cold-adapted influenza A and B virus vaccines. Viral Immunol 2002; 15: 295–323.

Murphy BR, Kasel JA, Chanock RM. Association of serum anti-neuraminidase antibody with resistance to influenza in man. N Engl J Med 1972; 286: 1329–1332.

Murphy BR, Sly DL, Tierney EL, Hosier NT, Massicot JG, London WT, Chanock RM, Webster RG, Hinshaw VS. Reassortant virus derived from avian and human influenza A viruses is attenuated and immunogenic in monkeys. Science 1982; 218: 1330–1332.

Nakajima K, Desselberger U, Palese P. Recent human influenza A (H1N1) viruses are closely related genetically to strains isolated in 1950. Nature 1978; 274: 334–339.

Nicholson KG, Colegate AE, Podda A, Stephenson I, Wood J, Ypma E, Zambon MC. Safety and antigenicity of non-adjuvanted and MF59-adjuvanted influenza A/Duck/Singapore/97 (H5N3) vaccine: a randomised trial of two potential vaccines against H5N1 influenza. Lancet 2001; 357: 1937–1943.

OIE. Update on Avian Influenza in Animals (Type H5). 2006. http://www.oie.int/downld/avian%20influenza/AA1-Asia-htm.

O'Neill RE, Talon J, Palese P. The influenza virus NEP (NS2 protein) mediates the nuclear export of viral ribonucleoproteins. Embo J 1998; 17: 288–296.

Panigrahy B, Senne DA, Pedersen JC. Avian influenza virus subtypes inside and outside the live bird markets, 1993–2000: a spatial and temporal relationship. Avian Dis 2002; 46: 298–307.

Parrish CR, Kawaoka Y. The origins of new pandemic viruses: the acquisition of new host ranges by canine parvovirus and influenza A viruses. Annu Rev Microbiol 2005; 59: 553–586.

Peiris JS, Guan Y, Markwell D, Ghose P, Webster RG, Shortridge KF. Cocirculation of avian H9N2 and contemporary "human" H3N2 influenza A viruses in pigs in south-eastern China: potential for genetic reassortment? J Virol 2001; 75: 9679–9686.

Peiris JS, Yu WC, Leung CW, Cheung CY, Ng WF, Nicholls JM, Ng TK, Chan KH, Lai ST, Lim WL, Yuen KY, Guan Y. Re-emergence of fatal human influenza A subtype H5N1 disease. Lancet 2004; 363: 617–619.

Peiris M, Yuen KY, Leung CW, Chan KH, Ip PL, Lai RW, Orr WK, Shortridge KF. Human infection with influenza H9N2. Lancet 1999; 354: 916–917.

Perdue ML, Latimer J, Greene C, Holt P. Consistent occurrence of hemagglutinin variants among avian influenza virus isolates of the H7 subtype. Virus Res 1994; 34: 15–29.

Perdue ML, Latimer JW, Crawford JM. A novel carbohydrate addition site on the hemagglutinin protein of a highly pathogenic H7 subtype avian influenza virus. Virology 1995; 213: 276–281.

Perdue ML, Suarez DL. Structural features of the avian influenza virus hemagglutinin that influence virulence. Vet Microbiol 2000; 74: 77–86.

Perez DR, Lim W, Seiler JP, Yi G, Peiris M, Shortridge KF, Webster RG. Role of quail in the interspecies transmission of H9 influenza A viruses: molecular changes on HA that correspond to adaptation from ducks to chickens. J Virol 2003; 77: 3148–3156.

Puthavathana P, Auewarakul P, Charoenying PC, Sangsiriwut K, Pooruk P, Boonnak K, Khanyok R, Thawachsupa P, Kijphati R, Sawanpanyalert P. Molecular characterization of the complete genome of human influenza H5N1 virus isolates from Thailand. J Gen Virol 2005; 86: 423–433.

Puzelli S, Di Trani L, Fabiani C, Campitelli L, De Marco MA, Capua I, Aguilera JF, Zambon M, Donatelli I. Serological analysis of serum samples from humans exposed to avian H7 influenza viruses in Italy between 1999 and 2003. J Infect Dis 2005; 192: 1318–1322.

Reid AH, Fanning TG, Hultin JV, Taubenberger JK. Origin and evolution of the 1918 "Spanish" influenza virus hemagglutinin gene. Proc Natl Acad Sci USA 1999; 96: 1651–1656.

Reid AH, Taubenberger JK. The origin of the 1918 pandemic influenza virus: a continuing enigma. J Gen Virol 2003; 84: 2285–2292.

Reid AH, Taubenberger JK, Fanning TG. The 1918 Spanish influenza: integrating history and biology. Microbes Infect 2001; 3: 81–87.

Rogers GN, D'Souza BL. Receptor binding properties of human and animal H1 influenza virus isolates. Virology 1989; 173: 317–322.

Rogers GN, Paulson JC, Daniels RS, Skehel JJ, Wilson IA, Wiley DC. Single amino acid substitutions in influenza haemagglutinin change receptor binding specificity. Nature 1983; 304: 76–78.

Rota PA, Wallis TR, Harmon MW, Rota JS, Kendal AP, Nerome K. Cocirculation of two distinct evolutionary lineages of influenza type B virus since 1983. Virology 1990; 175: 59–68.

Rott R, Orlich M, Scholtissek C. Correlation of pathogenicity and gene constellation of influenza A viruses. III. Non-pathogenic recombinants derived from highly pathogenic parent strains. J Gen Virol 1979; 44: 471–477.

Russell CJ, Webster RG. The genesis of a pandemic influenza virus. Cell 2005; 123: 368–371.

Scholtissek C. Pigs as the "mixing vessel" for the creation of new pandemic influenza A viruses. Med Princ Pract 1990; 2: 65–71.

Scholtissek C, Rohde W, Von Hoyningen V, Rott R. On the origin of the human influenza virus subtypes H2N2 and H3N2. Virology 1978a; 87: 13–20.

Scholtissek C, Vallbracht A, Flehmig B, Rott R. Correlation of pathogenicity and gene constellation of influenza A viruses. II. Highly neurovirulent recombinants derived from non-neurovirulent or weakly neurovirulent parent virus strains. Virology 1979; 95: 492–500.

Scholtissek C, von Hoyningen V, Rott R. Genetic relatedness between the new 1977 epidemic strains (H1N1) of influenza and human influenza strains isolated between 1947 and 1957 (H1N1). Virology 1978b; 89: 613–617.

Senne DA, Panigrahy B, Kawaoka Y, Pearson JE, Suss J, Lipkind M, Kida H, Webster RG. Survey of the hemagglutinin (HA) cleavage site sequence of H5 and H7 avian influenza viruses: amino acid sequence at the HA cleavage site as a marker of pathogenicity potential. Avian Dis 1996; 40: 425–437.

Seo SH, Hoffmann E, Webster RG. Lethal H5N1 influenza viruses escape host anti-viral cytokine responses. Nat Med 2002; 8: 950–954.

Sharp GB, Kawaoka Y, Jones DJ, Bean WJ, Pryor SP, Hinshaw V, Webster RG. Coinfection of wild ducks by influenza A viruses: distribution patterns and biological significance. J Virol 1997; 71: 6128–6135.

Shaw MW, Xu X, Li Y, Normand S, Ueki RT, Kunimoto GY, Hall H, Klimov A, Cox NJ, Subbarao K. Reappearance and global spread of variants of influenza B/Victoria/2/87 lineage viruses in the 2000–2001 and 2001–2002 seasons. Virology 2002; 303: 1–8.

Shek LP, Lee BW. Epidemiology and seasonality of respiratory tract virus infections in the tropics. Paediatr Respir Rev 2003; 4: 105–111.

Shinya K, Ebina M, Yamada S, Ono M, Kasai N, Kawaoka Y. Avian flu: influenza virus receptors in the human airway. Nature 2006; 440: 435–436.

Shortridge KF. Poultry and the influenza H5N1 outbreak in Hong Kong, 1997: abridged chronology and virus isolation. Vaccine 1999; 17(Suppl 1): S26–S29.

Shortridge KF, Stuart-Harris CH. An influenza epicentre? Lancet 1982; 2: 812–813.

Simonsen L. The global impact of influenza on morbidity and mortality. Vaccine 1999; 17(Suppl 1): S3–S10.

Solorzano A, Webby RJ, Lager KM, Janke BH, Garcia-Sastre A, Richt JA. Mutations in the NS1 protein of swine influenza virus impair anti-interferon activity and confer attenuation in pigs. J Virol 2005; 79: 7535–7543.

Steinhauer DA. Role of hemagglutinin cleavage for the pathogenicity of influenza virus. Virology 1999; 258: 1–20.

Steinhauer DA, Holland JJ. Rapid evolution of RNA viruses. Annu Rev Microbiol 1987; 41: 409–433.

Stephenson I, Bugarini R, Nicholson KG, Podda A, Wood JM, Zambon MC, Katz JM. Cross-reactivity to highly pathogenic avian influenza H5N1 viruses after vaccination with nonadjuvanted and MF59-adjuvanted influenza A/Duck/Singapore/97 (H5N3) vaccine: a potential priming strategy. J Infect Dis 2005; 191: 1210–1215.

Stephenson I, Nicholson KG, Colegate A, Podda A, Wood J, Ypma E, Zambon M. Boosting immunity to influenza H5N1 with MF59-adjuvanted H5N3 A/Duck/Singapore/97 vaccine in a primed human population. Vaccine 2003a; 21: 1687–1693.

Stephenson I, Nicholson KG, Gluck R, Mischler R, Newman RW, Palache AM, Verlander NQ, Warburton F, Wood JM, Zambon MC. Safety and antigenicity of whole virus and subunit influenza A/Hong Kong/1073/99 (H9N2) vaccine in healthy adults: phase I randomised trial. Lancet 2003b; 362: 1959–1966.

Stevens J, Blixt O, Glaser L, Taubenberger JK, Palese P, Paulson JC, Wilson IA. Glycan microarray analysis of the hemagglutinins from modern and pandemic influenza viruses reveals different receptor specificities. J Mol Biol 2006; 355: 1143–1155.

Stiver G. The treatment of influenza with antiviral drugs. CMAJ 2003; 168: 49–56.

Sturm-Ramirez KM, Ellis T, Bousfield B, Bissett L, Dyrting K, Rehg JE, Poon L, Guan Y, Peiris M, Webster RG. Reemerging H5N1 influenza viruses in Hong Kong in 2002 are highly pathogenic to ducks. J Virol 2004; 78: 4892–4901.

Sturm-Ramirez KM, Hulse-Post DJ, Govorkova EA, Humberd J, Seiler P, Puthavathana P, Buranathai C, Nguyen TD, Chaisingh A, Long HT, Naipospos TS, Chen H, Ellis TM, Guan Y, Peiris JS, Webster RG. Are ducks contributing to the endemicity of highly pathogenic H5N1 influenza virus in Asia? J Virol 2005; 79: 11269–11279.

Suarez DL. Overview of avian influenza DIVA test strategies. Biologicals 2005; 33: 221–226.

Suarez DL, Perdue ML, Cox N, Rowe T, Bender C, Huang J, Swayne DE. Comparisons of highly virulent H5N1 influenza A viruses isolated from humans and chickens from Hong Kong. J Virol 1998; 72: 6678–6688.

Suarez DL, Schultz-Cherry S. Immunology of avian influenza virus: a review. Dev Comp Immunol 2000; 24: 269–283.

Subbarao EK, London W, Murphy BR. A single amino acid in the PB2 gene of influenza A virus is a determinant of host range. J Virol 1993; 67: 1761–1764.

Subbarao K, Chen H, Swayne D, Mingay L, Fodor E, Brownlee G, Xu X, Lu X, Katz J, Cox N, Matsuoka Y. Evaluation of a genetically modified reassortant H5N1 influenza A virus vaccine candidate generated by plasmid-based reverse genetics. Virology 2003; 305: 192–200.

Subbarao K, Katz JM. Influenza vaccines generated by reverse genetics. Curr Top Microbiol Immunol 2004; 283: 313–342.

Subbarao K, Klimov A, Katz J, Regnery H, Lim W, Hall H, Perdue M, Swayne D, Bender C, Huang J, Hemphill M, Rowe T, Shaw M, Xu X, Fukuda K, Cox N. Characterization of an avian influenza A (H5N1) virus isolated from a child with a fatal respiratory illness. Science 1998; 279: 393–396.

Subbarao K, Murphy BR, Fauci AS. Development of effective vaccines against pandemic influenza. Immunity 2006a; 24: 5–9.

Subbarao, K, Swayne, DE, Olsen, CW. Epidemiology and Control of Human and Animal Influenza. In: Influenza Virology Current Topics (Kawaoka Y, editor). Norfolk, England: Caister Academic Press; 2006b, pp. 229–280.

Swayne DE. Vaccines for list A poultry diseases: emphasis on avian influenza. Dev Biol (Basel) 2003; 114: 201–212.

Szucs T. The socio-economic burden of influenza. J Antimicrob Chemother 1999; 44(Suppl B): 11–15.

Taubenberger JK, Reid AH, Lourens RM, Wang R, Jin G, Fanning TG. Characterization of the 1918 influenza virus polymerase genes. Nature 2005; 437: 889–893.

Thompson WW, Shay DK, Weintraub E, Brammer L, Cox N, Anderson LJ, Fukuda K. Mortality associated with influenza and respiratory syncytial virus in the United States. JAMA 2003; 289: 179–186.

To KF, Chan PK, Chan KF, Lee WK, Lam WY, Wong KF, Tang NL, Tsang DN, Sung RY, Buckley TA, Tam JS, Cheng AF. Pathology of fatal human infection associated with avian influenza A H5N1 virus. J Med Virol 2001; 63: 242–246.

Tran TH, Nguyen TL, Nguyen TD, Luong TS, Pham PM, Nguyen VC, Pham TS, Vo CD, Le TQ, Ngo TT, Dao BK, Le PP, Nguyen TT, Hoang TL, Cao VT, Le TG, Nguyen DT, Le HN, Nguyen KT, Le HS, Le VT, Christiane D, Tran TT, Menno de J, Schultsz C, Cheng P, Lim W, Horby P, Farrar J. Avian influenza A (H5N1) in 10 patients in Vietnam. N Engl J Med 2004; 350: 1179–1188.

Treanor JJ, Hayden FG, Vrooman PS, Barbarash R, Bettis R, Riff D, Singh S, Kinnersley N, Ward P, Mills RG. Efficacy and safety of the oral neuraminidase inhibitor oseltamivir in treating acute influenza: a randomized controlled trial. US Oral Neuraminidase Study Group. JAMA 2000; 283: 1016–1024.

Treanor JJ, Wilkinson BE, Masseoud F, Hu-Primmer J, Battaglia R, O'Brien D, Wolff M, Rabinovich G, Blackwelder W, Katz JM. Safety and immunogenicity of a recombinant hemagglutinin vaccine for H5 influenza in humans. Vaccine 2001; 19: 1732–1737.

Tumpey TM, Basler CF, Aguilar PV, Zeng H, Solorzano A, Swayne DE, Cox NJ, Katz JM, Taubenberger JK, Palese P, Garcia-Sastre A. Characterization of the reconstructed 1918 Spanish influenza pandemic virus. Science 2005; 310: 77–80.

Tweed SA, Skowronski DM, David ST, Larder A, Petric M, Lees W, Li Y, Katz J, Krajden M, Tellier R, Halpert C, Hirst M, Astell C, Lawrence D, Mak A. Human illness from avian influenza H7N3, British Columbia. Emerg Infect Dis 2004; 10: 2196–2199.

Uiprasertkul M, Puthavathana P, Sangsiriwut K, Pooruk P, Srisook K, Peiris M, Nicholls JM, Chokephaibulkit K, Vanprapar N, Auewarakul P. Influenza A H5N1 replication sites in humans. Emerg Infect Dis 2005; 11: 1036–1041.

Ungchusak K, Auewarakul P, Dowell SF, Kitphati R, Auwanit W, Puthavathana P, Uiprasertkul M, Boonnak K, Pittayawonganon C, Cox NJ, Zaki SR, Thawatsupha P, Chittaganpitch M, Khontong R, Simmerman JM, Chunsutthiwat S. Probable person-to-person transmission of avian influenza A (H5N1). N Engl J Med 2005; 352: 333–340.

USAHA. Report of the Committee on Transmissible Diseases of Poultry and Other Avian Species. Criteria for determining that an AI virus isolation causing an outbreak must be considered for eradication. In: 98th Annual Meeting U.S. Animal Health Association. Richmond, VA: U.S. Animal Health Association; 1994; p. 522.

van der Goot JA, Koch G, de Jong MC, van Boven M. Quantification of the effect of vaccination on transmission of avian influenza (H7N7) in chickens. Proc Natl Acad Sci USA 2005; 102: 18141–18146.

van Riel D, Munster VJ, de Wit E, Rimmelzwaan GF, Fouchier RA, Osterhaus AD, Kuiken T. H5N1 virus attachment to lower respiratory tract. Science 2006; 312: 399.

Vines A, Wells K, Matrosovich M, Castrucci MR, Ito T, Kawaoka Y. The role of influenza A virus hemagglutinin residues 226 and 228 in receptor specificity and host range restriction. J Virol 1998; 72: 7626–7631.

Webby RJ, Perez DR, Coleman JS, Guan Y, Knight JH, Govorkova EA, McClain-Moss LR, Peiris JS, Rehg JE, Tuomanen EI, Webster RG. Responsiveness to a pandemic alert: use of reverse genetics for rapid development of influenza vaccines. Lancet 2004; 363: 1099–1103.

Webby RJ, Webster RG. Emergence of influenza A viruses. Philos Trans R Soc Lond B Biol Sci 2001; 356: 1817–1828.

Webby RJ, Woolcock PR, Krauss SL, Walker DB, Chin PS, Shortridge KF, Webster RG. Multiple genotypes of nonpathogenic H6N2 influenza viruses isolated from chickens in California. Avian Dis 2003; 47: 905–910.

Webster RG, Bean WJ, Gorman OT, Chambers TM, Kawaoka Y. Evolution and ecology of influenza A viruses. Microbiol Rev 1992; 56: 152–179.

Webster RG, Geraci J, Petursson G, Skirnisson K. Conjunctivitis in human beings caused by influenza A virus of seals. N Engl J Med 1981; 304: 911.

Webster RG, Guan Y, Peiris M, Walker D, Krauss S, Zhou NN, Govorkova EA, Ellis TM, Dyrting KC, Sit T, Perez DR, Shortridge KF. Characterization of H5N1 influenza viruses that continue to circulate in geese in southeastern China. J Virol 2002; 76: 118–126.

Webster RG, Yakhno M, Hinshaw VS, Bean WJ, Murti KG. Intestinal influenza: replication and characterization of influenza viruses in ducks. Virology 1978; 84: 268–278.

WHO. Recommended laboratory tests to identify influenza A/H5 virus in specimens from patients with an influenza-like illness. 2004.

WHO. Avian influenza: assessing the pandemic threat. 2005.

WHO. Advice on use of oseltamivir, 2006a. http://www.who.int/csr/disease/avian_influenza/guidelines/useofoseltaniviv2006_03_17A.pdf.

WHO. Cumulative Number of Confirmed Human Cases of Avian Influenza A/(H5N1) Reported to WHO. 2006b. http://www.who.int/csr/disease/avian_influenza/country/cases_table_2006_08_03/en/index.html.

Wong SS, Yuen KY. Avian influenza virus infections in humans. Chest 2006; 129: 156–168.

Xu X, Smith CB, Mungall BA, Lindstrom SE, Hall HE, Subbarao K, Cox NJ, Klimov A. Intercontinental circulation of human influenza A (H1N2) reassortant viruses during the 2001–2002 influenza season. J Infect Dis 2002; 186: 1490–1493.

Xu X, Subbarao K, Cox NJ, Guo Y. Genetic characterization of the pathogenic influenza A/Goose/Guangdong/1/96 (H5N1) virus: similarity of its hemagglutinin gene to those of H5N1 viruses from the 1997 outbreaks in Hong Kong. Virology 1999; 261: 15–19.

Yen HL, Monto AS, Webster RG, Govorkova EA. Virulence may determine the necessary duration and dosage of oseltamivir treatment for highly pathogenic A/Vietnam/1203/04 influenza virus in mice. J Infect Dis 2005; 192: 665–672.

Yuen KY, Chan PK, Peiris M, Tsang DN, Que TL, Shortridge KF, Cheung PT, To WK, Ho ET, Sung R, Cheng AF. Clinical features and rapid viral diagnosis of human disease associated with avian influenza A H5N1 virus. Lancet 1998; 351: 467–471.

Zakstelskaja LJ, Yakhno MA, Isacenko VA, Molibog EV, Hlustov SA, Antonova IV, Klitsunova NV, Vorkunova GK, Burkrinskaja AG, Bykovsky AF, Hohlova GG, Ivanova VT, Zdanov VM. Influenza in the USSR in 1977: recurrence of influenza virus A subtype H1N1. Bull World Health Organ 1978; 56: 919–922.

Zamarin D, Garcia-Sastre A, Xiao X, Wang R, Palese P. Influenza virus PB1-F2 protein induces cell death through mitochondrial ANT3 and VDAC1. PLoS Pathog 2005; 1: e4.

Zhdanov VM, Lvov DK, Zakstelskaya LY, Yakhno MA, Isachenko VI, Braude NA, Reznik VI, Pysina TV, Andreyev VP, Podchernyaeva RY. Return of epidemic A1 (H1N1) influenza virus. Lancet 1978; 1: 294–295.

Emerging Viruses in Human Populations
Edward Tabor (Editor)
DOI 10.1016/S0168-7069(06)16006-1

The Emerging West Nile Virus: From the Old World to the New

Theresa L. Smith

Division of Vector-Borne Infectious Diseases, National Center for Infectious Diseases, Centers for Disease Control and Prevention, Department of Health and Human Services, 3150 Rampart Rd, Fort Collins, CO 80521, USA

Introduction

West Nile virus (WNV) is a flavivirus (genus *Flavivirus*, family *Flaviviridae*) in the Japanese encephalitis (JE) antigenic complex of viruses (Calisher, 1988). The JE antigenic complex includes arboviruses found throughout Africa, Asia, Australia, Europe, and the Americas. These viruses are predominantly pathogens of nonhuman animals, but JE virus, Murray Valley encephalitis virus, St. Louis encephalitis virus (SLEV), and WNV also cause neurologic disease in humans. WNV was first isolated from the blood of a febrile patient in the West Nile district of northern Uganda in 1937 during research on yellow fever (Smithburn et al., 1940). Since then, not only has our understanding of the virus and its geography, transmission, and clinical aspects of infection changed, but also the virus, its geography, transmission, and clinical aspects have changed. The possibility of change in the spectrum of human disease caused by WNV is difficult to assess due to the differences in clinical tools and the changes in geography, and therefore populations affected, that have occurred.

The virus

WNV is a spherical virus of 45–50 nm diameter. Its positive-sense, single-stranded RNA is 11,000–12,000 nucleotides long, encoding 7 nonstructural (NS1, NS2a, NS2b, NS3, NS4a, NS4b, and NS5) and 3 structural (core protein C, envelope E, and pre-membrane prM) proteins (Fig. 1) (Petersen and Roehrig, 2001). The RNA is enclosed in an icosahedral nucleocapsid made of 12 kDa capsid protein building blocks (Petersen and Roehrig, 2001). In turn, the capsid lies within a host-derived membrane envelope altered by two viral membrane glycoproteins, E, and prM (Fig. 2). WNV seasonally causes inapparent infection, a febrile syndrome called

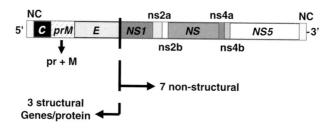

Fig. 1 Genomic structure of WNV, showing 3 structural proteins, C-capsid, M-membrane, and E-envelope; and 7 nonstructural proteins (Petersen and Roehrig, 2001). (For colour version: see Colour Section on page 349).

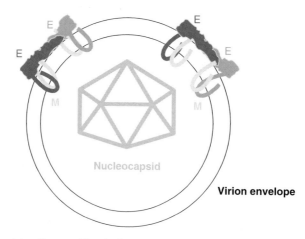

Fig. 2 Flavivirus virion diagram. The single stranded RNA is enclosed in the nucleocapsid, which in turn is surrounded by an envelope containing E-glycoproteins (E) and integral membrane proteins (M) (Petersen and Roehrig, 2001). (For colour version: see Colour Section on page 350).

West Nile fever (WNF), or neuroinvasive disease, at a ratio of approximately 110 asymptomatic infections and 30 WNF cases for each neuroinvasive infection (Tsai et al., 1998; CDC, 2001; Mostashari et al., 2001).

Based on the E-glycoprotein, phylogenetic lineages have been determined for WNV isolates collected worldwide from diagnostic specimens, outbreak investigations, and ecologic studies (Fig. 3) (Lanciotti et al., 1999; Murgue et al., 2001b). Based on these lineages, the original emergence of WNV as a distinct flavivirus is calculated to have occurred approximately 1000 years ago (Galli et al., 2004). Subsequently, two WNV lineages developed. Lineage 1 is responsible for epidemic WNV transmission both within and outside of Africa and includes the Kunjin virus subtype of Australiasia. Lineage 2 has been associated with enzootic cycles in Africa. Both lineages may be found in some African countries. In addition, WNV strains of multiple phylogenetic profiles within lineage 1 have been isolated in many countries (Hammam and Price, 1966; Deardorff et al., 2006).

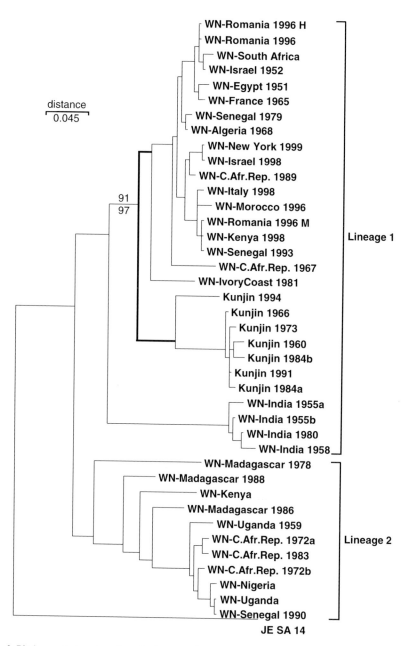

Fig. 3 Phylogenetic tree based on E-glycoprotein nucleic acid sequence data (Lanciotti et al., 1999).

The 1999 emergence of WNV disease in the United States (US) involved a strain related to a lineage 1 strain previously found in a goose in Israel in 1998 (Lanciotti et al., 1999). In the US, WNV has caused larger epidemics than seen previously, occurring across a larger area (O'Leary et al., 2004). Large-scale evaluations of North American WNV strains (Davis et al., 2005) also have identified a less virulent strain, found in Mexico (Davis et al., 2004; Deardorff et al., 2006). Of possibly greater importance is the emergence of a WNV strain that appears to have increased infectivity for mosquitoes (Ebel et al., 2004).

Geography

Historical aspects of the virus distribution

WNV was first found in Uganda in 1937 (Smithburn et al., 1940) and was subsequently found in other African and Asian countries (Smithburn, 1942, 1953; Smithburn et al., 1954). Antibody studies led to an understanding of the geographic range of WNV and sometimes provided isolates of WNV from only mildly symptomatic persons (Smithburn et al., 1940; Melnick et al., 1951). Outbreak investigations also yielded geographic, virologic, and clinical information (Bernkopf et al., 1953). Large regional follow-up serosurveys in central Africa, begun in 1939, found anti-WNV seropositivity rates of 1.4% (in part of the Belgian Congo) to 46.4% (in the White Nile area of Sudan). In Egypt in 1950, greater than 90% of those studied who were over 40 years of age had antibodies to WNV (Melnick et al., 1951). Ecologic studies expanded both the known geographic range and led to an increased understanding of the ecologic niche of WNV (Work et al., 1955; Hurlbut et al., 1956). Molecular studies showed Kunjin virus to be a part of the WNV lineage 1 (Lanciotti et al., 1999). Through these and similar studies, WNV was found to be widespread in Africa, southern Europe, Australia, and southwest Asia (Solomon and Mallewa, 2001; Campbell et al., 2002).

WNV was not detected in the Western hemisphere until 1999, when an apparent outbreak of disease due to SLEV in the greater New York City area was noted to have clinical features in humans and birds that were unusual for SLEV (CDC, 1999). Since reaching the Western hemisphere, WNV has spread to all of the contiguous US states, Canada, Mexico (Blitvich et al., 2003; Lorono-Pino et al., 2003), the Caribbean (Dupuis et al., 2003, 2005), and South and Central America (Davis et al., 2005) (Fig. 4). Although the method of spread of WNV to the US is unclear (Calisher, 2000), it is clear that the US strains are closely related to WNV found in Israel, and that the virus found in the US and Israel have high avian virulence in common (Petersen and Roehrig, 2001).

Current distribution of WNV

Although evidence of WNV infections initially came from predominantly rural areas (Smithburn et al., 1940; Smithburn and Jacobs, 1942; Melnick et al., 1951; Olejnik, 1952; Bernkopf et al., 1953; Dick, 1953; Smithburn, 1953; Goldblum et al.,

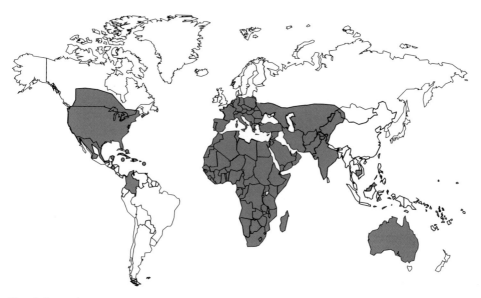

Fig. 4 Approximate global distribution of West Nile virus. (For colour version: see Colour Section on page 350).

1954; Smithburn et al., 1954; Radt, 1955; Weinbren, 1955), recent outbreaks have included metropolitan areas of Canada, France, Romania, Russia, and the US, with large numbers of people infected because of the population densities in the cities (Campbell et al., 2001; Lopez, 2002; Mirza et al., 2003; Del Giudice et al., 2004; Fedorova et al., 2004; Watson et al., 2004; Feki et al., 2005; Gingrich and Williams, 2005; Mandalakas et al., 2005; Palmisano et al., 2005; Shaman et al., 2005; Shcherbakova et al., 2005; Willis, 2005; Wilson et al., 2005). In the Eastern hemisphere, it is unclear whether urban outbreaks reflect a change in the viral ecology, or an improvement in diagnosis. The 1996 outbreak in Romania was associated with substandard housing (Han et al., 1999; Campbell et al., 2001). Many areas, such as Algeria, Israel, Italy, and Morocco, continue to have rural WNV outbreaks, suggesting that any changes in the epidemiology of WNV in urban areas are not due to changes in the virus itself (Chastel et al., 1995; Murgue et al., 2001a; Green et al., 2005; Schuffenecker et al., 2005). In 2003, it was found that lineage 2, previously only seen in Africa, emerged in Hungary (Bakonyi et al., 2006) in an enzootic cycle.

Transmission

Historical aspects of the ecology

Enzootic, and ultimately, epidemic transmission of WNV depend on a bird–mosquito–bird pattern of transmission. After early recognition that mosquitoes are

WNV vectors (Philip and Smadel, 1943; Kitaoka, 1950; Goldwasser and Davies, 1953), ecologic studies of WNV in Egypt revealed the enzootic cycle involving mosquito vectors and bird amplifying hosts, and the occurrence of dead-end infections in humans and horses (Work et al., 1953; Work et al., 1955).

Not all mosquito species are equally likely to transmit WNV. Mosquitoes commonly found to be infected with WNV include largely ornithophilic species in the genus *Culex* (Taylor et al., 1953; Davies and Yoshpe-Purer, 1954; Tahori et al., 1955; Hurlbut, 1956) as well as largely mammalophilic species in the genus *Aedes* (Philip and Smadel, 1943; Kitaoka, 1950; Turell et al., 2005). Only amplifying hosts, such as birds, develop sufficient viremia for transmission of WNV to feeding mosquitoes. Following an "extrinsic" incubation period, the mosquito can infect birds that it feeds on (Hurlbut, 1956). In contrast, if an infected mosquito feeds on an animal not capable of developing high-titer WNV viremia, the virus will be unable to infect a subsequently feeding mosquito, resulting in infections of dead-end hosts such as humans (Taylor et al., 1953; Work et al., 1953, 1955; Hurlbut, 1956). Some ticks are capable of becoming infected and transmitting WNV, but are apparently not an important part of the ecology of WNV (Hurlbut, 1956).

Historically, the only known modes of WNV transmission to humans were mosquito-borne, which accounted for the vast majority of infections, and laboratory-acquired, which accounted for a few infections, mainly thought to have been spread by the airborne route (Smithburn et al., 1940; Hamilton and Taylor, 1954; Nir, 1959). Therefore, avoidance of mosquitoes has been the mainstay for preventing human WNV disease (Philip and Smadel, 1943).

Modern aspects of ecology

More recently, as WNV has spread to new geographic areas with previously unaffected birds and different mosquito vectors, our understanding of WNV ecology has expanded. Mosquito species transmitting WNV vary by region (Bell et al., 2005; Gingrich and Williams, 2005; Godsey Jr, 2005). For example, in the US, *Cx. pipiens, Cx. tarsalis*, and *Cx. quinquefasciatus* are each important regional WNV vectors. *Cx. pipiens* predominates in the East, *Cx. tarsalis* in the Midwest and West, and *Cx. quinquefasciatus* in the Southeast (Hayes et al., 2005a). Other animals besides birds may develop sufficiently high-titer viremia to infect feeding mosquitoes, including alligators (Klenk et al., 2004) and rabbits (Tiawsirisup et al., 2005). Bird-to-bird transmission of WNV also can occur (Langevin et al., 2001; Komar et al., 2003). The WNV strain recently circulating in Israel and North America causes higher avian mortality than previously observed (Bin et al., 2001; Swayne et al., 2001). In the US, this strain has caused significant avian mortality, especially among members of *Corvidae* (e.g., crows, jays, and magpies) (Brault et al., 2004; Yaremych et al., 2004). Since spreading in North America, at least one strain of WNV has developed increased mosquito infectivity (Ebel et al., 2004).

Although the vast majority of WNV infections are mosquito-borne, other modes of transmission have also been recognized more recently. Conjunctival exposure to viremic blood can result in infection (Fonseca et al., 2005), and the laboratory environment continues to be a source of a few WNV infections, including through percutaneous inoculation (CDC, 2002c). During the large and unprecedented WNV epidemics that have occurred in the US in recent years, several novel modes of WNV transmission were recognized. Transmission by blood transfusion (CDC, 2002b), organ transplantation (CDC, 2002e), intrauterine exposure (CDC, 2002a), and possibly by breast feeding (CDC, 2002d) were newly recognized during the 2002 WNV epidemic.

The recognition that WNV can be transmitted by infected blood donations led to the rapid development of *in vitro* assays for screening blood donations. As stated above, this mode of transmission was first recognized in 2002, when 23 persons contracted WNV disease within 4 weeks of receipt of a blood product from one of 16 donors found to have had West Nile viremia at the time of donation (Pealer et al., 2003). In response to these events, beginning in 2003 blood donations in the US were screened for the presence of WNV RNA (CDC, 2003). Subsequently, WNV has also been found in the blood supply of Canada (Cameron et al., 2005) and Mexico (Sanchez-Guerrero et al., 2006).

WNV transmission through organ transplantation was first recognized in 2002, having occurred because an organ donor had previously received a contaminated blood transfusion (Iwamoto et al., 2003). Despite the reduction in transmission of WNV by transfusion due to screening tests and the expectation that transmission by transplantation would also become less likely, transmission of WNV by organ donation was documented to have occurred again in 2005 (CDC, 2005), apparently after a mosquito-borne infection of the organ donor.

The evidence for intrauterine transmission of WNV prompted the development of a registry for women who had become infected with WNV while pregnant (O'Leary et al., 2006). Possible transmission through breast milk has been documented once.

Despite these newly recognized modes of human-to-human WNV transmission, the vast majority of infections are still mosquito-borne, as shown by its continued seasonality (O'Leary et al., 2004). Prevention of human WNV infections still relies upon avoidance of mosquitoes (Hayes and Gubler, 2006); specifically, remaining indoors at dawn and dusk when *Culex* are more likely to bite, wearing light colored clothing that covers the arms and legs, and use of insect repellent on skin and clothing. Effective insect repellents, U.S. Environmental Protection Agency-registered, now include *N,N*-diethyl-*m*-toluamide (DEET), oil of lemon eucalyptus, and picaradin for skin, and permethrin for clothing (Fradin and Day, 2002; Barnard and Xue, 2004).

Clinical aspects of WNV infection

Historical

Initial laboratory studies in mice and primates revealed WNV to be neurotropic (Smithburn et al., 1940). Based on early observations, human WNV disease seemed to fall into two categories: a mild, self-limited, febrile disease called "West Nile fever" and seen mostly in children and young adults (Olejnik, 1952; Goldblum et al., 1954), and rare cases of West Nile meningitis or encephalitis seen mainly in older patients (Smithburn and Jacobs, 1942; Bernkopf et al., 1953). A review of early reports shows that relatively little has changed regarding the known clinical spectrum of WNV disease. Outbreaks in Israel, Egypt, and France documented a clinical spectrum similar to that seen today (Leffkowitz, 1942; Olejnik, 1952; Bernkopf et al., 1953; Goldblum et al., 1954; Hamilton and Taylor, 1954; Southam and Moore, 1954; Hurlbut et al., 1956; Spigland et al., 1958; Panthier et al., 1968; Murgue et al., 2001a,b).

Illness due to WNV was described in these outbreaks as having a 3–6-day incubation period followed by systemic symptoms such as fever, headaches, chills, malaise, diaphoresis, weakness, drowsiness, or lymphadenopathy. Pharyngitis and conjunctivitis were also sometimes observed. Dermatologic manifestations sometimes included a short-lived, truncal, nonpruritic, maculopapular rash. Gastrointestinal symptoms occurred in some patients, including anorexia, nausea, vomiting, abdominal pain, or diarrhea. Muscular symptoms included chest, back and limb pain, or pain on movement of the eyes. Although symptoms resolved within a week in the majority of patients, some experienced a mild relapse after their symptoms improved, and many had a convalescence marked by fatigue that lasted for weeks. The lymphadenopathy usually took 1–2 months to resolve. WNV was recovered from the blood only during the first few days of illness.

When encephalitis occurred, symptoms and signs included decreased level of consciousness, from drowsiness to near-coma; altered deep tendon reflexes, usually initially hyperactive, and later diminished; extrapyramidal disorders, such as involuntary muscle twitching, seizures, or cranial nerve palsies. A long convalescence with fatigue commonly occurred, especially in adults.

The current view of the WNV clinical spectrum

Symptoms and signs

More recent expansion of our understanding of WNV disease has focused on rarer, more severe outcomes. For instance, it is clear that neurologic involvement of the spinal cord, characterized by anterior myelitis, may occur with or without overt encephalitis. In a recent evaluation of a cohort of 27 patients with WNV-associated anterior myelitis, all 24 patients who were evaluated at one-year of follow-up had some improvement in strength. Unfortunately, three patients had died, and initial involvement of the respiratory muscles was related to poor outcome (Sejvar et al., 2005). Patients presenting with possible WNV-associated anterior myelitis must be differentiated from those with WNV-associated Guillain–Barré syndrome, a newly recognized entity (Ahmed et al., 2000). Extrapyramidal disorders due to WNV can involve involuntary muscle twitching, tremor, myoclonus, and Parkinsonism (Sejvar et al., 2003). Although rare, hepatitis, myocarditis, nephritis, pancreatitis, and splenomegaly can occur (Perelman and Stern, 1974; Mathiot et al., 1990; Omalu et al., 2003). Ocular involvement (Bakri and Kaiser, 2004), specifically multifocal chorioretinitis, is a hallmark of WNV disease with meningitis or encephalitis, and it was found to have 88% sensitivity and 100% specificity for identifying WNV infection among those presenting with possible WNV meningitis or encephalitis (Abroug et al., 2006).

More severe outcomes of WNV disease increase with advancing age (Panthier et al., 1968; Weinberger et al., 2001). Interestingly, more severe outcomes of WNV disease are associated with a history of organ transplantation (Kumar et al., 2004). One case of persistent WNV infection in an immunocompromised patient without evidence of a humoral response to WNV (Penn et al., 2006) underscores the importance of antibody development to the clearance of WNV (Diamond et al., 2003). Excess mortality has been documented in the 2 years following WNV disease among men (compared to women), among patients over 85 years of age, among diabetics, and among those with dementia (Green et al., 2005). Different outbreaks appear to vary in terms of certain clinical features such as mortality and frequency of the rash (Chowers et al., 2001; Petersen and Roehrig, 2001). Possible explanations include differences in population age distribution and intensity of surveillance.

Diagnosis

Diagnostic tests for WNV infection usually rely on serology, as the viremia is short-lived once symptoms begin and is rarely found in patients presenting with encephalitis. Enzyme immunoassays (EIA) for IgM and IgG (Tardei et al., 2000) are useful, especially the relatively specificity of WNV IgM. Plaque-reduction neutralization tests measure virus-specific neutralizing antibody titer. The presence of IgM antibody to WNV in both acute- and convalescent-phase sera (for specificity) and the presence of IgG antibody to WNV in later samples, along with a fourfold or greater rise in titers of neutralizing antibody, are considered necessary for documenting a recent infection. Because flaviviruses are notoriously cross-reactive in serologic tests, serologic tests for infection with WNV or another flavivirus must be conducted in conjunction with a geographically appropriate battery of assays to detect flaviviruses or their antigens in comparative tests (e.g., to distinguish between WNV and SLEV infections in the US). Recently, IgG avidity using enzyme-linked immunosorbent assays (ELISA) has been proposed as a method to differentiate recent from remote infections (Fox et al., 2006), but this approach has not been standardized.

Evidence of neuroinvasive WNV disease can be seen in magnetic resonance imaging (MRI) studies, which can reveal hyperintense signals in the basal ganglia, pons, substantia nigra, thalamus, and/or anterior horns (Maschke et al., 2004). Although these MRI images are not diagnostic for WNV disease, nor are they universally present in WNV neurologic involvement, the presence of these lesions can help exclude herpes encephalitis, the most common cause of sporadic encephalitis. For patients with symptoms that could be attributable to either anterior myelitis or Guillain–Barré syndrome, electromyography can differentiate axonal neuropathy seen in anterior myelitis from demyelinating neuropathy seen in Guillain–Barré syndrome (Ahmed et al., 2000).

Treatment of WNV disease

Treatment of WNV disease is supportive. Both WNF and WNV neurologic disease can be painful, requiring analgesia. Rehydration may be required after severe nausea and vomiting. Patients with encephalitis may require hospitalization for airway protection and seizure management. Investigational therapeutic options currently undergoing clinical trials include ribavirin, intravenous immunoglobulin from donors in areas of high WNV endemicity, and alpha interferon (Hayes et al., 2005b).

Conclusions

WNV has undergone alterations in viral genetics and spread geographically. In Mexico and the US, it has spread across a continent inhabited by a predominantly immunologically WNV-naïve human population, but in a continent with ample pre-adapted mosquito vectors and vertebrate amplifying hosts. This situation has led to large epidemics that in turn led to the recognition of the rarer clinical manifestations and modes of transmission of this virus. The clinical spectrum and diagnostic findings in WNV diseases have been clarified, and will likely continue to be refined as new epidemics occur. We can expect WNV to continue to find ecologic niches where it can be enzootically maintained, and because of this, also to continue to affect human populations.

Acknowledgments

The author thanks Grant L. Campbell, Duane J. Gubler, Robert S. Lanciotti, Anthony A. Marfin, Lyle Petersen, and John T. Roehrig for the use of their illustrations.

References

Abroug F, Ouanes-Besbes L, Letaief M, Ben Romdhane F, Khairallah M, Triki H, Bouzouiaia N. A cluster study of predictors of severe West Nile virus infection. Mayo Clin Proc 2006; 81: 12–16.

Ahmed S, Libman R, Wesson K, Ahmed F, Einberg K. Guillain–Barre syndrome: an unusual presentation of West Nile virus infection. Neurology 2000; 55: 144–146.

Bakonyi T, Ivanics E, Erdelyi K, Ursu K, Ferenczi E, Weissenbock H, Nowotny N. Lineage 1 and 2 strains of encephalitic West Nile virus, Central Europe. Emerg Infect Dis 2006; 12: 618–623.

Bakri SJ, Kaiser PK. Ocular manifestations of West Nile virus. Curr Opin Ophthalmol 2004; 15: 537–540.

Barnard DR, Xue RD. Laboratory evaluation of mosquito repellents against *Aedes albopictus*, *Culex nigripalpus*, and *Ochierotatus triseriatus* (Diptera: *Culicidae*). J Med Entomol 2004; 41: 726–730.

Bell JA, Mickelson NJ, Vaughan JA. West Nile virus in host-seeking mosquitoes within a residential neighborhood in Grand Forks, North Dakota. Vector Borne Zoonotic Dis 2005; 5: 373–382.

Bernkopf H, Levine S, Nerson R. Isolation of West Nile virus in Israel. J Infect Dis 1953; 93: 207–218.

Bin H, Grossman Z, Pokamunski S, Malkinson M, Weiss L, Duvdevani P, Banet C, Weisman Y, Annis E, Gandaku D, Yahalom V, Hindyieh M, Shulman L, Mendelson E. West Nile fever in Israel 1999–2000: from geese to humans. Ann N Y Acad Sci 2001; 951: 127–142.

Blitvich BJ, Fernandez-Salas I, Contreras-Cordero JF, Marlenee NL, Gonzalez-Rojas JI, Komar N, Gubler DJ, Calisher CH, Beaty BJ. Serologic evidence of West Nile virus infection in horses, Coahuila State, Mexico. Emerg Infect Dis 2003; 9: 853–856.

Brault AC, Langevin SA, Bowen RA, Panella NA, Biggerstaff BJ, Miller BR, Nicholas K. Differential virulence of West Nile strains for American crows. Emerg Infect Dis 2004; 10: 2161–2168.

Calisher CH. Antigenic classification and taxonomy of flaviviruses (family *Flaviviridae*) emphasizing a universal system for the taxonomy of viruses causing tick-borne encephalitis. Acta Virol 1988; 32: 469–478.

Calisher CH. West Nile virus in the New World: appearance, persistence, and adaptation to a new econiche—an opportunity taken. Viral Immunol 2000; 13: 411–414.

Cameron C, Reeves J, Antonishyn N, Tilley P, Alport T, Eurich B, Towns D, Lane D, Saldanha J. West Nile virus in Canadian blood donors. Transfusion 2005; 45: 487–491.

Campbell GL, Ceianu CS, Savage HM. Epidemic West Nile encephalitis in Romania: waiting for history to repeat itself. Ann N Y Acad Sci 2001; 951: 94–101.

Campbell GL, Marfin AA, Lanciotti RS, Gubler DJ. West Nile virus. Lancet Infect Dis 2002; 2: 519–529.

CDC. Outbreak of West Nile-like viral encephalitis—New York, 1999. MMWR Morb Mortal Wkly Rep 1999; 48: 845–849.

CDC. Human West Nile virus surveillance—Connecticut, New Jersey, and New York, 2000. MMWR Morb Mortal Wkly Rep 2001; 50: 265–268.

CDC. Intrauterine West Nile virus infection—New York, 2002. MMWR Morb Mortal Wkly Rep 2002a; 51: 1135–1136.

CDC. Investigation of blood transfusion recipients with West Nile virus infections. MMWR Morb Mortal Wkly Rep 2002b; 51: 823.

CDC. Laboratory-acquired West Nile virus infections—United States, 2002. MMWR Morb Mortal Wkly Rep 2002c; 51: 1133–1135.

CDC. Possible West Nile virus transmission to an infant through breast-feeding—Michigan, 2002. MMWR Morb Mortal Wkly Rep 2002d; 51: 877–878.

CDC. West Nile virus infection in organ donor and transplant recipients—Georgia and Florida, 2002. MMWR Morb Mortal Wkly Rep 2002e; 51: 790.

CDC. Detection of West Nile virus in blood donations—United States, 2003. MMWR Morb Mortal Wkly Rep 2003; 52: 769–772.

CDC. West Nile virus infections in organ transplant recipients—New York and Pennsylvania, August–September, 2005. MMWR Morb Mortal Wkly Rep 2005; 54: 1021–1023.

Chastel C, Bailly-Choumara H, Bach-Hamba D, Le Lay G, Legrand MC, Le Goff F, Vermeil C. Tick-transmitted arbovirus in Maghreb. Bull Soc Pathol Exot 1995; 88: 81–85.

Chowers MY, Lang R, Nassar F, Ben-David D, Giladi M, Rubinshtein E, Itzhaki A, Mishal J, Siegman-Igra Y, Kitzes R, Pick N, Landau Z, Wolf D, Bin H, Mendelson E, Pitlik SD, Weinberger M. Clinical characteristics of the West Nile fever outbreak, Israel, 2000. Emerg Infect Dis 2001; 7: 675–678.

Davies AM, Yoshpe-Purer Y. Observation on the biology of West Nile virus, with special reference to its behaviour in the mosquito *Aedes aegypti*. Ann Trop Med Parasitol 1954; 48: 46–54.

Davis CT, Beasley DW, Guzman H, Siirin M, Parsons RE, Tesh RB, Barrett AD. Emergence of attenuated West Nile virus variants in Texas, 2003. Virology 2004; 330: 342–350.

Davis CT, Ebel GD, Lanciotti RS, Brault AC, Guzman H, Siirin M, Lambert A, Parsons RE, Beasley DW, Novak RJ, Elizondo-Quiroga D, Green EN, Young DS, Stark LM, Drebot MA, Artsob H, Tesh RB, Kramer LD, Barrett AD. Phylogenetic analysis of North American West Nile virus isolates, 2001–2004: evidence for the emergence of a dominant genotype. Virology 2005; 342: 252–265.

Deardorff E, Estrada-Franco J, Brault AC, Navarro-Lopez R, Campomanes-Cortes A, Paz-Ramirez P, Solis-Hernandez M, Ramey WN, Davis CT, Beasley DW, Tesh RB, Barrett AD, Weaver SC. Introductions of West Nile virus strains to Mexico. Emerg Infect Dis 2006; 12: 314–318.

Del Giudice P, Schuffenecker I, Vandenbos F, Counillon E, Zellet H. Human West Nile virus, France. Emerg Infect Dis 2004; 10: 1885–1886.

Diamond MS, Sitati EM, Friend LD, Higgs S, Shrestha B, Engle M. A critical role for induced IgM in the protection against West Nile virus infection. J Exp Med 2003; 198: 1853–1862.

Dick GW. Epidemiological notes on some viruses isolated in Uganda; Yellow fever, Rift Valley fever, Bwamba fever, West Nile, Mengo, Semliki forest, Bunyamwera, Ntaya, Uganda S and Zika viruses. Trans R Soc Trop Med Hyg 1953; 47: 13–48.

Dupuis II AP, Marra PP, Kramer LD. Serologic evidence of West Nile virus transmission, Jamaica, West Indies. Emerg Infect Dis 2003; 9: 860–863.

Dupuis II AP, Marra PP, Reitsma R, Jones MJ, Louie KL, Kramer LD. Serologic evidence for West Nile virus transmission in Puerto Rico and Cuba. Am J Trop Med Hyg 2005; 73: 474–476.

Ebel GD, Carricaburu J, Young D, Bernard KA, Kramer LD. Genetic and phenotypic variation of West Nile virus in New York, 2000–2003. Am J Trop Med Hyg 2004; 71: 493–500.

Fedorova MV, Lopatina iu V, Khutoretskaia NV, Lazorenko VV, Platonov AE. [The study of mosquito fauna (Diptera, *Culicidae*) in Volgograd city in light of the outbreak of West Nile fever in Volgograd region, 1999]. Parazitologiia 2004; 38: 209–218.

Feki I, Marrakchi C, Ben Hmida M, Belahsen F, Ben Jemaa M, Maaloul I, Kanoun F, Ben Hamed S, Mhiri C. Epidemic West Nile virus encephalitis in Tunisia. Neuroepidemiology 2005; 24: 1–7.

Fonseca K, Prince GD, Bratvold J, Fox JD, Pybus M, Preksaitis JK, Tilley P. West Nile virus infection and conjunctival exposure. Emerg Infect Dis 2005; 11: 1648–1649.

Fox JL, Hazell SL, Tobler LH, Busch MP. Immunoglobulin G avidity in differentiation between early and late antibody responses to West Nile virus. Clin Vaccine Immunol 2006; 13: 33–36.

Fradin MS, Day JF. Comparative efficacy of insect repellents against mosquito bites. N Engl J Med 2002; 347: 13–18.

Galli M, Bernini F, Zehender G. Alexander the Great and West Nile virus encephalitis. Emerg Infect Dis 2004; 10: 1332–1333.

Gingrich JB, Williams GM. Host-feeding patterns of suspected West Nile virus mosquito vectors in Delaware, 2001–2002. J Am Mosq Control Assoc 2005; 21: 194–200.

Godsey Jr. MS. West Nile virus-infected mosquitoes, Louisiana, 2002. Emerg Infect Dis 2005; 11: 1401–1406.

Goldblum N, Sterk VV, Paderski B. West Nile fever; the clinical features of the disease and the isolation of West Nile virus from the blood of nine human cases. Am J Hyg 1954; 59: 89–103.

Goldwasser RA, Davies AM. Transmission of a West Nile-like virus by *Aedes aegypti*. Trans R Soc Trop Med Hyg 1953; 47: 336–337.

Green MS, Weinberger M, Ben-Ezer J, Bin H, Mendelson E, Gandacu D, Kaufman Z, Dichtiar R, Sobel A, Cohen D, Chowers MY. Long-term death rates, West Nile virus epidemic, Israel, 2000. Emerg Infect Dis 2005; 11: 1754–1757.

Hamilton PK, Taylor RM. Report of clinical case of West Nile virus infection probably acquired in the laboratory. Am J Trop Med Hyg 1954; 3: 51–53.

Hammam HM, Price WH. Further observations on geographic variation in the antigenic character of West Nile and Japanese B viruses. Am J Epidemiol 1966; 83: 113–122.

Han LL, Popovici F, Alexander Jr. JP, Laurentia V, Tengelsen LA, Cernescu C, Gary Jr. HE, Ion-Nedelcu N, Campbell GL, Tsai TF. Risk factors for West Nile virus infection and meningoencephalitis, Romania, 1996. J Infect Dis 1999; 179: 230–233.

Hayes EB, Gubler DJ. West Nile virus: epidemiology and clinical features of an emerging epidemic in the United States. Annu Rev Med 2006; 57: 181–194.

Hayes EB, Komar N, Nasci RS, Montgomery SP, O'leary DR, Campbell GL. Epidemiology and transmission dynamics of West Nile virus disease. Emerg Infect Dis 2005a; 11: 1167–1173.

Hayes EB, Sejvar JJ, Zaki SR, Lanciotti RS, Bode AV, Campbell GL. Virology, pathology, and clinical manifestations of West Nile virus disease. Emerg Infect Dis 2005b; 11: 1174–1179.

Hurlbut HS. West Nile virus infection in arthropods. Am J Trop Med Hyg 1956; 5: 76–85.

Hurlbut HS, Rizk F, Taylor RM, Work TH. A study of the ecology of West Nile virus in Egypt. Am J Trop Med Hyg 1956; 5: 579–620.

Iwamoto M, Jernigan DB, Guasch A, Trepka MJ, Blackmore CG, Hellinger WC, Pham SM, Zaki S, Lanciotti RS, Lance-Parker SE, Diazgranados CA, Winquist AG, Perlino CA, Wiersma S, Hillyer KL, Goodman JL, Marfin AA, Chamberland ME, Petersen LR. Transmission of West Nile virus from an organ donor to four transplant recipients. N Engl J Med 2003; 348: 2196–2203.

Kitaoka M. Experimental transmission of the West Nile virus by the mosquito. Jpn Med J (Natl Inst Health Jpn) 1950; 3: 77–81.

Klenk K, Snow J, Morgan K, Bowen R, Stephens M, Foster F, Gordy P, Beckett S, Komar N, Gubler D, Bunning M. Alligators as West Nile virus amplifiers. Emerg Infect Dis 2004; 10: 2150–2155.

Komar N, Langevin S, Hinten S, Nemeth N, Edwards E, Hettler D, Davis B, Bowen R, Bunning M. Experimental infection of North American birds with the New York 1999 strain of West Nile virus. Emerg Infect Dis 2003; 9: 311–322.

Kumar D, Drebot MA, Wong SJ, Lim G, Artsob H, Buck P, Humar A. A seroprevalence study of West Nile virus infection in solid organ transplant recipients. Am J Transplant 2004; 4: 1883–1888.

Lanciotti RS, Roehrig JT, Deubel V, Smith J, Parker M, Steele K, Crise B, Volpe KE, Crabtree MB, Scherret JH, Hall RA, Mackenzie JS, Cropp CB, Panigrahy B, Ostlund E, Schmitt B, Malkinson M, Banet C, Weissman J, Komar N, Savage HM, Stone W, Mcnamara T, Gubler DJ. Origin of the West Nile virus responsible for an outbreak of encephalitis in the northeastern United States. Science 1999; 286: 2333–2337.

Langevin SA, Bunning M, Davis B, Komar N. Experimental infection of chickens as candidate sentinels for West Nile virus. Emerg Infect Dis 2001; 7: 726–729.

Leffkowitz M. An unknown epidemic infectious disease. Harefuah J Palest Jew Med Ass 1942; 22: 3–4.

Lopez W. West Nile virus in New York City. Am J Public Health 2002; 92: 1218–1221.

Lorono-Pino MA, Blitvich BJ, Farfan-Ale JA, Puerto FI, Blanco JM, Marlenee NL, Rosado-Paredes EP, Garcia-Rejon JE, Gubler DJ, Calisher CH, Beaty BJ. Serologic evidence of West Nile virus infection in horses, Yucatan State, Mexico. Emerg Infect Dis 2003; 9: 857–859.

Mandalakas AM, Kippes C, Sedransk J, Kile JR, Garg A, Mcleod J, Berry RL, Marfin AA. West Nile virus epidemic, northeast Ohio, 2002. Emerg Infect Dis 2005; 11: 1774–1777.

Maschke M, Kastrup O, Forsting M, Diener HC. Update on neuroimaging in infectious central nervous system disease. Curr Opin Neurol 2004; 17: 475–480.

Mathiot CC, Georges AJ, Deubel V. Comparative analysis of West Nile virus strains isolated from human and animal hosts using monoclonal antibodies and cDNA restriction digest profiles. Res Virol 1990; 141: 533–543.

Melnick JL, Paul JR, Riordan JT, Barnett VH, Goldblum N, Zabin E. Isolation from human sera in Egypt of a virus apparently identical to West Nile virus. Proc Soc Exp Biol Med 1951; 77: 661–665.

Mirza H, Cross S, Mileno M. First case of West Nile infection in Rhode Island. Med Health R I 2003; 86: 213–215.

Mostashari F, Bunning ML, Kitsutani PT, Singer DA, Nash D, Cooper MJ, Katz N, Liljebjelke KA, Biggerstaff BJ, Fine AD, Layton MC, Mullin SM, Johnson AJ, Martin DA, Hayes EB, Campbell GL. Epidemic West Nile encephalitis, New York, 1999: results of a household-based seroepidemiological survey. Lancet 2001; 358: 261–264.

Murgue B, Murri S, Triki H, Deubel V, Zeller HG. West Nile in the Mediterranean basin: 1950–2000. Ann N Y Acad Sci 2001a; 951: 117–126.

Murgue B, Murri S, Zientara S, Durand B, Durand JP, Zeller H. West Nile outbreak in horses in southern France, 2000: the return after 35 years. Emerg Infect Dis 2001b; 7: 692–696.

Nir YD. Airborne West Nile virus infection. Am J Trop Med Hyg 1959; 8: 537–539.

O'leary DR, Kuhn S, Kniss KL, Hinckley AF, Rasmussen SA, Pape WJ, Kightlinger LK, Beecham BD, Miller TK, Neitzel DF, Michael SF, Campbell GL, Lanciotti RS, Hayes EB. Birth outcomes following West Nile virus infection of pregnant women in the United States: 2003–2004. Pediatrics 2006; 117: 537–545.

O'leary DR, Marfin AA, Montgomery SP, Kipp AM, Lehman JA, Biggerstaff BJ, Elko VL, Collins PD, Jones JE, Campbell GL. The epidemic of West Nile virus in the United States, 2002. Vector Borne Zoonotic Dis 2004; 4: 61–70.

Olejnik E. Infectious adenitis transmitted by *Culex molestus*. Bull Res Counc Isr 1952; 2: 210–211.

Omalu BI, Shakir AA, Wang G, Lipkin WI, Wiley CA. Fatal fulminant pan-meningopolioencephalitis due to West Nile virus. Brain Pathol 2003; 13: 465–472.

Palmisano CT, Taylor V, Caillouet K, Byrd B, Wesson DM. Impact of West Nile virus outbreak upon St. Tammany Parish Mosquito Abatement District. J Am Mosq Control Assoc 2005; 21: 33–38.

Panthier R, Hannoun C, Beytout D, Mouchet J. [Epidemiology of West Nile virus. Study of a center in Camargue. 3.-Human diseases]. Ann Inst Pasteur (Paris) 1968; 115: 435–445.

Pealer LN, Marfin AA, Petersen LR, Lanciotti RS, Page PL, Stramer SL, Stobierski MG, Signs K, Newman B, Kapoor H, Goodman JL, Chamberland ME. Transmission of West Nile virus through blood transfusion in the United States in 2002. N Engl J Med 2003; 349: 1236–1245.

Penn RG, Guarner J, Sejvar JJ, Hartman H, Mccomb RD, Nevins DL, Bhatnagar J, Zaki SR. Persistent neuroinvasive West Nile virus infection in an immunocompromised patient. Clin Infect Dis 2006; 42: 680–683.

Perelman A, Stern J. Acute pancreatitis in West Nile Fever. Am J Trop Med Hyg 1974; 23: 1150–1152.

Petersen LR, Roehrig JT. West Nile virus: a reemerging global pathogen. Emerg Infect Dis 2001; 7: 611–614.

Philip CB, Smadel JE. Transmission of West Nile virus by infected *Aedes albopictus*. Proc Soc Exp Biol 1943; 53: 49–50.

Radt P. Clinical observations on patients with West Nile fever during outbreaks of the disease in 1950–1953. Harefuah 1955; 49: 41–44.

Sanchez-Guerrero SA, Romero-Estrella S, Rodriguez-Ruiz A, Infante-Ramirez L, Gomez A, Villanueva-Vidales E, Garcia-Torres M, Dominguez AM, Vazquez JA, Calderon ED, Valiente-Banuet L, Linnen JM, Broulik A, Harel W, Marin YLRA. Detection of West Nile virus in the Mexican blood supply. Transfusion 2006; 46: 111–117.

Schuffenecker I, Peyrefitte CN, El Harrak M, Murri S, Leblond A, Zeller HG. West Nile virus in Morocco, 2003. Emerg Infect Dis 2005; 11: 306–309.

Sejvar JJ, Bode AV, Marfin AA, Campbell GL, Ewing D, Mazowiecki M, Pavot PV, Schmitt J, Pape J, Biggerstaff BJ, Petersen LR. West Nile virus-associated flaccid paralysis. Emerg Infect Dis 2005; 11: 1021–1027.

Sejvar JJ, Haddad MB, Tierney BC, Campbell GL, Marfin AA, Van Gerpen JA, Fleischauer A, Leis AA, Stokic DS, Petersen LR. Neurologic manifestations and outcome of West Nile virus infection. JAMA 2003; 290: 511–515.

Shaman J, Day JF, Stieglitz M. Drought-induced amplification and epidemic transmission of West Nile virus in southern Florida. J Med Entomol 2005; 42: 134–141.

Shcherbakova SA, Bil'ko EA, Kliueva EV, Danilov AN, Plotnikova EA, Tarasov MA, Chekashov VN, Udovikov AI, Kniazeva TV, Shilov MM, Samoilova LV, Khramov VN, Kazakova LV, Kuklev EV, Kulichenko AN. [The ecology and prevalence of arboviruses on the territory of the Saratov Region]. Zh Mikrobiol Epidemiol Immunobiol 2005; 5: 27–30.

Smithburn KC. Differentiation of the West Nile virus from the viruses of St. Louis encephalitis and Japanese B encephalitis. J Immunol 1942; 44: 25–31.

Smithburn KC. Immunity to neurotropic viruses, especially those of the Japanese-B-West Nile group, among indigenous residents of India. Fed Proc 1953; 12: 460.

Smithburn KC, Hughes TP, Burke AW, Paul JH. A neurotropic virus isolated from the blood of a native of Uganda. Am J Trop Med 1940; 20: 471–492.

Smithburn KC, Jacobs HR. Neutralization-tests against neurotropic viruses with sera collected in central Africa. J Immunol 1942; 44: 9–23.

Smithburn KC, Taylor RM, Rizk F, Kader A. Immunity to certain arthropod-borne viruses among indigenous residents of Egypt. Am J Trop Med Hyg 1954; 3: 9–18.

Solomon T, Mallewa M. Dengue and other emerging flaviviruses. J Infect 2001; 42: 104–115.

Southam CM, Moore AE. Induced virus infections in man by the Egypt isolates of West Nile virus. Am J Trop Med Hyg 1954; 3: 19–50.

Spigland I, Jasinska-Klingberg W, Hofshi E, Goldblum N. [Clinical and laboratory observations in an outbreak of West Nile fever in Israel in 1957]. Harefuah 1958; 54: 275–280 (English & French abstracts 280–281).

Swayne DE, Beck JR, Smith CS, Shieh WJ, Zaki SR. Fatal encephalitis and myocarditis in young domestic geese (*Anser anser domesticus*) caused by West Nile virus. Emerg Infect Dis 2001; 7: 751–753.

Tahori AS, Sterk VV, Goldblum N. Studies on the dynamics of experimental transmission of West Nile virus by *Culex molestus*. Am J Trop Med Hyg 1955; 4: 1015–1027.

Tardei G, Ruta S, Chitu V, Rossi C, Tsai TF, Cernescu C. Evaluation of immunoglobulin M (IgM) and IgG enzyme immunoassays in serologic diagnosis of West Nile virus infection. J Clin Microbiol 2000; 38: 2232–2239.

Taylor RM, Hurlbut HS, Dressler HR, Spangler EW, Thrasher D. Isolation of West Nile virus from *Culex* mosquitoes. J Egypt Med Assoc 1953; 36: 199–208.

Tiawsirisup S, Platt KB, Tucker BJ, Rowley WA. Eastern cottontail rabbits (*Sylvilagus floridanus*) develop West Nile virus viremias sufficient for infecting select mosquito species. Vector Borne Zoonotic Dis 2005; 5: 342–350.

Tsai TF, Popovici F, Cernescu C, Campbell GL, Nedelcu NI. West Nile encephalitis epidemic in southeastern Romania. Lancet 1998; 352: 767–771.

Turell MJ, Dohm DJ, Sardelis MR, Oguinn ML, Andreadis TG, Blow JA. An update on the potential of North American mosquitoes (Diptera: *Culicidae*) to transmit West Nile virus. J Med Entomol 2005; 42: 57–62.

Watson JT, Jones RC, Gibbs K, Paul W. Dead crow reports and location of human West Nile virus cases, Chicago, 2002. Emerg Infect Dis 2004; 10: 938–940.

Weinberger M, Pitlik SD, Gandacu D, Lang R, Nassar F, Ben David D, Rubinstein E, Izthaki A, Mishal J, Kitzes R, Siegman-Igra Y, Giladi M, Pick N, Mendelson E, Bin H, Shohat T. West Nile fever outbreak, Israel, 2000: epidemiologic aspects. Emerg Infect Dis 2001; 7: 686–691.

Weinbren MP. The occurrence of West Nile virus in South Africa. S Afr Med J 1955; 29: 1092–1097.

Willis J. Metro Atlanta responds to West Nile virus: a coordinated public health response. Ethn Dis 2005; 15: S49–S51.

Wilson SD, Varia M, Lior LY. West Nile virus: the buzz on Ottawa residents' awareness, attitudes and practices. Can J Public Health 2005; 96: 109–113.

Work TH, Hurlbut HS, Taylor RM. Isolation of West Nile virus from hooded crow and rock pigeon in the Nile delta. Proc Soc Exp Biol Med 1953; 84: 719–722.

Work TH, Hurlbut HS, Taylor RM. Indigenous wild birds of the Nile delta as potential West Nile virus circulating reservoirs. Am J Trop Med Hyg 1955; 4: 872–888.

Yaremych SA, Warner RE, Mankin PC, Brawn JD, Raim A, Novak R. West Nile virus and high death rate in American crows. Emerg Infect Dis 2004; 10: 709–711.

Emerging Viruses in Human Populations
Edward Tabor (Editor)

DOI 10.1016/S0168-7069(06)16007-3

Monkeypox Virus Infections

Kurt D. Reed

Emerging Infectious Disease Laboratory, Marshfield Clinic Research Foundation, 1000 N. Oak Avenue, Marshfield, WI 54449, USA

Introduction

Monkeypox is an uncommon viral zoonosis caused by a member of the genus *Orthopoxvirus* (Breman, 2000). The disease is important to public health because the monkeypox virus (MPV) has a close genetic relationship to another orthopox-virus, variola virus (smallpox virus), and is capable of causing a clinical syndrome that resembles that caused by variola virus. Other important orthopoxviruses causing infections in humans include vaccinia virus (used for smallpox vaccination) and cowpox virus.

MPV was named as such because it was first recognized in association with nine outbreaks of vesicular exanthems among captive primates in laboratories and zoos during the 1950s and 1960s (Arita and Henderson, 1968; Arita et al., 1972). The first cases of human disease caused by this virus were reported in 1970 in Zaire (now the Democratic Republic of Congo). Prior cases of human monkeypox un-doubtedly occurred in central Africa but most likely were confused with smallpox. Since its initial recognition, monkeypox has been documented to occur sporadically in humans throughout central and western Africa, and is considered by some to be the most important orthopoxvirus now that smallpox has been eradicated.

Renewed interest in human monkeypox was generated by the unexpected emergence of the disease in the midwestern U.S. associated with the importation of infected rodents from western Africa (Reed et al., 2004). Additional interest has focused on MPV because it is considered to be a potential agent of bioterrorism.

Description of the agent

MPV is a large, complex, double-stranded DNA virus of the chordopoxvirus fam-ily. MPV is endemic in central and western Africa and is a classic zoonosis acquired through contact with infected rodents and squirrels. Secondary spread from person to person can occur among close contacts, but this occurs much less frequently than with smallpox virus. Two genetic clades of MPV are recognized, a Congo basin-derived clade associated with 2–10% mortality in unvaccinated individuals, and a west African clade associated with milder illness and very low mortality (Chen et al., 2005; Likos et al., 2005).

Epidemiology of MPV infections

Human monkeypox has probably occurred in central and western Africa for hundreds, if not thousands, of years but was overshadowed by smallpox until variola virus was eradicated in central Africa in the late 1960s. Unlike variola virus, MPV is a zoonotic pathogen. However, there is surprisingly little detailed information on the enzootic cycle of MPV in nature. Humans and monkeys are generally considered incidental hosts and the reservoirs that amplify the virus in natural settings are probably rodents or squirrels that inhabit the sub-Saharan rain forests (Khodakevich et al., 1988). Laboratory studies indicate MPV has a broad host range and can infect numerous species of small mammals. Field studies from the Democratic Republic of Congo have shown that rope squirrels and tree squirrels (*Funisciurus* and *Heliosciurus* spp., respectively) and Gambian giant rats (*Cricetomys* spp.) that inhabit agricultural areas have high seroprevalence rates for MPV and seem to be important in sustaining viral transmission in agricultural areas (Khodakevich et al., 1986).

Epidemiologic studies during 1970–1979 documented 47 cases of human monkeypox worldwide. Most of these cases ($n = 38$) occurred in the Democratic Republic of Congo with the remainder in the western African countries of Gabon, the Ivory Coast, Liberia, Nigeria, and Sierra Leone. Cases in the Democratic Republic of Congo were highly associated with animal contact and seven of the 47 cases (14.9%) were fatal. Secondary transmission occurred among 7.5% of family members (Breman et al., 1980).

Over the years there has been great concern that monkeypox might have the potential to emerge from central Africa and replace smallpox as a global health problem, but this appears to be unlikely. World Health Organization (WHO) surveillance between 1981 and 1986 in the Democratic Republic of Congo revealed that >70% of cases were associated with an animal source of infection; the remainder were due to secondary transmission. Most cases occurred in children and the mean age was 4.4 years. Although the rate of secondary transmission was several times higher than that observed during the 1970s, in no instance did the chain of transmission go beyond four generations, suggesting that MPV has low potential for epidemic spread (Jezek et al., 1986; Jezek and Fenner, 1988). Stochastic modeling of MPV transmission supported that conclusion (Jezek et al., 1987a). More recently, extended person-to-person transmission of MPV was observed in a hospital in the Democratic Republic of Congo where up to six sequential transmission cycles were hypothesized to have occurred (Learned et al.,

2005). This pattern of sustained transmission suggests that MPV may have the capacity to adapt to the human host more than that been previously observed.

The number of reported cases of human monkeypox declined after formal WHO surveillance ended in 1986. From 1986 to 1992, only 13 cases were reported in the medical literature and none were reported from 1993 to 1995 (Heymann et al., 1998). This trend suddenly reversed in 1996–1997 when more than 500 cases of suspected monkeypox were reported in the Kasai-Oriental province of Democratic Republic of Congo. This outbreak was associated with a low fatality rate (1–5%) and high person-to-person transmission (78%) compared to previous outbreaks. Since many of these suspected cases were not laboratory confirmed, some authors have speculated that the majority of cases were actually due to varicella rather than MPV (Hutin et al., 2001). From 1998 to 2002, greater than 1200 cases of monkeypox were reported to the Democratic Republic of Congo Ministry of Health. Of those cases that were laboratory confirmed, patient's age ranged from 10 months to 38 years (mean of 16.5 years) (Kebela, 2004). Active and passive surveillance for monkeypox continues on the African continent but is hampered by political unrest and lack of adequate public health resources.

In May and June of 2003, human MPV infections were identified for the first time in the western hemisphere (Reed et al., 2004). In total, 72 cases were reported, with 37 confirmed by laboratory testing. Epidemiologic investigation indicated that nearly all of the patients had been exposed directly or indirectly to ill prairie dogs (*Cynomys* spp.) that had been kept or sold as pets. Two of the patients were parents of other patients, who had provided direct care to their infected children and could possibly have acquired MPV by person-to-person transmission.

The prairie dogs had been housed with rodents that were part of a large shipment of animals imported from Ghana in western Africa. The shipment included rope squirrels, tree squirrels, Gambian giant rats, brushtail porcupines (*Atheurus* spp.), dormice (*Graphiurus* spp.), and striped mice (*Hybomys* spp.). Laboratory testing revealed that at least one Gambian giant rat, two rope squirrels, and three dormice were infected with MPV. Some of the infected rodents were sold to a pet distributor in the Chicago area, to which they were transported in association with prairie dogs. The exposed (and infected) prairie dogs were then sold to the index patient and others at pet "swap meets" in Wisconsin, Illinois, Indiana, and Ohio. Cases were also reported in Kansas and Missouri (MMWR, 2003).

Most of the patients in the U.S. outbreak had mild, self-limited disease in comparison to the more severe illness reported among African patients. The milder illness can be explained in part by the fact that many of the adults who were infected had previously received smallpox vaccination. In addition, the strain of MPV associated with the U.S. outbreak was of west African origin and is known to be less virulent than the Congo basin-derived strains. Of 69 patients for whom data are available, 18 were hospitalized. No deaths were reported. Two pediatric patients had serious clinical illness; one child had severe encephalitis requiring treatment in an intensive care unit for 14 days and the other had diffuse pox lesions and painful cervical and tonsillar lymphadenopathy and oropharyngeal lesions (Anderson et al., 2003; Huhn et al., 2005).

A significant concern during the outbreak in the U.S. was the possibility that MPV infection could spread to North American rodent populations and establish a zoonotic sylvan cycle of infection. To date, extensive investigations of that possibility have provided no evidence that MPV extended into local rodent populations as a result of the 2003 outbreak in humans and prairie dogs sold as pets.

Clinical features

The first human MPV infection was recognized in 1970 in a 9-month-old child living in Zaire, not long after smallpox was considered to have been eradicated from that country (Ladnyj et al., 1972). Over the next decade, clinical manifestations of MPV infection remained poorly defined, because fewer than 50 cases were documented. Initial descriptions suggested that the disease resembled smallpox in terms of morbidity and mortality, but that it was distinct in having low transmissibility between humans (Breman et al., 1980).

Observational studies of human monkeypox in central and western Africa during the 1980s revealed that MPV infection had an incubation period of 10–14 days and a period of infectivity during the first week of rash. MPV enters the body through skin abrasions, the upper respiratory tract mucosa, or by ingestion. During primary viremia the virus migrates to regional lymph nodes and then disseminates throughout the body. A prodrome of fever and malaise typically occurs 1–2 days prior to the onset of a rash and is associated with lymphadenopathy in around 90% of cases. The distribution of lymphadenopathy is variable and can include submandibular, cervical, axillary, and inguinal areas. It is important to note that smallpox is rarely associated with significant lymphadenopathy, making this a key distinguishing clinical feature between the two diseases.

The rash caused by MPV begins as papular lesions of 1–5 mm in diameter that progress through vesicular, pustular, and crusted stages over a period of 14–21 days (Fig. 1). The crusts eventually slough off, leaving depressed scars. Case descriptions from Africa emphasize a centrifugal pattern of spread that becomes generalized over time. However, a centripetal distribution of the rash, similar to that seen in chickenpox, has been described in a few cases (Jezek et al., 1987b).

Several unique clinical manifestations were noted among patients infected during the 2003 outbreak of monkeypox in the U.S. These included focal hemorrhagic necrosis, particularly at the sites of bites or scratches, and erythematous flares that may have been more apparent on light skin (Reed et al., 2004). The list of differential diagnoses for the rash lesions of monkeypox is long and includes smallpox, chickenpox, orf another name for contagious ecthyma. It is a parapoxvirus infection of sheep and goats that is transmissible to man, milker's nodule, erythema multiforme, drug eruptions, rickettsialpox, and eczema herpeticum.

Extracutaneous manifestations of MPV infection include cough, pharyngitis, a feeling of chest tightness, nausea, diarrhea, myalgia, and back pain. Complications

Inoculation lesions

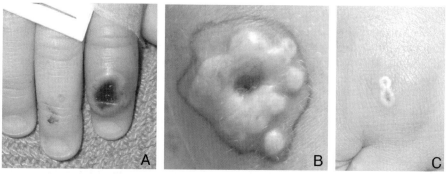

Dissemination lesions

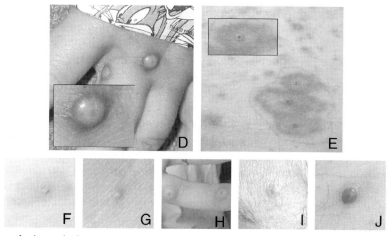

Evolution of primary lesions

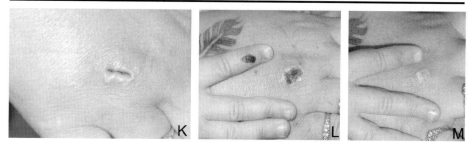

Fig. 1 Cutaneous lesions of human monkeypox. The top panels show primary inoculation lesions at the site of a prairie dog bite (A) or scratch (B and C). The middle panels show the variation of the appearance of disseminated lesions of monkeypox ranging from smallpox-like (D) to varicella-like (E–J). The lower panels (K–M) document the progression of a primary lesion from the pustular stage through scarring. (For colour version: see Colour Section on page 351).

can include secondary infections of skin and soft tissue (20%), pneumonitis (12%), ocular involvement (5%), and rarely, encephalitis (<1%) (Nalca et al., 2005).

Prior smallpox vaccination modulates the clinical course of human monkeypox disease in a number of aspects. In general, patients who were previously vaccinated against smallpox experience a milder illness and have lower morbidity and mortality. The rash of MPV infection tends to be more pleomorphic in individuals vaccinated against smallpox and more closely resembles the rash of chickenpox.

Laboratory diagnosis

Human monkeypox is a reportable disease; state and local health departments should be notified immediately of any suspected cases. Although the history and clinical characteristics can be helpful in differentiating between monkeypox and other causes of vesiculopustular eruptions, it is highly desirable that all cases be confirmed by laboratory testing. During the 2003 U.S. outbreak, the Centers for Disease Control and Prevention (CDC) recommended the following laboratory criteria for diagnosing human monkeypox cases: (1) isolation of MPV in culture; (2) demonstration of MPV DNA by PCR testing in a clinical sample; (3) electron microscopic evidence of an orthopoxvirus in the absence of exposure to another orthopoxvirus; and (4) immunohistochemical evidence of an orthopoxvirus in tissue in the absence of exposure to another orthopoxvirus.

MPV grows well in established cell lines and embryonated chicken eggs. Cell lines that MPV grows in include rhesus-monkey kidney, rabbit kidney, MRC-5, RD, B-SC-40, and Vero cells. Cytopathic effect usually occurs within 1–4 days and includes plaques of elongated and rounded cells with prominent cytoplasmic bridging and formation of syncytium. When MPV is grown in embryonated chicken eggs, it produces small, opaque, hemorrhagic pocks on the chorioallantoic membranes of the chicken egg that are distinct from lesions produced by other orthopoxviruses.

Samples from suspected cases of MPV infection that are appropriate for virus isolation include biopsies and touch preparations refer to pressing a glass slide against the lesion so that adherent cellular material can be stained and viewed under a microscope of skin lesions, lymph nodes, oropharyngeal swabs, and whole blood during the prodromal stage (Damon and Esposito, 2003). MPV-infected clinical samples can be handled safely by laboratory personnel who have received smallpox vaccination within the past 10 years and who use strict biosafety level 2 containment. As a practical consideration, most diagnostic laboratories in the U.S. have limited experience with isolating orthopoxviruses from clinical specimens and should refer specimens from suspected cases to their state health laboratory or to the CDC.

A number of molecular diagnostic tests are available to aid in the definitive diagnosis of MPV infections. DNA-based tests, such as PCR with restriction endonuclease digestion or sequencing of the hemagglutinnin gene (HA), can confirm the identity of an orthopoxvirus to the species level and can be accomplished in just a few hours. This method is based on the use of primers EACP1 and EACP2 (for Old World orthopoxviruses) or NACP1 and NACP2 (for New World orthopoxviruses) (Damon and Esposito, 2003). Additional PCR protocols target the A-type inclusion body protein or B cytokine response modifier (Ropp et al., 1995; Meyer et al., 1997; Meyer et al., 1998).

Electron microscopy (EM) is an important front-line method for the laboratory diagnosis of poxvirus infections because it is a simple technique that can rapidly exclude varicella virus (chickenpox), a herpesvirus, from the differential diagnosis (Hazelton and Gelderblom, 2003; Curry et al., 2006). Transmission EM of tissue biopsies reveals virions with dumbbell-shaped inner cores highly characteristic of poxviruses. However, this technique does not distinguish between orthopoxviruses and the other genera of poxviruses. When vesicle fluid or tissue culture supernatants are examined by EM of specimens negatively stained with phosphotungstic acid or another heavy metal, orthopoxviruses have a distinctive brick-shaped appearance with regularly spaced threadlike ridges on the exposed surfaces. In contrast, parapoxviruses appear ovoid with spiraling criss-cross surface projections. Negative stain EM of cell culture supernatants provided the first clues that the 2003 U.S. outbreak was due to an orthopoxvirus (Reed et al., 2004).

The histopathology of monkeypox skin lesions mirrors the clinical progression of these lesions. Early lesions contain ballooning degeneration of basal keratinocytes and spongiosis of a mildly acanthotic epidermis. These progress to full thickness necrosis of a markedly acanthotic epidermis containing few viable keratinocytes. A mixed inflammatory infiltrate and progressive exocytosis with the keratinocyte necrosis appear, involving the superficial and deep vascular plexes, eccrine units, and follicles. Multinucleated syncytial keratinocytes and hyaline intracytoplasmic inclusions appear, reflecting the presence of virus in the cells.

The histologic differential diagnosis includes herpes simplex, varicella, and other poxviruses. EM can be used to distinguish between herpesvirus and poxvirus infections. Immunohistochemistry with anti-orthopoxvirus antibodies can be useful to detect viral antigen within the keratinocytes of lesions in the epidermis, in the follicular and eccrine epithelium, and in scattered dermal macrophages (Bayer-Garner, 2005). The histologic, ultrastructural, and immunohistochemical appearance of MPV infection are shown in Fig. 2.

Use of serologic tests to identify MPV infection is difficult because of the close antigenic relationships among the various orthopoxviruses. Neutralization tests, hemagglutination inhibition assays, and ELISAs are available to detect orthopox antibodies in patients' sera, but the sensitivity of these assays ranges from 50% to 95%. Currently, there is no widely available serologic test that is sensitive and specific for identifying MPV infections (Damon and Esposito, 2003). However, serological testing has proven useful in epidemiologic studies. A retrospective study of individuals potentially exposed to MPV in the 2003 U.S. outbreak revealed three cases of asymptomatic infection that occurred in persons who had been vaccinated against smallpox decades earlier (Hammarlund et al., 2005).

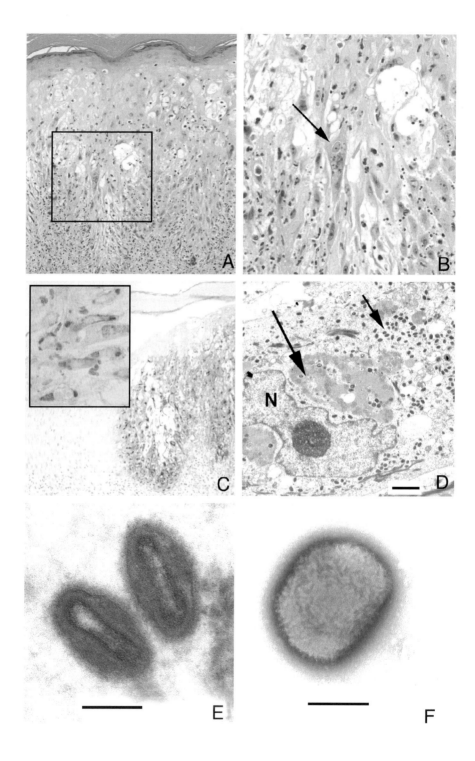

Prevention of MPV infections

Vaccination with vaccinia virus (smallpox vaccine) is highly protective (around 85%) against MPV infection. Post-exposure smallpox vaccination is indicated for persons who are at high risk of MPV infection, including those investigating animal or human monkeypox cases, health care workers caring for infected patients, and laboratory workers who handle specimens that may contain MPV. Vaccination within 4 days after initial close contact with a confirmed monkeypox case is recommended by CDC and should be considered up to 14 days after exposure. Vaccinia immune globulin may be considered as a prophylactic for exposed persons with impaired T-cell function who would not be candidates for vaccination (Di Giulio and Eckburg, 2004).

Treatment of MPV infections

Treatment of severe illness with vaccinia immune globulin should be considered but no data are available documenting sensitivity in treating human monkeypox. There are no antiviral drugs approved for treating monkeypox. Cidofovir is a broad-spectrum antiviral drug with known *in vitro* activity against cytomegalovirus and many other DNA viruses, including MPV. Although clinical experience with the use of cidofovir in human monkeypox infections is limited, antiviral treatment with that agent was more effective than post-exposure smallpox vaccination in the cynomolgus monkey (*Macaca fascicularis*) model (Stittelaar et al., 2006).

Transmission of MPV within hospitals has been described but the overall risk appears low. CDC recommends a combination of precautions, including standard, contact, and large droplet precautions for infection control purposes. Airborne precautions for small aerosolized droplets ($<5\mu m$ in size) should be implemented whenever possible. All laboratory specimens should be handled in a biological safety cabinet (Fleischauer et al., 2005).

Fig. 2 Histological, ultrastructural, and immunohistochemical appearance of MPV infection. Panel A: Scattered degenerating and necrotic keratinocytes are shown within the epidermis along with a moderate inflammatory cell infiltrate in the superficial dermis (hematoxylin and eosin). Panel B: Higher magnification of the boxed area shows multinucleated cells (long arrow) and eosinophilic viral inclusion bodies. Panel C: Strong immunoreactivity for orthopoxvirus antigen is present in the epidermis. Panel D: Transmission electron microscopy shows virions within the cytoplasm of a keratinocyte, including immature forms undergoing assembly (long arrow) and mature forms (short arrow). Panel E: High magnification shows the characteristic dumbbell-shaped inner core of poxviruses. Panel F: Negative staining of a virion from cell culture shows the brick-shaped particle with regularly spaced, threadlike ridges on the exposed surface. (For colour version: see Colour Section on page 352).

Conclusions

The 2003 U.S. outbreak of MPV was a sobering reminder of the impact that emerging infectious diseases can have on the public health. That emergence of monkeypox in North America was linked directly to the importation of rodents from West Africa and subsequent co-mingling of these animals with animals native to North America. On June 11, 2003, the CDC and the Food and Drug Administration issued a joint order prohibiting the importation of all African rodents into the U.S. The order also banned within the U.S. any sale, distribution, transport, or release into the environment of prairie dogs and six specific genera of African rodents. On November 4, 2003 the joint order was replaced by an interim final rule that maintained the importation ban. Animals can still be imported for scientific, exhibition, or educational purposes with a valid permit issued by CDC.

Although the close genetic relationship between MPV and smallpox has raised concern about potential for use of MPV as an agent of bioterrorism, the low secondary attack rate and generally self-limited illness associated with MPV in humans makes its use as a weapon unlikely. This situation could change dramatically if genetic engineering were used to increase the transmissibility and virulence of the pathogen to humans, a change that remains only theoretical at present.

References

Anderson JG, Frenkel LD, Homann S, Guffey J. A case of severe monkeypox disease in an American child: emerging infections and changing professional values. Pediatr Infect Dis J 2003; 22: 1093.

Arita L, Henderson DA. Smallpox and monkeypox in non-human primates. Bull World Health Organ 1968; 39: 277.

Arita LR, Gispen S, Kalter S, Wah LT, Marennikova SS, Netter R, Tagaya I. Outbreaks of monkeypox and serological surveys in non-human primates. Bull World Health Organ 1972; 46: 625.

Bayer-Garner IB. Monkeypox virus: histologic, immunohistochemical and electron-microscopic findings. J Cutan Pathol 2005; 32: 28.

Breman JG. Monkeypox: an emerging infection for humans? In: Emerging Infections 4 (Scheld MW, Craig WA, Hughes JM, editors). Washington, DC: ASM Press; 2000; p. 45.

Breman JG, Kalisa R, Steniowski MV, Zanotto E, Gromyko AI, Arita I. Human monkeypox, 1970–79. Bull World Health Organ 1980; 58: 165.

Chen N, Li G, Liszewski MK, Atkinson JP, Jahrling PB, Feng Z, Schriewer J, Buck C, Wang C, Lefkowitz EJ, Esposito JJ, Harms T, Damon IK, Roper RL, Upton C, Buller RML. Virulence differences between monkeypox virus isolates from West Africa and the Congo basin. Virology 2005; 340: 46.

Curry A, Appleton H, Dowsett B. Application of transmission electron microscopy to the clinical study of viral and bacterial infections: present and future. Micron 2006; 37: 91.

Damon IK, Esposito JJ. Poxviruses that infect humans. In: Manual of Clinical Microbiology (Murray PR, Barron EJ, Jorgensen JH, Pfaller MA, Yolken RH, editors). 8th ed. Washington, DC: ASM Press; 2003.

Di Giulio DB, Eckburg PB. Human monkeypox: an emerging zoonosis. Lancet Infect Dis 2004; 4: 199.

Fleischauer AT, Kile JC, Davidson M, Fischer M, Karem KL, Teclaw R, Messersmith H, Pontones P, Beard BA, Braden ZH, Cono J, Sejvar JJ, Khan AS, Damon I, Kuehnert MJ. Evaluation of human-to-human transmission of monkeypox from infected patients to health care workers. Clin Infect Dis 2005; 40: 689.

Hammarlund E, Lewis MW, Carter SV, Amanna I, Hansen SG, Strelow LI, Wong SW, Yoshihara P, Hanifin JM, Slifka MK. Multiple diagnostic techniques identify previously vaccinated individuals with protective immunity against monkeypox. Nat Med 2005; 11: 1005.

Hazelton PR, Gelderblom HR. Electron microscopy for rapid diagnosis of infectious agents in emergent situations. Emerg Infect Dis 2003; 9: 294.

Heymann DL, Szczeniowski M, Esteves K. Re-emergence of monkeypox in Africa: a review of the past six years. Br Med Bull 1998; 54: 693.

Huhn GD, Bauer AM, Yorita K, Graham MB, Sejvar J, Likos A, Damon IK, Reynolds MG, Kuehnert MJ. Clinical characteristics of human monkeypox, and risk factors for severe disease. Clin Infect Dis 2005; 41: 1742.

Hutin YJ, Williams RJ, Malfait P, Pebody R, Loparev VN, Ropp SL, Rodriquez M, Knight JC, Tshioko FK, Khan AS, Szczeniowski MV, Esposito JJ. Outbreak of human monkeypox, Democratic Republic of Congo, 1996 to 1997. Emerg Infect Dis 2001; 7: 434

Jezek Z, Arita I, Mutombo M, Dunn C, Nakano JH, Szczeniowski M. Four generations of probable person-to-person transmission of human monkeypox. Am J Epidemiol 1986; 123: 1004.

Jezek Z, Fenner F. Human monkeypox. In: Monographs in Virology (Melnick JL, editor). vol. 17. Basel, Switzerland: Karger, 1988.

Jezek Z, Grab B, Dixon H. Stochastic model for interhuman spread of monkeypox. Am J Epidemiol 1987a; 126: 1082.

Jezek Z, Szczeniowski M, Paluku KM, Jutombo M. Human monkeypox: clinical features in 282 patients. J Infect Dis 1987b; 156: 293.

Kebela B. Le profi épidémiologique de monkeypox en RDC, 1998–2002. Bulletin Épidémiologique de la République Democratique du Congo 2004; 29: 2.

Khodakevich L, Jezek Z, Messinger D. Isolation of monkeypox virus from wild squirrel infected in nature. Lancet 1986; 1: 98.

Khodakevich L, Jezek Z, Messinger D. Monkeypox virus: ecology and public health significance. Bull World Health Organ 1988; 66: 747.

Ladnyj ID, Ziegler P, Kima E. A human infection caused by monkeypox virus in Basankusu Territory, Democratic Republic of Congo. Bull World Health Organ 1972; 46: 593.

Learned LA, Reynolds MG, Wassa DW, Li Y, Olson VA, Karem K, Stempora LL, Braden ZH, Kline R, Likos A, Libama F, Moudzeo H, Bolanda JD, Tarangonia P, Boumandoki P, Formenty P, Harvey JM, Damon IK. Extended interhuman transmission of monkeypox in a hospital community in the Republic of the Congo, 2003. Am J Trop Med Hyg 2005; 73: 428.

Likos AM, Sammons SA, Olson VA, Frace AM, Li Y, Olsen-Rasmussen M, Davidson W, Galloway R, Khristova ML, Reynolds MG, Zhao H, Carroll DS, Curns A, Formenty P, Espisito JJ, Regnery RL, Damon IK. A tale of two clades: monkeypox viruses. J Gen Virol 2005; 86: 2661.

Meyer H, Ropp SL, Esposito JJ. Gene for A-type inclusion body protein is useful for a polymerase chain reaction assay to differentiate orthopoxviruses. J Virol Methods 1997; 64: 217.

Meyer H, Ropp SL, Esposito JJ. Poxviruses. In: Diagnostic Virology Protocols, Vol. 12 of Methods in Molecular Medicine (Stephenson JR, Warnes A, editors). Totowa, NJ: Humana Press; 1998 p. 199.

MMWR. Update: multistate outbreak of monkeypox—Illinois, Indiana, Kansas, Missouri, Ohio, and Wisconsin. Morb Mortal Wkly Rep 2003; 52, 642.

Nalca A, Rimoin AW, Bavari S, Whitehouse CA. Reemergence of monkeypox: prevalence, diagnostics, and countermeasures. Clin Infect Dis 2005; 41: 1765.

Reed KD, Melski JW, Graham MB, Regnery RL, Sotir MJ, Wegner MV, Kazmierczak JJ, Stratman EJ, Li Y, Fairley JA, Swain GR, Olson VA, Sargent EK, Kehl SC, Frace MA, Kline R, Foldy SL, Davis JP, Damon IK. The detection of monkeypox in humans in the Western Hemisphere. N Engl J Med 2004; 350: 342.

Ropp SL, Jin Q, Knight JC, Massung RF, Esposito JJ. PCR strategy for identification and differentiation of smallpox and other orthopoxviruses. J Clin Microbiol 1995; 33: 2069.

Stittelaar KJ, Neyts J, Naesens L, van Amerongen G, van Lavieren RF, Holy A, De Clercq E, Niesters HG, Fries E, Maas C, Mulder PG, van der Zeijst BA, Osterhaus AD. Antiviral treatment is more effective than smallpox vaccination upon lethal monkeypox virus infection. Nature 2006; 439: 745.

Emerging Viruses in Human Populations
Edward Tabor (Editor)

DOI 10.1016/S0168-7069(06)16008-5

Hantaviruses in the Old and New World

J. Clement, P. Maes, M. Van Ranst

Hantavirus Reference Centre, Laboratory of Clinical and Epidemiological Virology, Rega Institute, Katholieke Universiteit Leuven, Minderbroedersstraat 10, B3000 Leuven, Belgium.

Introduction

Hantavirus is a genus in the *Bunyaviridae* family, comprising more than 30 different hantavirus (HTV) species. HTV is the only haemorrhagic fever virus with a ubiquitous, worldwide distribution, including the temperate regions of the northern hemisphere. Increased risk of HTV disease occurs through exposure to excreta of wild (or laboratory) rodents, which are the main carriers of HTV in nature. Until 1993, the majority of known HTV serotypes affected the kidney as the primary target organ, explaining why the disease was first called "nephropathia epidemica" (NE) in the western world. Today, the most commonly used name for this disease is "haemorrhagic fever with renal syndrome" (HFRS), which is the official WHO name for it. This term is now mainly used for describing disease caused by the Hantaan virus (HTNV), an HTV in Asia and Eastern Russia, where the clinical picture is often more severe than that caused by the Puumala virus (PUUV), which is the prevalent form in Europe. Sin Nombre virus (SNV), however, isolated after a 1993 epidemic in the USA, seems to affect primarily the lungs, where it causes a viral form of adult respiratory distress syndrome (ARDS), now called hantavirus pulmonary syndrome, or "HPS" (Duchin et al., 1994; Hjelle et al., 1995).

Although only recently recognized, HTVs are not "new" viruses, since phylogenetic studies show that they are the product of millions of years of co-evolution with their respective rodent hosts. This explains the differences between HTVs of the New and the Old World, but also some common features.

It is worth noting that humans are an evolutionary "dead-end" for HTV infection, since the pronounced immunological response in man after a hantaviral infection often leads to killing of the infecting virus. In some severe clinical cases however the infected human host is killed by the infection.

Historical background

The first description of the so-called "Songo-fever", later called "Epidemic haemorrhagic fever" (EHF) dates back to the early 1930s, when Japanese troops invaded Manchuria (northern China) and suffered 12,600 cases of a then-unknown disease with fever. During the Korean War (1951–1953), Western medicine was suddenly confronted for the first time with an unknown acute febrile illness with multi-organ dysfunction (mainly shock, acute renal failure [ARF], and haemorrhage), with a mortality rate between 10% and 15%, and affecting over 3000 United Nations troops (Earle, 1954). Despite an enormous investigative effort by a special Haemorrhagic Fever Commission of the US Army, it was not until 1976 that Lee and co-workers discovered a virus-specific antigen in the lungs of a Korean striped field mouse (*Apodemus agrarius Coreae*), a discovery that led to the isolation and characterization of the responsible agent in 1977 (Lee et al., 1978). This first prototype agent was called HTNV, after the river Hantaan, which runs near the 38th parallel between North and South Korea, where most of the cases were recorded, and where HTNV-infected rodents were trapped.

The first clinical description of NE in Europe was in 1934 in Sweden, where a "kidney disease with peculiar symptoms"(Myhrman, 1934) and a "nephritis simulating an acute abdomen"(Zetterholm, 1934) were independently reported. German troops in Finnish Lapland suffered thousands of cases of "Feldnephritis" during World War II (Stuhlfauth, 1943). A virus in the lungs of the red bank vole (*Clethrionomys glareolus*), collected in Puumala, Finland (PUUV strain) and Sweden (Hällnäs strain) (Niklasson and LeDuc, 1984), was shown to react with antiserum from European patients with NE and from Korean patients with HFRS. Thus, exactly half a century after its first clinical description in Scandinavia, the virus causing NE was successfully adapted to Vero E6 cell culture and appeared to be related to the Korean prototype HTNV.

Hantaviruses, their rodent hosts, and routes of transmission

Hantaviruses

HTVs are the only non-arthropod-borne viruses in the *Bunyaviridae* family, in contrast to the other human and animal *Bunyaviridae* pathogens, such as Crimean–Congo haemorrhagic fever (CCHF) virus, transmitted by ticks, the sandfly fever viruses (phleboviruses), causing Toscana meningo-encephalitis virus and Pappataci fever, transmitted by sandflies, and Rift Valley fever (RFV) virus, transmitted by mosquitos. Both CCHF and sandfly fever viruses are present in Southern Europe and can mimic HTV disease. Like all other *Bunyaviridae*, HTVs have a lipid envelope, and contain a negative-sense tripartite RNA genome. HTVs are notoriously difficult to culture, and hence have less risk of use for bioterrorism (Clement, 2003a). Owing to their lipid coating, HTVs are sensitive to heat, acid pH, detergents, formalin, lipid solvents, and chlorite (bleach) solutions.

Each HTV serotype has its own principal rodent vector, its own geographic distribution, and its own more-or-less specific clinical expression. All have rodent hosts belonging to the *Muridae* family, consisting of the subfamilies *Arvicolinae* (voles), *Murinae* (Old World rats and mice), or *Sigmodontinae* (New World rats and mice) (Fig. 1). Seoul virus (SEOV) is the only HTV spread worldwide, by murine wild (and laboratory) rats.

Certain HTVs have a known pathogenicity for humans (shown in Table 1). The chronology of their discovery is noteworthy:

1. The first clinically important HTVs to be isolated (HTNV and SEOV) were found in the early 1980s in the Far East, followed (with the exception for PUUV) by the isolation of European species more than a decade later. HTNV

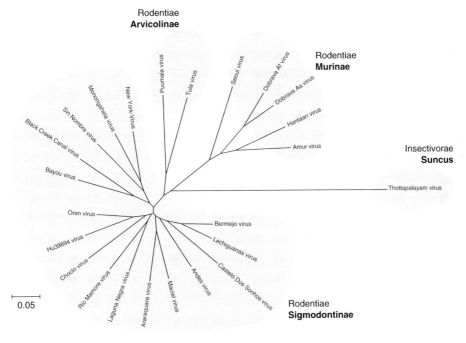

Fig. 1 Neighbour joining phylogenetic tree based on the S segment of hantaviruses known to be pathogenic (except Thottapalayam virus) and for which an S segment sequence was available. The virus groups carried by the *Rodentiae* family Arvicolinae, Sigmodontinae and Murinae, and by the *Insectivorae* family Suncus are indicated. Genbank accession numbers of the S segment nucleotide sequences: Amur virus (AB127997), Andes virus (NC003466), Araraquara virus (AF307325), Bayou virus (L36929), Black Creek Canal virus (L39949), Bermejo virus (AF482713), Castelo Dos Sonhos virus (AF307324), Choclo virus (DQ285046), Dobrava virus Aa strain (AJ009773), Dobrava virus Af strain (AJ131673), Hantaan virus (AB127998), Hu39694 virus (AF482711), Laguna Negra virus (AF005727), Lechiguanas virus (AF482714), Maciel virus (AF482716), Monongahela virus (U32591), New York virus (U09488), Orán virus (AF482715), Puumala virus (NC005224), Rio Segundo virus (U18100), Seoul virus (AY273791), Sin Nombre virus (NC005216), Thottapalayam virus (AY526097), and Tula virus (NC005227).

Table 1

Pathogenic hantavirus genotypes known up to 2005

Hantavirus serotype	First isolation or genotyping	Main rodent vector (geographic locale)	Human illness	Type of spread
1. **Hantaan (HTNV)**	1978	*Apodemus agrarius mantchuricus* (striped field mouse) (Asia, Eastern Russia and Southern Europe)	Severe: KHF, EHF, HFRS	Rural
2. **Puumala (PUUV)**	1980	*Clethrionomys glareolus* (bank vole) (Europe and Western Russia)	Mild: NE	Rural
3. Seoul (**SEOV**)	1982	*Rattus norvegicus* (Norway or brown rat) *Rattus rattus* (black rat) (worldwide)	Intermediate: HFRS	Urban and rural
4. **Dobrava (DOBV-Af)**	1992	*Apodemus flavicollis* (yellow-necked field mouse) (Balkans, Central and Eastern Europe, Middle-East)	Very severe: HFRS	Rural
5. **Sin Nombre virus (SNV)**	1993	*Peromyscus maniculatus* (deer mouse) (Canada and USA)	HPS	Rural
6. Juquitiba (JUQV)	1993	Unknown (Brazil)	HPS	Rural
7. **Tula (TULV)**	1994	*Microtus arvalis* (common vole) (Central and Eastern Europe)	HFRS	Rural
8. **New York (NYV)**	1995	*Peromyscus leucopus* (white-footed mouse) (Canada and Eastern USA)	HPS	Rural
9. **Black Creek Canal (BCCV)**	1995	*Sigmodon hispidus* (hispid cotton rat) (Eastern and Southern USA to Venezuela, Peru)	HPS	Rural
10. **Bayou (BAYV)**	1995	*Oryzomys palustris* (marsh rice rat) (Louisiana)	HPS	Rural
11. **Monongahela (MONV)**	1996	*P. maniculatus nubiterrae* (forest form) (cloudland deer mouse) (Canada and Eastern USA)	HPS	Rural

Table 1 (*continued*)

Hantavirus serotype	First isolation or genotyping	Main rodent vector (geographic locale)	Human illness	Type of spread
12. **Andes** (**ANDV**)	1996	*Oligoryzomys longicaudatus* (southern) (long-tailed rice rat) (Argentina, Chile, Uruguay)	HPS	Rural and urban
13. **Rio Mamoré** (**RMV**)	1997	*Oligoryzomys microtis* (small-eared rice rat) (Bolivia and Peru)	HPS	Rural
14. **Laguna Negra** (**LNV**)	1997	*Calomys laucha* (white paunch mouse) (Paraguay and Bolivia)	HPS	Rural
15. Hu 39694	1997	Unknown (Central Argentina)	HPS	Rural
16. **Dobrava-Aa** (**DOBV-Aa**)	1997	*Apodemus agrarius agrarius* (striped field mouse) (East and Central Europe)	HFRS	Rural
17. Orán (ORNV)	1998	*Oligoryzomys longicaudatus* (northern) (long-tailed rice rat) (Northern and Western Argentina)	HPS	Rural
18. Lechiguanas (LECHV)	1998	*Oligoryzomys flavescens* (yellow pygmy rice rat) (Central Argentina)	HPS	Rural
19. Araraquara (ARAV)	1999	Unknown (Brazil)	HPS	Rural
20. Castelo dos Sonhos (CASV)	1999	Unknown (Brazil)	HPS	Rural
21. Amur (AMRV)	2000	*Apodemus peninsulae* (Korean field mouse) (Far Eastern Russia)	HFRS	Rural
22. Far East (FEV)	2000	*Apodemus peninsulae* (Korean field mouse) (Far Eastern Russia)	HFRS	Rural
23. Choclo (CHOV)	2000	*Oligoryzomys fulvescens* (fulvous pygmy rice rat) (Panama)	HPS	Rural
24. Bermejo (BMJV)	2002	*Oligoryzomys chacoensis* (chacoan pygmy rice rat) (Central Argentina, Bolivia)	HPS	Rural

Note: Genotypes in bold are those of which at least one (rodent or human) virus isolate exists; others were detected by PCR. EHF: epidemic haemorrhagic fever; HFRS: haemorrhagic fever with renal syndrome; HPS: hantavirus pulmonary syndrome; KHF: Korean haemorrhagic fever; and NE: nephropathia epidemica.

and SEOV today remain the most important HTVs, representing more than 90% of reported cases. Mixed epidemics of HTNV and SEOV are a major public health problem in China, and have been so recognized since the 1930s; their peak incidence of 115,985 sero-confirmed cases (fatality rate 2.2%) occurred in 1986. The average number of cases in China during the past decade was still high, with about 50,000 cases per year, despite the successful introduction of programs to trap rats and to begin vaccination of the population (Clement et al., 1998).

2. The first HTV described in the Americas (SNV, 1993) was discovered almost a decade after the first European HTV (PUUV, 1984). Although the number of HPS cases in South America each year is now greater than the number of North American HPS cases, all together they amount to not more than a 100 reported cases per year, whereas European NE cases consist of at least a 1000 per year, and East Asian HFRS cases consist of more than 10,000 cases per year. However, the number of publications about HTVs grew exponentially after America was first confronted with HPS in 1993.

Several "new" HTV serotypes have recently been discovered. Dobrava virus (DOBV) is a "newer" murine European HTV serotype with a documented presence in the Balkans, Russia, and Central Europe. In addition to the serotype DOBV-Af, isolated from a yellow-necked wood mouse (*Apodemus flavicollis*) captured in the 1980s in Dobrava, Slovenia, a second but distinct DOBV strain, called DOBV-Aa, has been isolated (Table 1). DOBV-Aa is also called Saaremaa virus (SAAV) by some Scandinavian authors, and may be in fact the same virus, although the debate is not closed (Klempa et al., 2003a; Sironen et al., 2005). The SAAV strain was isolated in 1999 from a striped field mouse (*A. agrarius*) in Estonia (Nemirov et al., 1999), and was later shown to have the potential to infect humans (Lundkvist et al., 2002). However, in typical cases of HFRS, the infecting agent SAAV could never be clearly differentiated from the previously described DOBV (Clement et al., 2003b). In contrast, an HFRS case in Germany was the first to be linked definitively to DOBV-Aa by molecular methods (Klempa et al., 2004). Moreover, most DOBV cases of HFRS in Central Europe may in fact be caused by the DOBV-Aa strain (Klempa et al., 2005). Tula virus (TULV), isolated from European common voles (*Microtus* spp.) until recently had no known pathogenic potential for humans. In 2003, however, an HFRS case with both renal and pulmonary involvement associated with TULV infection was documented in Germany for the first time (Klempa, 2003B).

Rodent hosts

The phylogeny and epidemiology of HTVs are closely linked to those of their respective rodent reservoirs, to a degree almost unique in zoonotic diseases (Clement and Van Ranst, 2000a). The phylogeny of the greater than 30 HTV species now recognized is almost perfectly mirrored by the phylogeny of their respective rodent hosts, confirming a very narrow co-evolution between rodent and virus during millions of years (Table 1; Fig. 1). This close virus–rodent relationship also defines the current geographic repartition of HTVs worldwide. Each rodent species has its preferred habitat in a biotope, defined by climatic conditions and food supply. As in all other zoonoses, the recognition of the responsible vector is important for a better understanding of the dynamics of the disease, for its prevention, and for the diagnostic and epidemiological value of studies comparing rodent and human tissues with modern biomolecular tools such as polymerase chain reaction (PCR) (Clement et al., 1998).

For instance, the preferred habitat of the red bank vole (*Clethrionomys glareolus*), the natural reservoir in Europe of PUUV, is limited to mixed forests of deciduous broadleaf trees (beeches and oaks) and pine trees, present in most of Europe and the southern part of Siberia. Moreover, the bank vole is one of the most common small mammals in these forested regions (Clement et al., 1994a). This arvicoline rodent feeds mainly on oak and beech seeds. In temperate Western and Central Europe, the so-called "mast years" of forest trees that occur following exceptionally warm and humid summers, can produce high to very high seed crops, resulting in an up to 10-fold higher local bank vole population. This in turn can lead to occasional human outbreaks of NE (Clement et al., 1994b). The mixed forest habitat, however, is replaced in Central and North Siberia by the tundra, and in southern Europe by the drier so-called "Mediterranean shrub", explaining why so few NE cases are reported in Siberia, Spain, Portugal, Italy, and Greece.

American HTV strains that cause HPS are carried by another common wild rodent, the deer mouse (*Peromyscus maniculatus*). It can also be carried by other species of the New World *Sigmodontinae* subfamily, which are absent in Eurasia (Childs et al., 1994; Hjelle et al., 1995).

Thottapalayam virus (TPMV) is the only HTV isolated from a non-rodent, hence its unique place on the dendrogram (Fig. 1). It was isolated in 1964 near Vellore in Southern India from a shrew, *Suncus murinus*, which is an insectivore, not a rodent (Clement et al., 2000b). This is the only indigenous HTV documented so far in India. To date, no human pathogenicity for TPMV has been shown (and it is therefore not listed in Table 1). Interestingly, PUUV may be a cause of fatal Indian cases of HTV infection with both kidney and lung involvement (see below), although the bank vole is not found in India. IgG and IgM reactions to a PUUV antigen in an immunoblot were found in these Indian patients (Clement et al., 2000b, 2006). These observations suggest the fascinating possibility of cross-reactions of PUUV with TPMV or with a yet-unknown HTV strain in India.

Simultaneous natural infection with more than one HTV species in a single rodent species has not been demonstrated so far. Even when two different HTVs (e.g. HTNV and DOBV-Aa, see Table 1) appear to be carried by the same rodent species (*Apodemus agrarius*), this unusual situation actually occurs because the two HTV species are in fact carried by two different subspecies of the same rodent population, in this case *A. agrarius mantchuricus* for HTNV and *A. agrarius agrarius* for SAAV or DOBV-Aa. In this case, the genetic difference between the two HTVs is more important than between the rodent carriers. This is best explained by a switchover during the long evolution of HTVs to adapt to carriage by one rodent species to carriage by another genetically more distant rodent (sub) species.

Transmission

HTV is transmitted to humans by rodent excretions and aerosols thereof, consisting of infectious respiratory and urinary droplets from apparently healthy rodent carriers. It is likely that infected rodents excrete infectious virus in saliva, urine, faeces, and from their lungs, for the duration of their lives. The survival time of HTV from these excretions in the environment is not known. Whereas most patients with proven HTV disease actually can recall sighting rodents, whether in Europe (Clement et al., 1994c, 1996; Van Loock et al., 1999) or in the US (Zeitz et al., 1995), prior physical contact with rodents is almost never reported (Dournon et al., 1984), except in the case of laboratory-acquired infections (Desmyter et al., 1983; Dournon et al., 1984). Epidemiological studies of farm workers in China (Xu et al., 1985) and of shepherds and woodcutters in Greece (Antoniadis et al., 1987) revealed a high infection rate among individuals sleeping on the ground. This was also observed in a case-control study among US military in the region of Ulm (southern Germany) after a 1990 outbreak of NE during a winter field exercise (Clement et al., 1996). This Ulm outbreak was remarkable for its very high attack rate in a single unit encamped on vole-infested ground, for its almost equal male-to-female infection rate, and for the fact that in the neighbouring city of Ulm not a single civilian case of NE was reported during the same winter. Thus, campers and trekkers are at increased risk when sleeping among rodent burrows, even in mountain regions of southern Europe where bank voles are rare (Keyaerts et al., 2004). This risk may even be greater when sleeping in confined spaces that are infested with rodents (e.g. caravans, mountain refuges, hunter lodges, fisher cabins, in both the Americas [Zeitz et al., 1995] and in Europe [Van Loock et al., 1999]).

Person-to-person transmission of HTV appears to be extremely rare. It was reported for the first time during an HPS outbreak in southwest Argentina in 1996, involving 16 cases (Wells et al., 1997; Toro et al., 1998), and caused by ANDV (south lineage). Noticeably, ANDV is also the only American HTV to be isolated from human serum (Galeno et al., 2002) and is one of the very few HTVs that can cause lethal disease resembling HPS in an animal model (in the Syrian golden hamster) (Hooper et al., 2001).

Person-to-person transmission of ANDV (Cent BsAs lineage) may also have occurred in 4 clusters of HPS in the province of Buenos Aires, Argentina (Martinez et al., 2005), based on epidemiological and genetic data. Prolonged and close contact in confined spaces (a 14-h bus trip seated near the index case of HPS) may have been necessary for person-to-person transmission. If confirmed, this is reassuring for the safety of personnel caring for infected patients.

The many clinical faces of HTV infections: HFRS-HPS and NE-HPS, and their pathogenesis

Clinical presentation

Fever with myalgia, headache, and general malaise, followed by abdominal symptoms such as nausea, vomiting, and diarrhoea are the presenting symptoms both in Old and New World infections, indistinguishable from a "bad flu" lasting 3–5 days. Often accompanied by high leukocytosis, this tableau may simulate a surgical condition, as first suggested in the early European reports (Myhrman, 1934; Zetterholm, 1934). After this prodromal period, organ involvement is heralded in HFRS by back pain, oliguria (or anuria); in HPS, a dry, non-productive cough can evolve into severe dyspnoea. Radiologic studies reveal swollen kidneys in HFRS and interstitial pulmonary oedema or bilateral lung infiltrates in HPS, and third-space fluid accumulation (pleuritis, ascites, pericarditis) in both.

In HPS, rapidly progressive, non-cardiogenic pulmonary oedema and severe hypotension (systolic BP ≤ 85 mm Hg) can follow. During the first years of experience with HPS, about 50% of patients died within the first 48 h of hospitalization from uncorrected hypoxia and/or from intractable shock, even with intensive care including assisted ventilation (Duchin et al., 1994; Hjelle et al., 1995). Pathological findings consist of pulmonary congestion, interalveolar oedema, and minimal or moderate interstitial immunoblast infiltrates in the lung (Hjelle et al., 1995; Zaki et al., 1995). In New World forms, cardiac involvement appears to play an often-decisive role, hence the recently proposed name of "HPCS" instead of the currently used HPS. Typical haematological anomalies are absolute leukocytosis, and the "diagnostic triad" of a left shift, presence of immunoblasts, and thrombocytopenia (Hjelle et al., 1995).

The clinical presentation of the European variant, NE caused by the PUUV serotype, is mostly mild. Symptoms and signs consist of sudden fever, often severe back pain (due to acute interstitial nephritis with renal swelling), rapidly progressive ARF, and particularly thrombocytopenia (which is found in more than 75% of the cases, if assessed early enough after the onset of symptoms) (Clement et al., 1995, 1998; Colson et al., 1995). Early and marked proteinuria is found in almost all NE and HFRS cases, but is also encountered in most American HPS cases (Enria et al., 2000). In contrast, early ophthalmologic symptoms (eye pain, conjunctival injection, blurred vision, cheimosis, acute glaucoma, etc.) are detected in about 25% of NE cases (Clement et al., 1994b; Colson et al., 1995), but have rarely been reported so far in New World HTV cases. However, conjunctival injection has been observed in South American ANDV infections (Enria et al., 2000; Peters and Khan, 2002).

Haemorrhagic symptoms in NE (i.e. in the West) are rare (≤ 20% of cases) and minor (petechiae, nose bleeding), in contrast to the more severe disease caused by HTNV and DOBV-Af in the Far East and in the Balkans, respectively, where severe haemorrhagic complications and shock often lead to death (Gligic et al., 1992; Avsic-Zupanc et al., 1994). Haemorrhagic necrosis of the pituitary gland

(Sheehan's syndrome), of the adrenals, or of the right atrium have also been mentioned as complications in severe HTNV-induced infections, but are extremely rare in NE. In severe NE cases, renal swelling can be so intense that spontaneous "internal rupture" with perinephric haemorrhage ensues (Clement et al., 2001). Indeed, most symptoms are mild and self-limited in NE; complete restoration of normal kidney function within 2–3 weeks is the rule. Except for ophthalmologic symptoms and the rare haemorrhagic complications, the symptoms of NE are often non-specific or even totally absent (subclinical forms). Except during an epidemic, the diagnosis can only be confirmed by serological tests.

NE has a good prognosis, with a mortality rate of only 0.1%. The fatality rate of HPS, which was 50% in 1993, has now decreased to 20% or lower (Enria et al., 2000; Peters and Khan, 2002); these figures are equal to mortality rates in the most severe outbreaks of HTNV or DOBV in the Old World. The decrease in mortality rate probably represents increased recognition of milder cases and improved medical care. As with every emerging disease, the most severe cases were recognized first, and milder or even asymptomatic cases were recognized later.

As predicted (Clement et al., 1997), there was found to be overlap of the range of symptoms in both the Eastern and Western hemispheres. Cases of HPS with kidney involvement (Enria et al., 2000) and HFRS cases with lung involvement (Stuart et al., 1996; Klempa et al., 2003; Launay et al., 2003) were eventually recognized. A series of European forms of NE was reported, presenting with an HPS-like non-cardiogenic acute pulmonary oedema (Clement et al., 1994d). In unusual cases, these forms may also need mechanical ventilation and dialysis (Clement et al., 1994b,d; Stuart et al., 1996). Even "diagnostic" immunoblasts have now been reported in a European NE case (Keyaerts et al., 2004).

Pathogenesis

The reasons for the "organ preference" (lung or kidney) of HTV are far from clear, but immunohistochemical studies show a preferential, and often abundant, presence of viral antigen in human pulmonary capillary endothelial cells in SNV infections, and a mainly renal endothelial presence in HTNV and PUUV infections. However, there is no evidence of a viral cytopathic effect either in tissue specimens or cell culture, nor are viral inclusions seen (Zaki et al., 1995). The pathogenesis of organ dysfunction is poorly understood, but a constant feature is a "capillary leak", leading to interstitial oedema in the kidney or lung, fluid accumulation (pleural, pericardial, peritoneal), haemoconcentration, and eventually multiple organ failure. Mechanisms appear to be related to immunological pathways, determined by host factors, and probably resulting in a disturbed interplay of mediators of inflammation (NO, cyto-, and chemokines) and their receptors in the endothelium (Maes et al., 2004b). Virus-induced apoptosis appears to be minimal or absent.

Laboratory diagnosis and differential diagnosis

Laboratory diagnosis

Serology

The earliest methods for serodiagnosis of HTV infections (in the 1970s and 1980s) were immunofluorescent assays (IFA) for the detection of specific hantaviral antibodies against lung cells of rodents infected with HTNV and/or SEOV. These methods were quickly replaced by the use of Vero E6 cells (African green monkey kidney cells), infected with various HTV strains (Clement et al., 1995). This technique is still used but is limited by the need for an experienced laboratory technician and the occurrence of positive reactions due to many cross-reacting antibodies to other related HTVs.

Enzyme-linked immunosorbent assays (ELISA), in general used since the 1990s, use either native purified antigens, recombinant nucleocapsid proteins (rNp), or even truncated rNp as antigen sources (Kallio-Kokko et al., 1998; Maes et al., 2004a). ELISA is automated and allows an easy distinction between IgG and IgM antibodies, essential for the clinical diagnosis of a recent infection (Niklasson et al., 1990). IgG antibodies may persist lifelong, whereas IgM antibodies indicate recent infection but may take up to 2 weeks to appear (Kallio-Kokko et al., 1998; Galeno et al., 2002); IgM antibodies can even remain false negative in exceptional circumstances, such as after a therapeutic plasma exchange (Keyaerts et al., 2004). Several variants of immunoblot assays are more specific, such as the stripe immuno assay (SIA), useful for New World HTV infections (Hjelle et al., 1997) and potentially for HTV infections in the Old World as well (Hujakka et al., 2003).

For serotyping infections by genetically related HTVs (e.g. HTNV vs. SEOV, DOBV vs. SAAV), the most specific test and the "gold standard" is the cumbersome plaque reduction neutralization test (PRNT) or its modern variants. But even in this very specific test, cross-reactions can occur, particularly in IgM detection during the first weeks after infection (Lundkvist et al., 1997).

Molecular biology

PCR followed by sequencing can identify the genotype of the infecting HTV with extreme precision. PCR was used to characterize the characterization of the "new" SNV in the US in 1993, before the virus was isolated (Nichol et al., 1993). Sequencing of the PCR fragments from both patients and suspected rodent reservoirs can identify the epidemiological connection, providing an essential step to a better understanding of HTVs. Genotyping also permits identification of "new" species of HTVs in human cases (e.g. Hu39694, Araraquara, etc., see Table 1). However, PCR can only yield positive results if the serum sample contains sufficient viral RNA to be detected, i.e. only in recent cases in which the samples have been handled and stored appropriately, and in sera only when there are persistent high degrees of viraemia. The presumably low degree of PUUV viraemia in mild European NE cases vs. the high degree of SNV(-like) viraemia in severe American cases of HPS could explain why PCR for HTVs is more useful in the Americas than in Europe.

Immunohistochemistry (IHC)

This technique allows staining of a suspected hantaviral antigen in tissue samples, making it the ideal tool for retrospective diagnosis of HTV infections in historically conserved biopsies. The absence, however, of a stainable antigen is no proof that a HTV infection did not occur. For instance, PUUV antigen is frequently absent from kidney biopsies of confirmed NE cases (Clement et al., 1995).

Clinical and laboratory differential diagnosis

Almost all emerging or re-emerging infections, bacterial or viral, but particularly zoonoses, may be complicated by symptoms resembling ARDS; for HTV infections in the New World, HPS may resemble ARDS as well. The "diagnostic triad" of a left shift, presence of immunoblasts, and thrombocytopenia on the blood smear indicates the presence of HPS, particularly if lung infiltrates are present on X-ray, and if haematocrit is elevated, indicating plasma leakage. It is striking to see that most zoonoses can also cause renal compromise, which can confuse the diagnosis of HTV renal disease.

Dengue haemorrhagic fever and scrub typhus can mimic HFRS, but the great imitator of HFRS is without doubt leptospirosis (Clement et al., 1997, 1998, 1999). The wild rat that transmits leptospirosis is found nearly everywhere, and all symptoms, laboratory anomalies, and even kidney biopsies in leptospirosis are virtually identical to those of HFRS. It is important to differentiate HFRS, and particularly with SEOV-induced HFRS, from leptospirosis (Clement et al., 1997, 1998, 1999). In cases of ARF with thrombocytopenia, excluding leptospirosis and screening for HTV with an arvicoline and a murine antigen (including also SEOV), it was possible to demonstrate the first documented HTV infections respectively in the Netherlands (Koolen et al., 1989; Osterhaus et al., 1989), in the New World (Hinrichsen et al., 1993), in Northern Ireland (McKenna et al., 1994), and in India (Clement et al., 2000b, 2006). It is of interest that Northern Ireland and India are both regions where bank voles are absent and where the wild rat is the only known local reservoir for pathogenic HTVs. To further complicate the diagnosis, severe and even lethal pulmonary and cardiac involvement can occur in leptospirosis as well as in HTV infection (Yersin et al., 2000). Dual infections with both leptospirosis and SEOV after a rat contact have been described (Kudesia et al., 1988).

Rat-bite fever (RBF), a worldwide zoonosis, is often forgotten in the differential diagnosis of fever and general malaise after contact with a rat (Clement and Van Ranst, 2000a). RBF, caused by a bacterium, *Streptobacillus moniliformis*, and occurs most often after a rat bite or ingestion of food contaminated by rats.

Symptoms include rash, arthropathy, and multiple abscess formation; all symptoms rare or absent in HTV disease (Clement et al., 2003c).

What to treat and not to treat

There are no effective treatments for HTV infections except ribavirin, a nucleoside analogue, and that should be given only early and intravenously in the clinical course. Thus, its use is limited to quickly recognized (e.g. during an epidemic) and severe forms of disease. In practice, this is applicable only for outbreaks of severe HTNV disease in Korea and China, where encouraging results have been obtained (Huggins et al., 1991). However, in a small field study in the US, no beneficial effect could be demonstrated with ribavirin in HPS (Mertz et al., 2004).

The main treatment of severe HPS or HFRS case is purely supportive, including mechanical ventilation or even extra-corporeal membrane oxygenation for HPS and haemodialysis for HFRS. These are aimed at controlling the consequences of interstitial oedema, the key pathological feature of all HTV infections.

In HFRS acute dialysis is rarely needed. In NE, dialysis is now required in fewer than 5% of cases in most European series (Colson et al., 1995; Clement et al., 1998). Although a very rapid deterioration of kidney function is seen, a rapid and spontaneous recovery also occurs, most often within 2 weeks. Hyperkalaemia, severe uraemia, and hypertension are rarely encountered, and the only true indication for dialysis is fluid overload in cases with anuria. However, this is a complication that can often be avoided with careful fluid management.

Steroids have no proven benefit in HPS or HPRS, despite isolated case reports of the so-called hastened recovery with steroids. In the largest retrospective study conducted in 60 patients with biopsy-proven acute interstitial nephritis (of which HTV nephropathy is a form), no beneficial effect of steroids was found (Clarkson et al., 2004).

Recombinant vaccines for HTV are being developed, but none are available at present. The only effective means of prophylaxis against HTV infection consists of reduced exposure to rodents and their aerosolized excreta.

References

Antoniadis A, LeDuc J, Daniel-Alexiou S. Clinical and epidemiological aspects of haemorrhagic fever with renal syndrome (HFRS) in Greece. Eur J Epidemiol 1987; 3: 295–301.

Avsic-Zupanc T, Poljak M, Furlan P, Kaps R, Xiao SY, Leduc JW. Isolation of a strain of a Hantaan virus from a fatal case of hemorrhagic fever with renal syndrome in Slovenia. Am J Trop Med Hyg 1994; 51: 393–400.

Childs JE, Ksiazek TG, Spiropoulou CF, Krebs JW, Morzunov S, Maupin GO, Gage KL, Rollin PE, Sarisky J, Enscore RE, et al. Serologic and genetic identification of *Peromyscus maniculatus* as the primary rodent reservoir for a new hantavirus in the southwestern United States. J Infect Dis 1994; 169: 1271–1280.

Clarkson MR, Giblin L, O'Connell FP, O'Kelly P, Walshe JJ, Conlon P, O'Meara Y, Dormon A, Campbell E, Donohoe J. Acute interstitial nephritis: clinical features and response to corticosteroid therapy. Nephrol Dial Transplant 2004; 19: 2778–2783.

Clement J. Viral bioterrorism—hantaviruses. Antiviral Res 2003a; 57: 121–127.

Clement J, Colson P, Mc Kenna P. Hantavirus pulmonary syndrome in New England and Europe. N Eng J Med 1994d; 331: 545–546 Discussion 547-8.

Clement J, Frans J, Van Ranst M. Human Tula virus infection or rat-bite fever? Eur J Clin Microbiol Infect Dis 2003c; 22: 332–333.

Clement J, Heyman P, Mc Kenna P, Colson P, Avsic-Zupanc T. The hantaviruses of Europe: from the bedside to the bench. Emerg Infect Dis 1997; 3: 205–211.

Clement J, Hinrichsen S, Crescente J, Bigaignon G, Yersin C, Muthusethupathi M, Nainan G, Terpstra W, Hartskeerl R, Lundkvist A, Van Ranst M. Hantavirus-induced hemorrhagic fever with renal syndrome (HFRS) has to be considered in the differential diagnosis of leptospirosis-suspected cases in the New and the Old World. Am J Trop Med Hyg 1999; 61: 316–317.

Clement J, Lameire N, Keyaerts E, Maes P, Van Ranst M. Hantavirus infections in Europe. Lancet Infect Dis 2003b; 3: 752–754.

Clement J, Maes P, Muthusethupathi M, Nainan G, Van Ranst M. First evidence of fatal hantavirus nephropathy in India, mimicking leptospirosis, Nephrol Dial Transplant 2006; 21: 826–827.

Clement J, Mc Kenna P, Avsic-Zupanc T, Skinner CR. Rat-transmitted HVD in Sarajevo. Lancet 1994c; 344: 131.

Clement J, Mc Kenna P, Colson P, Damoiseaux P, Penalba C, Halin P, Lombart D. Hantavirus epidemic in Europe. Lancet 1994b; 343: 114.

Clement J, McKenna P, Groen J, Osterhaus A, Colson P, Vervoort T, van der Groen G, Lee HW. Epidemiology and laboratory diagnosis of hantavirus (HTV) infections. Acta Clin Belg 1995; 50: 9–19.

Clement J, Mc Kenna P, Leirs H, Verhagen R, Lefevre A, Song G, Tkachenko E, van der Groen G. Hantavirus infections in rodents. In: Virus Infections of Rodents and Lagomorphs (Horzinek, editor), 5th Volume in a series "Virus Infections in Vertebrates" (Osterhaus AD, editor). Amsterdam: Elsevier Science BV; 1994a; pp. 295–316.

Clement J, Mc Kenna P, van der Groen G, Vaheri A, Peters CJ. Hantaviruses. In: Zoonoses. Biology, Clinical Practice, and Public Health Control (Palmer SR, Soulsby L, Simpson DIH, editors). Oxford, UK: Oxford University Press; 1998; pp. 331–352.

Clement J, Muthusethupathi M, Nainan G, Van Ranst M. First fatal cases of hantavirus nephropathy in India. Clin Infect Dis 2000b; 31: 315.

Clement J, Underwood P, Ward D, Pilaski J, LeDuc JW. Hantavirus outbreak during military manoeuvres in Germany. Lancet 1996; 347: 336.

Clement J, Van Ranst M. The role of rodents in emerging and re-emerging human infections. Infect Dis Rev 2000a; 2: 84–87.

Clement J, Van Ranst M, Lameire N. Hantavirus infection complicated with ARF and spontaneous perinephric haemorrhage. Nephron 2001; 89: 241–242.

Colson P, Damoiseaux Ph, Duvivier E, Lerecque P, Roger JM, Bouilliez DJ, Mc Kenna P, Clement J. Hantavirose dans l'Entre-Sambre-et-Meuse. Acta Clin Belg 1995; 50: 197–205.

Desmyter J, Johnson KM, Deckers C, LeDuc JW, Brasseur F, Van Ypersele de Strihou C. Laboratory rat associated outbreak of haemorrhagic fever with renal syndrome due to Hantaan-like virus in Belgium. Lancet 1983; 2: 1445–1448.

Dournon E, Morinière B, Matheson S, Girard PM, Gonzalez JP, Hirsch F, Mc Cormick JB. HFRS after a wild rodent bite in the Haute-Savoie and risk of exposure to Hantaan-like virus in a Paris laboratory. Lancet 1984; 1: 676–677.

Duchin JS, Koster FT, Peters CJ, Simpson GL, Tempest B, Zaki SR, Ksiazek TG, Rollin PE, Nichol S, Umland ET, Moolenaar RL, Reef SE, Nolte KB, Gallagher MM, Butler JC, Breiman R, et al. Hantavirus study group. Hantavirus pulmonary syndrome a clinical description of 17 patients with a newly recognized disease. N Engl J Med 1994; 330: 949–955.

Enria D, Briggiler A, Pini N, Levis S. Clinical Manifestations of New World Hantaviruses. In: Hantaviruses (Schmaljohn CS, Nichol ST, editors). Berlin: Springer; 2000; pp. 117–134.

Galeno H, Mora J, Villagra E, Fernandez J, Hernandez J, Mertz GJ, Ramirez E. First human isolate of hantavirus (Andes virus) in the Americas. Emerg Infect Dis 2002; 8: 657–661.

Gligic A, Dimkovic N, Xiao SY, Buckle GJ, Jovanovic D, Stojanovic R, Obradovic M, Diglisic G, Micic J, Asher D, LeDuc JW, Yanagihara R, Gajdusek DC. Belgrade virus: a new hantavirus causing severe hemorrhagic fever with renal syndrome in Yugoslavia. J Infect Dis 1992; 166: 113–120.

Hinrichsen S, Medeiros de Andrade A, Clement J, Leirs H, McKenna P, Matthys P, Neild G. Evidence of hantavirus infection in Brazilian patients from Recife with suspected leptospirosis. Lancet 1993; 341: 50.

Hjelle B, Jenison S, Torrez-Martinez N, Herring B, Quan S, Polito A, Pichuantes S, Yamada T, Morris C, Elgh F, Lee HW, Artsob H, Dinello R. Rapid and specific detection of Sin Nombre virus antibodies in patients with hantavirus pulmonary syndrome by a strip immunoblot assay suitable for field diagnosis. J Clin Microbiol 1997; 35: 600–608.

Hjelle B, Jenison SA, Goade DE, Green WB, Feddersen RM, Scott AA. Hantaviruses: clinical, microbiologic, and epidemiologic aspects. Crit Rev Clin Lab Sci 1995; 3(2): 469–508.

Hooper JW, Larsen T, Custer DM, Schmaljohn CS. A lethal disease model for hantavirus pulmonary syndrome. Virology 2001; 289: 6–14.

Huggins JW, Hsiang CM, Cosgriff TM, Guang MY, Smith JI, Wu ZO, LeDuc JW, Zheng ZM, Meegan JM, Wang QN, Oland DD, Gui XE, Gibbs PH, Yuan GH, Zhang TM. Prospective, double-blind, concurrent, placebo-controlled clinical trial of intravenous ribavirin therapy of hemorrhagic fever with renal syndrome. J Infect Dis 1991; 164: 1119–1127.

Hujakka H, Koistinen V, Kuronen I, Eerikainen P, Parviainen M, Lundkvist A, Vaheri A, Vapalahti O, Narvanen A. Diagnostic rapid tests for acute hantavirus infections: specific tests for Hantaan, Dobrava and Puumala viruses versus a hantavirus combination test. J Virol Methods 2003; 108: 117–122.

Kallio-Kokko H, Vapalahti O, Lundkvist A, Vaheri A. Evaluation of Puumala virus IgG and IgM enzyme immunoassays based on recombinant baculovirus-expressed nucleocapsid protein for early nephropathia epidemica diagnosis. Clin Diagn Virol 1998; 10: 83–90.

Keyaerts E, Ghijsels E, Lemey P, Maes P, Zachée P, Daelemans R, Vervoort T, Mertens G, Van Ranst M, Clement J. Plasma-exchange-associated IgM-negative hantavirus disease after a camping holiday in Southern France. Clin Infect Dis 2004; 38: 1350–1356.

Klempa B, Meisel H, Rath S, Bartel J, Ulrich R, Kruger DH. Occurrence of renal and pulmonary syndrome in a region of northeast Germany where Tula hantavirus circulates. J Clin Microbiol 2003b; 41: 4894–4897.

Klempa B, Schutt M, Auste B, Labuda M, Ulrichm R, Meisel H, Kruger DH. First molecular identification of human Dobrava virus infection in central Europe. J Clin Microbiol 2004; 42: 1322–1325.

Klempa B, Stanko M, Labuda M, Ulrich R, Meisel H, Kruger DH. Central European Dobrava hantavirus isolate from a striped field mouse (*Apodemus agrarius*). J Clin Microbiol 2005; 43: 2756–2763.

Koolen MI, Jansen JLJ, Assman KJM, Clement J, van Liebergen FJHM. A sporadic case of acute hantavirus nephropathy in The Netherlands. Neth J Med 1989; 35: 25–32.

Kudesia G, Christie P, Walker E, Pinkerton I, Lloyd G. Dual infection with leptospira and hantavirus. Lancet 1988; 1: 1397.

Launay D, Thomas Ch, Fleury D, Roueff S, Line ML, Droz D, Vanhille P. Pulmonary-renal syndrome due to hemorrhagic fever with renal syndrome: an unusual manifestation of Puumala virus infection in France. Clin Nephrol 2003; 59: 297–300.

Lee HW, Lee PW, Johnson KM. Isolation of the etiologic agent of Korean hemorrhagic fever. J Infect Dis 1978; 137: 298–308.

Lundkvist A, Hukic M, Horling J, Gilljam M, Nichol S, Niklasson B. Puumala and Dobrava viruses cause hemorrhagic fever with renal syndrome in Bosnia–Herzegovina: evidence of highly cross-neutralizing antibody responses in early patient sera. J Med Virol 1997; 53: 51–59.

Lundkvist A, Lindegren G, Brus Sjolander K, Mavtchoutko V, Vene S, Plyusnin A, Kalnina V. Hantavirus infections in Latvia. Eur J Clin Microbiol Infect Dis 2002; 21: 626–629.

Maes P, Clement J, Gavrilovskaya I, Van Ranst M. Hantaviruses: immunology, treatment and prevention. Viral Immunol 2004b; 17: 481–497.

Maes P, Keyaerts E, Clement J, Bonnet V, Robert A, Van Ranst M. Detection of Puumala hantavirus antibody with ELISA using a recombinant truncated nucleocapsid protein expressed in *Escherichia coli*. Viral Immunol 2004a; 17: 315–321.

Martinez VP, Bellomo C, San Juan J, Pinna D, Forlenza R, Elder M, Padula PJ. Person-to-person transmission of Andes virus. Emerg Infect Dis 2005; 11: 1848–1853.

McKenna P, Clement J, Matthys P, Coyle P, McCaughey C. Serological evidence of hantavirus disease in Northern Ireland. J Med Virol 1994; 43: 33–38.

Mertz GJ, Miedzinski L, Goade D, Pavia AT, Hjelle B, Hansbarger CO, Levy H, Koster FT, Baum K, Lindemulder A, Wang W, Riser L, Fernandez H, Whitley RJ, Collaborative Antiviral Study Group. Placebo-controlled, double-blind trial of intravenous ribavirin for the treatment of hantavirus cardiopulmonary syndrome in North America. Clin Infect Dis 2004; 39: 1307–1313.

Myhrman G. A kidney disease with peculiar symptoms. Nord Med 1934; 7: 793–794 (In Swedish).

Nemirov K, Vapalahti O, Lundkvist A, Vasilenko V, Golovljova I, Plyusnina A, Niemimaa J, Laakkonen J, Henttonen H, Vaheri A, Plyusnin A. Isolation and characterization of Dobrava hantavirus carried by the striped field mouse (*Apodemus agrarius*) in Estonia. J Gen Virol 1999; 80: 371–379.

Nichol ST, Spiropoulou CF, Morzunov S, Rollin PE, Ksiazek TG, Feldmann H, Sanchez A, Childs J, Zaki S, Peters CJ. Genetic identification of a hantavirus associated with an outbreak of acute respiratory illness. Science 1993; 262: 914–917.

Niklasson B, LeDuc JW. Isolation of the nephropathia epidemica agent in Sweden. Lancet 1984; I: 1012–1013.

Niklasson B, Tkachenko E, Ivanov AP, van der Groen G, Wiger D, Andersen HK, LeDuc J, Kjelsson T, Nystrom K. Haemorrhagic fever with renal syndrome: evaluation of ELISA for detection of Puumala-virus-specific IgG and IgM. Res Virol 1990; 141: 637–648.

Osterhaus ADME, Groen J, UytdeHaag FGCM, van Steenis G, van der Groen G, Clement J, Jordans JGM. Hantavirus nephropathy in the Netherlands. Lancet 1989; 2: 338–339.

Peters CJ, Khan AS. Hantavirus pulmonary syndrome: the new American hemorrhagic fever. Clin Infect Dis 2002; 34: 1224–1231.

Sironen T, Vaheri A, Plyusnin A. Phylogenetic evidence for the distinction of Saaremaa and Dobrava hantaviruses. Virol J 2005; 2: 90.

Stuart LM, Rice PS, Lloyd G, Beale RJ. A soldier in respiratory distress. Lancet 1996; 347: 30.

Stuhlfauth K. Nachtrag zu dem Bericht über ein neues schlammfieberähnliches Krankheitsbild bei Deutschen Truppen in Lappland. Dtsch Med Wochenschr 1943; 69: 439–443.

Toro J, Vega JD, Khan AS, Mills JN, Padula P, Terry W, Yadon Z, Valderrama R, Ellis BA, Parletic C, Cerda R, Zaki S, Shieh WJ, Meyer R, Tapia M, Mansilla C, Baro M, Vergara JA, Concha M, Calderon G, Enria D, Peters CJ, Ksiazek TG. An outbreak of hantavirus pulmonary syndrome, Chile, 1997. Emerg Infect Dis 1998; 4: 687–694.

Van Loock F, Thomas I, Clement J, Ghoos S, Colson P. A case-control study after a hantavirus outbreak in the South of Belgium: who is at risk? Clin Infect Dis 1999; 28: 834–839.

Wells RM, Sosa Estani S, Yadon ZE, Enria D, Padula P, Pini N, Mills JN, Peters CJ, Segura EL. An unusual hantavirus outbreak in southern Argentina: person-to-person transmission? Hantavirus pulmonary syndrome study group for Patagonia. Emerg Infect Dis 1997; 3: 171–174.

Xu ZY, Guo CS, Wu YL, Zhang XW, Liu K. Epidemiological studies of hemorrhagic fever with renal syndrome: analysis of risk factors and mode of transmission. J Infect Dis 1985; 152: 137–144.

Yersin C, Bovet P, Merien F, Clement J, Laille M, Van Ranst M, Perolat P. Pulmonary haemorrhage as a predominant cause of death in leptospirosis in Seychelles. Trans R Soc Trop Med Hyg 2000; 94: 71–76.

Zaki SR, Greer PW, Coffield LM, Goldsmith CS, Nolte KB, Foucar K, Feddersen RM, Zumwait RE, Miller GL, Khan AS, et al. Hantavirus pulmonary syndrome: pathogenesis of an emerging infectious disease. Am J Pathol 1995; 146: 552–579.

Zeitz PS, Butler JC, Cheek JE, Samuel MC, Childs JE, Shands LA, Turner RE, Voorhees RE, Sarisky J, Rollin PE, et al. A case-control study of hantavirus pulmonary syndrome during an outbreak in the Southwestern United States. J Infect Dis 1995; 171: 864–870.

Zetterholm SG. Acute nephritis simulating an acute abdomen. Svenska Lakartidningen 1934; 31: 425–429 (In Swedish).

Emerging Viruses in Human Populations
Edward Tabor (Editor)
DOI 10.1016/S0168-7069(06)16009-7

Nipah and Hendra Viruses

Vincent P. Hsu

*Clinical Performance Improvement and Infection Control, Florida Hospital, 601
E. Rollins St. Orlando, FL 32803, USA*

Introduction

Nipah and Hendra viruses are two zoonotic paramyxoviruses with an ability to cause fatal encephalitic and respiratory diseases in humans. Hendra virus was first identified in humans in Australia in 1994, with horses as the intermediate host. Nipah virus emerged in humans in 1998 in Malaysia, with pigs as the intermediate host. Nipah virus was later also identified in India and Bangladesh in 2001, with the flying fox (*Pteropus* spp.) as the natural host, although no intermediary animal host was found in more recent outbreaks there. A third zoonotic paramyxovirus, Menangle virus, was first identified in pigs, and will be discussed only briefly. Of the zoonotic paramyxoviruses, Nipah virus is responsible for the greatest number of human cases, with several hundred cases and at least 215 deaths reported, compared to Hendra virus, which has caused a handful of cases and 2 deaths, and Menangle, which has only caused self-limited illness in 2 individuals.

Classification, structure, and virology

Nipah and Hendra viruses are negative-sense, single-stranded RNA viruses in the *Paramyxoviridae* family, subfamily *Paramyxovirinae*. They are further categorized in the recently named genus *Henipavirus*, one of five genera in the subfamily (the others are *Respirovirus, Morbillovirus, Avulavirus,* and *Rubulavirus*) (Fig. 1). Other human pathogenic viruses exist in these other genera, such as measles, mumps, and parainfluenza viruses; Nipah and Hendra viruses, in the genus *Henipavirus*, and Menangle virus, in the genus *Rubalavirus*, are unique in that they are zoonotic and are viruses that have recently emerged in humans.

Nipah and Hendra viruses exhibit typical morphology of paramyxoviruses when examined by electron microscopy (EM), with a helical nucleocapsid structure

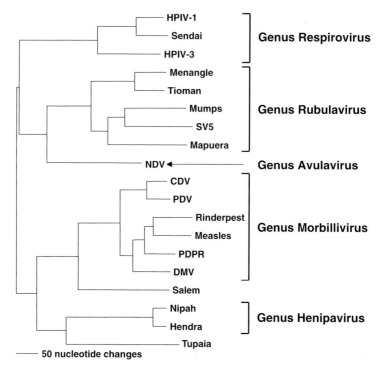

Fig. 1 Phylogenetic tree comparing Nipah and Hendra viruses within the paramyxovirus family. (HPIV = Human parainfluenza virus, SV5 = simian virus 5, NDV = Newcastle disease virus, CDV = canine distemper virus, PDV = Phocine distemper virus, DMV = dolphin morbillivirus)
Source: William J. Bellini, and Paul Rota, CDC. Used with permission.

surrounded by a membrane derived from the plasma membrane of the cell from which the viruses bud. Nucleocapsid filaments exhibit a typical 'herringbone' morphology, produced by the association of the nucleocapsid protein with genomic RNA (Murray et al., 1995b; Chua et al., 2000a; Halpin et al., 2000). In contrast to Nipah virus, which has only a single layer of surface projections, Hendra virus appears double-fringed, caused by projections on the surface of the viral envelope (Hyatt et al., 2001). Measurements by EM demonstrated that Nipah virus particles vary in size between 120 and 500 nm.

The determination of the nucleotide sequences of Nipah and Hendra viruses were completed soon after the Nipah outbreak in Malaysia in 1998 (Harcourt et al., 2000, 2001). Nipah and Hendra virus have 68–92% amino acid homology in the protein-coded regions and 40–67% nucleotide homology in the non-translated regions. Similar to other *Paramyxovirinae*, Nipah and Hendra viruses carry six genes that encode structural proteins, the nucleocapsid (N), phosphoprotein (P), matrix protein (M), fusion protein (F), glycoprotein (G), and the large polymerase (L), in that order. In addition, the P gene also encodes accessory proteins designated C, V, and W. The C protein appears to regulate viral RNA synthesis and may play a role as a virulence factor. The addition of a single nucleotide, G, allows expression of the V protein, while the addition of two Gs allow expression of the W protein (Harcourt et al., 2000). The N, P, and L proteins are associated with genomic RNA and form part of the RNA polymerase complex, while the M protein serves to maintain the virion structure, assembling between the envelope and nucleocapsid core. The V and W proteins appear to be virulence factors that act by blocking activation of an interferon-inducible promoter (Park et al., 2003). The two membrane glycoproteins are the F and G proteins. The fusion protein, F_0, is originally synthesized as an inactive precursor that requires cleavage by a host cell protease to become active subunits F_1 and F_2. These subunits mediate the fusion of the virion membrane with the plasma membrane of the host cell. The attachment protein, or glycoprotein, G, serves to mediate the binding of the virus to a cellular receptor, which has not yet been identified (Wang et al., 2001).

Strain variation Nipah viruses have been demonstrated. Genomic variation appears to be geographically distinct, with specific differences between human isolates from the outbreaks in Malaysia, India, and Bangladesh, and from bats in Cambodia (Harcourt et al., 2000; Harcourt, 2005; Reynes et al., 2005; Chadha et al., 2006). Although amino acid homologies between the Malaysia strain and Bangladesh strain were greater than 92%, the genome of the Bangladesh strain is 6 nucleotides longer than the Malaysian strain and demonstrated enough variation to be considered a new strain. Sequences obtained from the outbreak in India had a closer relation to the Bangladesh strain than the Malaysian strain, while the virus isolated in Cambodia demonstrated closer homology to the Malaysian strain. These observations support the finding that these viruses have natural reservoirs for evolving within distinct geographic areas.

Transcription and replication of the henipaviruses have not been studied because of the high level of laboratory safety that is required, but the evidence to date suggests that these viruses follow the same replication mechanisms as the other *Paramyxovirinae*. After binding and fusion of the G and F proteins, respectively, the ribonucleoprotein is released into the cell cytoplasm. Transcription of the N, P, and L proteins then occurs prior to production of new proteins, while new membrane glycoproteins are transported to the surface. The newly produced proteins assemble at the cytoplasm and are released via viral budding.

Several unique features differentiate the henipaviruses from the other *Paramyxovirinae* viruses. Antigenic cross-reactivity occurs between Hendra and Nipah viruses, but not with other paramyxoviruses. The viruses exhibit a much longer genomic length compared to other members (18.2 kb vs.15.5 kb), and have an unusually large P protein (Wang et al., 2000; Mayo, 2002). The cleavage of the F protein, a necessary step for all paramyxoviruses, occurs through a novel type of proteolytic cleavage that differs from that caused by known proteases (Moll et al., 2004). The G proteins of Nipah and Hendra virus do not have hemagglutinin and neuraminidase activity, features that are common to other paramyxoviruses (Yu et al., 1998; Wang et al., 2001). Lastly, it should be noted that Hendra and

Nipah viruses have a broad tropism, and are able to infect a broad range of animal species, a characteristic that is not typical of other paramyxoviruses.

Epidemiology

The epidemiology of Nipah and Hendra viruses has not been fully elucidated. A similarity exists between the epidemiology of each of these two viruses, such as the *Pteropus* fruit bat as the natural host for both viruses. For both Hendra and Nipah viruses, it is presumed that horses and pigs that have acted as an intermediary host to humans had been infected by indirect contact with pteropid bats endemic in these regions, although this has not been experimentally proven.

However, there are also differences in their epidemiology. Hendra virus was first described along the coastal regions of Australia, and to date has caused illnesses in 5 humans with 2 deaths, in infections that were acquired by close contact with ill horses infected with the virus (Table 1). Nipah virus infections in humans have been described in Malaysia, Singapore, Bangladesh, and India, and have been identified in bats in Cambodia and Thailand (Table 1). Until 2004, cases occurred only in clusters, but sporadic cases have been identified more recently through active surveillance (Anon., 2004b). Overall, Nipah virus has caused at least 215 human deaths to date. Direct contact with infected pigs was primarily responsible for the outbreak in Malaysia, although in Bangladesh the epidemiology was less well-defined, with some evidence for person-to-person transmission.

Description of Hendra virus outbreaks

In September 1994, a cluster of respiratory illnesses involving 18 horses and 2 humans was reported from the town of Hendra, a suburb of Brisbane, Australia. The first illness occurred in a pregnant mare that died, followed by 14 additional horse deaths. Within 1 week after the death of the index mare, a 49-year-old horse trainer and a 40-year-old stable hand who were closely involved in the care of the index mare (Murray et al., 1995a; Selvey et al., 1995) became ill with respiratory symptoms, and the trainer died after a 7-day illness. The stable hand recovered from mild respiratory symptoms after 6 weeks. An undescribed virus was isolated from several of the horses and from the kidney of the horse trainer who died; this virus was found to be distantly related to known morbilliviruses (Murray et al., 1995b). It was initially named equine morbillivirus and was subsequently renamed Hendra virus.

Sporadic cases of Hendra virus have continued to occur in horses and humans. In September 1995, a male farmer from Queensland, Australia was admitted to a hospital with fever, altered mental status, multiple seizures, and an initial diagnosis of meningitis (Anon., 1996; O'Sullivan et al., 1997). He died 25 days after admission. It was subsequently learned that the patient had been diagnosed with a self-limited episode of meningitis in August 1994, and that he had cared for two sick horses and assisted with their necropsies just prior to the onset of his first illness.

Table 1

Countries and regions where henipavirus infections have been identified

Virus	Country	Region (locality, if known)	Year	Affected species	Reference
Hendra	Australia	Queensland (Brisbane)	1994	Humans, horses	Murray et al. (1995a), Selvey et al. (1995)
		Queensland (Mackay)	1995	Human, horses	(Anon., 1996), O'Sullivan et al. (1997)
		Queensland, Northern Territories, New South Wales	1996, NA	Bats	Young et al. (1996), Paterson et al. (1998), Halpin et al. (2000)
		Queensland (Cairns)	1999	Horses	Field et al. (2000), Hooper et al. (2000)
		Queensland (Cairns, Townsville)	2004	Humans, horses	McCormack (2005)
	Papua New Guinea	Madang (Madang)	NA	Bats	Paterson et al. (1998)
Nipah	Malaysia	Perak, Negeri Sembilan, Selangor	1998–1999	Humans, pigs	(1999a; 1999b), Goh et al. (2000)
	Singapore	Singapore	1999	Humans	(Anon., 1999a, b)
	Cambodia	Various provinces	2000	Bats	Reynes et al. (2005)
	India	West Bengal (Siliguri)	2001	Humans	Chadha et al. (2006)
	Bangladesh	Meherpur (Chandpur)	2001	Humans	Hsu et al. (2004)
		Naogaon (Chalksita, Biljoania)	2003	Humans, bats	Hsu et al. (2004)
		Rajbari (Goalando)	2004	Humans, bats	(Anon., 2004b, c)
		Faridpur	2004	Humans	(Anon., 2004d)
	Thailand	Various provinces	2002–2004	Bats	Wacharapluesadee et al. (2005)

NA = not available.

Subsequent testing of cerebral spinal fluid obtained from the patient's first illness and from both ill horses confirmed that all were Hendra virus infections.

In 1999, a fatal case of Hendra virus infection occurred in a mare in Cairns, Queensland, Australia, but there was no recognized transmission to humans (Field et al., 2000; Hooper et al., 2000). In late 2004, two human cases of Hendra virus infection were reported in Cairns and Townsville, Queensland. Both illnesses were described as self-limited upper respiratory infections in female veterinarians who had each recently performed a postmortem examination of a horse that had been ill. Hendra virus was confirmed as the cause of death in one of those horses (McCormack, 2005).

Risk factors and transmission of Hendra virus

All reported human cases of Hendra virus infection have been associated with exposure to ill horses, most of which were also confirmed to have been infected with Hendra virus. The mode of transmission was attributed to exposure to horse respiratory droplets, but it appears that close and/or prolonged contact is necessary for transmission. After Hendra virus was first identified, subsequent surveillance among 296 other potential contacts failed to identify any other antibody positive individuals, suggesting that the threshold for infectivity is low (McCormack et al., 1999). There is no evidence for subclinical infection or human-to-human transmission of Hendra virus.

Description of Nipah virus outbreaks

Malaysia and Singapore

In late September 1998, a cluster of human illnesses characterized by encephalitic changes began appearing near the city of Ipoh in the Malaysian state of Perak, followed by a second cluster in December 1998 near the city of Sikamat in the state of Negri Sembilan. A third cluster, which ended up accounting for about 85% of all cases in Malaysia, began later that same month in the village of Sungai Nipah near the city of Bukit Pelandok, also in the state of Negri Sembilan, with a small number of cases confirmed from a third state, Selangor (Anon., 1999a). Most cases were in men who were working on pig farms, many in close contact with pigs. Some illnesses were observed in pigs 1–2 weeks before onset of the illness in humans. By February 1999, the outbreak in Perak had largely subsided, although it was not until early April that cases in Negri Sembilan began to decline. Altogether, a total of 265 Nipah virus encephalitis cases were confirmed, with 105 fatalities.

The outbreaks were facilitated by the movement of pigs between farms, and across the border with Singapore. In a 1-week period in March 1999, 11 abattoir workers in Singapore developed febrile illnesses that were confirmed to be due to Nipah virus infection, and all the affected workers had handled swine imported from Malaysia (Anon., 1999a). The outbreak in Singapore stopped after the pig importation from Malaysia was banned and the abattoirs were closed.

Because cases were associated with close contact with pigs, the disease was initially thought to be due to Japanese encephalitis, but another agent was sought after patients tested negative for that virus. Subsequent EM and immunofluorescence testing identified the etiologic agent as a Hendra-like virus. By early March 1999, the virus was determined to be a distinct paromyxovirus and was then named Nipah virus, after the village in Negri Sembilan where the first isolate was made from a fatal human case (Chua et al., 1999; Chua et al., 2000a). Measures taken to control the outbreak focused on culling pigs in the affected states; over 1 million pigs were eventually culled, with estimated economic losses between US$350 and $400 million mainly due to animal losses (Anon., 2004a). Other measures that were undertaken included a ban on transporting pigs within the country, education, use of personal protective equipment by persons exposed to pigs, and establishment of a national surveillance and control system to detect infected animals (Anon., 1999b). The last confirmed fatal case was reported in May 1999, and no cases have been reported from Malaysia or Singapore since 1999.

Through December 1999, a total of 283 cases of viral encephalitis with 109 fatalities and a case fatality rate of 38.5% were reported to the Malaysia Ministry of Health (Chua, 2003). However, these numbers reflected only symptomatic cases; the true number of persons infected with Nipah virus, although uncertain, is higher due to the fact that asymptomatic patients were largely unrecognized.

India

In January and February 2001, an outbreak of febrile illnesses occurred in the city of Siliguri, in the West Bengal region of India. Although initially reported as atypical measles, it has been retrospectively confirmed that Nipah virus was the most likely cause of the outbreak, with IgM and IgG antibodies to Nipah Virus detected in serum in 9 of 18 patients and a positive PCR in urine from 5 patients (Chadha et al., 2006). A total of 66 cases of Nipah virus encephalitis were identified with at least 43 deaths; all cases occurred in individuals over 15 years of age. No clear animal exposure was identified, but there was some evidence suggesting person-to-person and nosocomial transmission.

Bangladesh

In April and May 2001, a cluster of febrile neurologic illnesses with nine deaths was reported in a village in Meherpur District, Bangladesh. Preliminary testing of sera collected from survivors soon after the outbreak suggested that a Nipah-like virus might have been the cause. A similar outbreak of encephalitis was reported in January 2003 in Naogaon District with eight reported deaths. A later investigation concluded that these 17 deaths were probably due to Nipah virus encephalitis, with an additional eight encephalitis survivors having antibody to Nipah virus (Hsu et al., 2004). Clustering of cases occurred in several households, suggesting limited person-to-person transmission. No clear animal exposure was identified as a possible source for the disease, although two *Pteropus* bats in Naogaon were found to have antibodies to Nipah virus.

In January and February 2004, a cluster of encephalitic illnesses occurred in the Bangladesh district of Rajbari, followed by reports of other Nipah virus-associated illness in various other districts through March 2004 (Anon., 2004b). Altogether, 22 of 29 patients died. Nipah virus was isolated in this outbreak, which demonstrated a 95% homology with the Malaysian strain. A fourth outbreak occurred between

February and April 2004 in Faridpur District, with 27 fatalities from 36 total cases (Anon., 2004d). In this outbreak, it was observed that clusters of these cases occurred in households.

Risk factors and mechanisms of transmission of Nipah virus

Given the epidemiologic differences between cases in Malaysia, Bangladesh, and India, it is apparent that various factors play a role in the transmission of Nipah virus, including close exposure to intermediate zoonotic hosts, indirect contact with infected pteropid bats or exposure to their body secretions, and person-to-person transmission. In Malaysia and Singapore, direct contact with pigs, especially activities involving close contact, was the primary source of human Nipah virus infection (Parashar et al., 2000). Zoonotic transmission from pigs to humans probably occurred through respiratory droplets, given that infected pigs demonstrate both upper and lower respiratory vasculitis and have been shown in experimental studies to infect one another through the oral and respiratory route (Hooper and Williamson, 2000; Mohd Nor et al., 2000). Zoonotic transmission also appears to occur via close handling of infected tissue, as seen in the cases of infected abattoir workers (Paton et al., 1999).

Exposure to infected pigs accounted for most cases of Nipah virus in humans, but 8% of case patients stated had no direct contact with pigs (Parashar et al., 2000). Furthermore, no obvious zoonotic source of transmission has been found in any of the Bangladesh outbreaks. The observation that many infected individuals in Bangladesh were under 19 years of age and had no exposure to pigs or other animals, in contrast to the Malaysia outbreak has led to the hypothesis that infection might have occurred by indirect contact with fruit bats or their secretions. It was observed that in Goalanda, boys ate fruit collected from trees where fruit bats were presumably foraging (Anon., 2004c). Further epidemiologic studies and animal surveys of these outbreaks are currently ongoing.

Nipah virus has been isolated from urine and respiratory secretions of humans with Nipah virus infection during the Malaysia outbreaks, suggesting the possibility of person-to-person transmission. In Malaysia, no evidence of person-to-person transmission was found despite extensive searching; but several households in both the 2001 and 2004 outbreaks in Bangladesh exhibited family clustering of cases, suggesting that limited person-to-person transmission might have occurred (Hsu et al., 2004; Anon., 2004d). Person-to-person transmission was strongly suspected during the most recent outbreak in Faridpur District, of which studies are ongoing. Testing of high-risk health care workers with patient contact during the Malaysia and Bangladesh outbreaks revealed no evidence of nosocomial transmission (Mounts et al., 2001; Hsu et al., 2004). During the Siliguri outbreak, encephalitis cases developed among some hospital staff several days after the admission of patients with Nipah virus encephalitis, suggesting possible nosocomial transmission, but specific exposures were not assessed in affected individuals. Despite the high use of standard and respiratory precautions in Malaysia, only about 40% of health care workers in Bangladesh during the outbreaks used any type of barrier precaution. These findings taken together suggest that person-to-person transmission of Nipah virus can occur, but that the transmission is rather inefficient, and probably requires prolonged close contact.

Animal reservoirs

Fruit bats (order Chiroptera), specifically bats of the genus *Pteropus*, have been shown to be the natural reservoir for Nipah and Hendra virus. About 60 species of pteropid bats, also known as flying foxes, are known to exist; they are native to Asia (including throughout China) and Australia, ranging as far west as the east coast of Africa and as far east as the Pacific Islands (Koopman, 1992). The bats develop subclinical disease due to Nipah virus and are assumed to be the intermediate hosts for infections of humans, but this has not been experimentally shown (Williamson et al., 1998, 2000). Suspicion of bats as natural hosts for the zoonotic paramyxoviruses began after neutralizing antibodies to Hendra virus were found in 4 species of pteropid bats in Australia (Young et al., 1996). Hendra virus has since been isolated from reproductive tissue from *P. poliocephalus* and *P. alecto* (Halpin et al., 2000).

Hendra virus has been demonstrated in Australian bats from the northern city of Darwin down to Melbourne as well as in Papua New Guinea (Paterson et al., 1998). Extensive animal surveillance among other animals has not shown evidence of natural Hendra virus infection among horses or farm animals, or among more than 40 species of wildlife tested from Queensland (Rogers et al., 1996; Ward et al., 1996).

Antibodies to Nipah virus have been found in 9–25% of pteropid bats in Malaysia, Cambodia, Thailand, and Bangladesh, (Yob et al., 2001; Hsu et al., 2004; Reynes et al., 2005; Wacharapluesadee et al., 2005). Neutralizing antibodies to Nipah virus were found in *P. hypomelanus* and *P. vampyrus*, the two pteropid species in Peninsular Malaysia; in Cambodia, antibodies were found in a third species, *P. lylei*; while in Thailand, antibodies were present in all three species. In Bangladesh, *P. giagnteus* bats, a more common species in that region, were found to have neutralizing antibodies to Nipah virus. Neutralizing antibodies to Nipah virus have also been found in other frugivorous and insectivorous bat genera including *Eonycteris*, *Cynopterus*, *Scotophilus*, and *Hipposideros*, although in a lower proportion than in *Pteropus* spp. (Yob et al., 2001; Wacharapluesadee et al., 2005;) whether these bats are also considered natural hosts and the significance of these findings have yet to be determined. Isolation of Nipah virus from the bats has proven to be difficult, but the virus was isolated from 3 of 263 pooled bat urine samples in Malaysia, and 2 of 769 urine samples in Cambodia (Chua et al., 2002; Reynes et al., 2005).

Menangle virus

Menangle virus is a third zoonotic paramyxovirus, described only in New South Wales, Australia. Between April and September 1997, the number of live piglet births at a pig farm near Sydney was noted to decrease dramatically, accompanied by an increase in the number of deformed and stillborn piglets (Philbey et al., 1998). A novel virus, named Menangle, was isolated from affected piglets, characterized, and found to be in the genus *Rubulavirus*, a genus whose viruses are distantly related to Nipah and Hendra viruses (Bowden and Boyle, 2005) (Fig. 1). Of more than 250 persons with potential exposure to the infected pigs, 2 had antibodies to the virus, both of whom had a self-limited illness consisting of malaise, chills, and fever. Extensive serologic investigations ruled out other viruses (Chant et al., 1998). The entire Menangle virus genome was subsequently sequenced (Bowden and Boyle, 2005). As with Hendra and Nipah viruses, fruit bats are thought to be the primary reservoirs for Menangle virus.

Pathogenesis and clinical characteristics

Pathogenesis of Hendra virus infection

The incubation period of Hendra virus is not known, but illness onsets for the first two human cases began between 5 and 8 days after the known contact with the index case mare. Autopsies of these two human cases revealed disease in lung and brain tissue. One patient, with symptoms primarily of pneumonitis, had focal necrotizing alveolitis with giant cells, syncytial formation, and viral inclusions (Selvey et al., 1995). The other patient, with predominantly encephalitic symptoms, had leptomeningitis with lymphocyte and plasma cell infiltration (O'Sullivan et al., 1997). Necrosis of the neocortex, basal ganglia, and cerebellum, was seen, but the subcortical white matter was not affected. It is unclear how Hendra virus enters the CNS, but a guinea-pig model suggested evidence of invasion via the choroid plexus (Williamson et al., 2001). Multinucleated endothelial cells have been seen in the liver and spleen from patients with Hendra virus infections. Hendra virus has been detected by PCR in serum and CSF from humans, but it has only been isolated from kidneys.

In addition to natural Hendra virus infection in horses and humans, Hendra virus has been experimentally transmitted to cats and guinea pigs. In horses, the predominant pathological findings are in lungs, with pulmonary edema and congestion; histologically, interstitial pneumonia has been found with focal necrotizing alveolitis, along with syncytial formation affecting the vascular endothelium. In horses, cats, and guinea pigs, the virus has been isolated from spleen, kidney, urine, and serum (Westbury et al., 1996; Williamson et al., 2000).

Pathogenesis of Nipah virus infection

The exact incubation period of Nipah virus is uncertain; however, the period from last contact with pigs to onset of symptoms during the Malaysian outbreaks was <2 weeks in 92% of patients (mean = 10 days) (Chong et al., 2000; Goh et al., 2000). However, incubation periods up to 2 months have been reported, and in one case study, presumed Nipah virus encephalitis developed 4 months after exposure (Wong et al., 2001). It is unclear whether such unusual cases represent prolonged incubation periods or cases with late-onset encephalitis in initially asymptomatic individuals. The recent outbreaks in Bangladesh have not yielded further data regarding the incubation period.

Widespread vasculitis seen in patients is consistent with the viremia that appears to be the mechanism for spread to various organ systems. In humans and in the hamster animal model (Wong et al., 2002, 2003), it has been proposed that the virus enters the CSF as a result of vascular wall damage. In a porcine model, the data suggest that the virus invades the CNS directly through the cranial nerves (Weingartl et al., 2005). CNS involvement was seen in >90% of autopsies in the Malaysia outbreak, with both parenchymal necrosis and thrombotic vasculitis in the CNS, typically of the small vessels, characterized by varying degrees of segmental endothelial destruction, necrosis, and karyorrhexis (Wong et al., 2002). The lungs were the second most involved organ, with vasculitis seen in the lungs in 62% of cases, along with varying degrees of alveolar hemorrhage and pulmonary edema. Renal, cardiac, and splenic involvement is seen in lesser degrees, each associated with vasculitis, thrombosis, and necrosis (Chua et al., 2001). The occasional observation of syncytial multinucleated giant endothelial cells in the CNS and other organs is a distinct finding not usually seen in other types of viral encephalitis.

Nipah virus has been isolated from human CSF, throat and nasal swabs, and urine (Goh et al., 2000; Chua et al., 2001). Nipah virus has been shown experimentally to infect a variety of tissues from pigs, cats, dogs, and hamsters (Mohd Nor et al., 2000; Middleton et al., 2002; Wong et al., 2003). Most studies of the pathogenesis of Nipah virus have been conducted in pigs. Nipah virus infection is milder in pigs than in humans, often asymptomatic, with mortality from <1% to 5% (Mohd Nor et al., 2000). However, clinical disease in pigs can involve the respiratory system and CNS, and is known as porcine respiratory and encephalitis syndrome. Mild-to-severe lung injury is often present, with emphysema or hemorrhage, and evidence of consolidation. Histology of the lungs reveals interstitial pneumonia and syncytial cell formation with vasculitis, fibrinoid necrosis, and hemorrhage. In experimental infection of pigs, virus is present in nasal turbinates, trachea, lungs, cranial nerves, and olfactory epithelial cells (Weingartl et al., 2005).

Clinical manifestations

Clinical features of Hendra virus infection

It is difficult to delineate the clinical manifestations of a disease for which, to date, only three cases have been reported with detailed clinical information. No asymptomatic human infections have been observed, although asymptomatic Hendra virus infections have been noted in horses (Murray et al., 1995b).

The clinical features of Hendra virus infection involve the respiratory system or CNS, which range from a mild influenza-like illness to fatal pneumonia or encephalitis. In two of the three cases reported with detailed clinical descriptions, presenting symptoms included myalgia, headaches, lethargy, and vertigo (Selvey et al., 1995). One of the two was characterized by 6 weeks of lethargy, and otherwise normal physical and laboratory examinations. The other patient went on to develop nausea, vomiting, and respiratory failure. His chest X-ray had bilateral alveolar and interstitial infiltration. Initial laboratory abnormalities included thrombocytopenia, liver enzyme elevation, acidosis, and hypoxemia, but the white count and differential remained in the normal range. The third case developed a recurrent neurologic syndrome that began as a self-limited meningitis lasting about 2 weeks, followed 1 year later by an encephalitic syndrome consisting of fever, altered mental status (unconscious by day 7 of the encephalitis), focal and generalized tonic-clonic seizures, and death (O'Sullivan et al., 1997). Initial blood count, electrolytes, and liver function tests were normal, but there was a mononuclear pleocytosis in the CSF. MRI of the brain showed gray matter abnormalities that worsened as the illness progressed. Of the patients infected with Hendra virus who recovered, there have been no reports of residual neurologic or other clinical deficits.

Clinical features of Nipah virus infection

Nipah virus can cause asymptomatic infections in some patients; in the Malaysia and Singapore outbreaks between 17% and 45% of infections were asymptomatic. There has not been any evidence for asymptomatic infection in outbreaks in Bangladesh (Hsu et al., 2004). In a study of Malaysian house holds with symptomatic family members infected by Nipah virus, 6 of the 36 (17%) antibody positive individuals were asymptomatic (Tan et al., 1999). Parashar found that among symptomatic pig farmers and their families in Malaysia, 30 of 110 (27%) were asymptomatic (Parashar et al., 2000). In another study designed specifically to compare symptomatic versus asymptomatic Nipah virus infection among high risk groups in Singapore, 10 of 22 (45%) of those with Nipah virus antibodies were asymptomatic, with no neurologic or respiratory symptoms (Chan et al., 2002).

Nipah virus infection produces an encephalitic syndrome predominantly characterized by fever, headache, and neurologic signs. Fever is almost universal, followed by headache in 65–88% of patients (Chong et al., 2000; Goh et al., 2000). A reduced level of consciousness was seen in 55% of all infected individuals during the Malaysia outbreaks (Goh et al., 2000) and in >90% in the Bangladesh outbreaks (Hsu et al., 2004; Anon., 2004c). Vomiting and dizziness are reported as prominent clinical features, which could be secondary to neurologic dysfunction. Some neurological signs reflected brain stem abnormalities, including reduced or absent reflexes, variable reactive pupils, and doll's-eye reflexes. Other specific neurologic signs noted include myoclonus, tonic-clonic seizures, and nystagmus.

The respiratory system is the second most commonly affected system in Nipah virus infection. Cough, cold-like symptoms and dyspnea were the most common respiratory symptoms reported. Respiratory symptoms and abnormal chest x-rays were reported at a higher rate in the Bangladesh outbreaks compared with the Malaysia outbreaks (Anon., 2004c, d). This finding may explain why person-to-person transmission was found in Bangladesh but not in Malaysia. The gastrointintestinal system was much less commonly affected, with some reporting symptoms of abdominal pain, diarrhea, and constipation.

Laboratory and radiographic findings

Common hematologic abnormalities in Nipah virus infection include thrombocytopenia (30%) and leukopenia (11%). Elevated liver function tests are also seen in about 40% of patients, and hyponatremia is sometimes found. Hemoglobin, renal indices, and electrolytes other than sodium are usually normal. CSF white count and protein are elevated in about 75% of cases, although normal CSF white counts were reported in all cases in one outbreak (Chadha et al., 2006).

An initial IgM anti-Nipah virus antibody response was noted in about half of patients on day one of symptoms, rising to 100% from day 3–9 (Ramasundrum et al., 2000). Over half of patients exhibited positive IgG antibody after 2 weeks, and all became positive by day 17–25. However, the presence of antibody in serum or CSF did not influence the rate of isolation of virus from CSF, nor did it correlate with decreases in morbidity or mortality (Ramasundrum et al., 1999; Chua et al., 2000b).

Computed tomography of the head is normal, but MRI findings on T1-weighted imaging include multiple widespread small lesions in the white matter, mostly in the frontal and parietal lobes (Lee et al., 1999; Goh et al., 2000). The pons and cerebellum have also been affected (Lim et al., 2002). T2-weighted imaging demonstrates hyperintense lesions in gray matter and on fluid-attenuated inversion recovery sequences. Chest X-ray is abnormal in a varying number of patients, ranging from 6% to 72% in the Malaysia and Singapore outbreaks, consisting of mild interstitial infiltrates or alveolar consolidation in one or both lung fields (Paton et al., 1999; Chong et al., 2000; Goh et al., 2000;). In Bangladesh, a chest X-ray pattern seen in acute respiratory distress syndrome was interpreted and reported (Anon., 2004d).

Complications, relapse, and mortality

The exact prevalence of individuals with neurologic or psychiatric sequelae of Nipah virus encephalitis is uncertain, as study results vary and sample sizes are generally small. The largest study found 15% (14 of 110 individuals) with residual neurologic deficits (Goh et al., 2000). Higher percentages of residual neurologic, psychiatric, or cognitive symptoms have been reported in smaller studies (Lim et al., 2003; Ng et al., 2004). Neurologic sequelae have included residual cognitive deficits, verbal impairment, cranial nerve palsy, cerebellar abnormalities, and persistent vegetative state. Neuropsychiatric sequelae have included personality changes and major depression. Chronic fatigue syndrome has sometimes also been reported as a sequela of Nipah virus encephalitis.

Relapse occurs in 3–8% of patients, occasionally causing more severe clinical symptoms than the initial manifestation (Goh et al., 2000; Tan et al., 2002). Relapse occurs at a mean of 8 months after initial presentation. Late-onset encephalitis occurs in 3% of infected patients who were initially asymptomatic or non-encephalitic, and has been reported to occur as late as 4 months after initial infection (Goh et al., 2000; Wong et al., 2001). Clinical symptoms of relapsed and late-onset encephalitis are similar to those of initial encephalitis. However, focal MRI abnormalities of the cortical gray matter have also been present in patients with relapsed or late-onset encephalitis.

The overall mortality rate of symptomatic Nipah virus infection differs by country: 40% (105/265) in Malaysia, 9% (1/11) in Singapore, 74% (exact figures uncertain) in India, and 76% (66/87) in Bangladesh. It is uncertain whether these differences are due to virulence factors in the virus or whether they reflect the level or availability of supportive care in each country. Factors that predicted mortality included the presence of doll's-eye reflexes, tachycardia, high fever, hypertension, and a positive viral culture of the CSF (Chong et al., 2000; Chua et al., 2000b; Goh et al., 2000).

Laboratory diagnosis

Only a few laboratories worldwide have the capability for testing and confirming the presence of Hendra and Nipah viruses by virus isolation, immunohistochemistry, and molecular amplification. In addition, these viruses are classified as biosafety level 4 (BSL-4) agents and must be handled under strictest physical containment standards.

Viral isolation in cell culture from affected tissue is an important diagnostic methodology for these viruses, particularly when determining the etiology of a new outbreak (Daniels et al., 2001). Both Hendra and Nipah viruses grow well in Vero cells, and a cytopathic effect is usually noted within 3 days. Nipah virus has been isolated from human CSF, nasal and throat swabs, and urine (Chua et al., 1999; Goh et al., 2000). The virus has also been isolated from pigs and cats in a variety of tissue including lung, spleen, serum, and kidneys (Daniels et al., 2001; Middleton et al., 2002). Although Hendra virus has been isolated in humans only from kidney tissue, it has been isolated from serum, lung, spleen, and CNS tissue from a variety of animals including horses, cats, and guinea pigs (Murray et al., 1995a; Williamson et al., 1998, 2000, 2001). Immunostaining, neutralization techniques, PCR, and EM, including immunoelectron microscopy, are utilized for further identification of the virus.

Immunohistochemistry can be performed on preserved tissues allowing a diagnosis to be made retrospectively. It also has the advantage that testing can be done in the absence of a BSL-4 facility. A range of polycloncal and monoclonal antisera are used, but they are not available commercially. PCR methods and sequencing are necessary for genetic characterization of these viruses, especially with a suspected new outbreak in a geographically distinct area, as occurred in the Bangladesh outbreak (Harcourt, 2005). Nested primers coding for the M or N genes are most commonly used at present, although primers for the P gene were used in the initial outbreak in Malaysia and Singapore (Chua et al., 2000a; Daniels et al., 2001).

Serologic methods include neutralization tests and enzyme-linked immunosorbent assays (ELISA). The serum neutralization test is the accepted standard for serology, but it requires BSL-4 facilities, as cell cultures must be used to determine whether a cytopathic effect has occurred. The ELISA utilizes both indirect formats for IgG and antibody capture for detecting IgM antibodies for Hendra and Nipah viruses. To perform these tests, preparation of viral antigen has been used, but research is being done to express antigen utilizing individual viral proteins such as the N protein of both viruses (Bellini et al., 2002). These newer techniques allow ELISA preparation and testing to be done at facilities with BSL-2. This gives ELISA the advantage of being able to quickly detect antigen in a wider range of laboratory settings; the test is also more useful for rapid diagnosis for many cases in a suspected outbreak setting compared to serum neutralization. However, the sensitivity and specificity of the ELISA test are slightly inferior to serum neutralization tests.

Treatment, prevention, and control

Treatment for Hendra virus is supportive only. No effective antiviral therapy is known for Hendra virus. However, *in vitro*, ribavirin has been shown to have an inhibitory effect against RNA synthesis and the yield of Hendra virus (Wright et al., 2005).

Ribavirin and acyclovir have been used to treat Nipah virus infection. In Malaysia, ribavirin was administered orally or intravenously to 140 persons with Nipah virus encephalitis and compared to a group of 54 control patients who did not receive ribavirin. A total of 45 deaths in the treated group (32%) compared to 29 deaths in the control group (54%) suggested a 36% reduction in mortality with ribavirin administration (Chong et al., 2001). In Singapore, acyclovir was administered to all encephalitis patients during the Nipah outbreak (Paton et al., 1999; Bellini et al., 2002). Only one fatality occurred in Singapore, but the effect that the drug had on the course of disease is unclear.

Nipah and Hendra virus infections can theoretically be prevented by avoiding direct or indirect contact with fruit bats or fruit bat urine or droppings. Using precautionary measures such as gloves and masks may be considered in locations with fruit bats. Fruit or other products from trees where fruit bats roost should be carefully washed.

Because it is assumed that these viruses can spread through respiratory droplets or by contact, caution should be used when caring for an infected individual, including frequent handwashing, avoidance of direct contact with urine or salivary secretions, and wearing a mask. Although nosocomial transmission of the viruses is unlikely, contact and droplet precautions seem prudent when taking care of any patient with suspected Nipah or Hendra virus infection.

Surveillance is an important tool for early detection for illnesses caused by the henipaviruses. Surveillance for Hendra virus illness has been established in Australia, and surveillance for encephalitic disease has been implemented in Malaysia, Thailand, and Bangladesh. Clusters of respiratory or encephalitic illness in humans or in certain animals, occurring in geographic locations where *Pteropus* bats are known to be endemic, should raise awareness of the possibility of henipavirus infection. Thus, surveillance in animals such as horses and pigs is also important for the early detection of Nipah and Hendra virus infections.

No specific vaccine is available against Nipah or Hendra virus. However, active immunization against Nipah virus and passive transfer of antibody to Nipah virus have shown promising results in hamster models (Guillaume et al., 2004).

Ecologic aspects and future considerations

Ecologic changes, human demographics, and behavior patterns such as international travel, technology and industry, and microbial adaptation have all been factors that are thought to play a role in infectious disease emergence (Morse, 1995). For the henipaviruses, speculation has focused on environmental changes such as deforestation and hunting, which subsequently affected the roosting habitats of flying foxes and placed them in closer proximity to humans (Field et al., 2001; Daszak et al., 2004; Breed et al., 2005). It should be noted also that in Bangladesh, located at a more subtropical latitude, all Nipah outbreaks occurred in the first half of the year, suggesting that perhaps climate change or bat activities affected by seasonal change may also have played a role. Until a better understanding of the causes of these newly emergent viruses is obtained, future outbreaks are likely to recur. Research is continuing to identify the factors that have led to the emergence of Hendra and Nipah viruses in domestic animal and human populations.

Acknowledgments

The author would like to acknowledge Joel Montgomery and Umesh Parashar, both with the Centers for Disease Control and Prevention, for assistance and comments in reviewing this manuscript.

References

Anon. Another human case of equine morbillivirus disease in Australia, Emerg Infect Dis 1996; 2: 71–72.
Anon. Outbreak of Hendra-like virus—Malaysia and Singapore, 1998–1999. MMWR Morb Mortal Wkly Rep 1999a; 48: 265–269.

Anon. Update: outbreak of Nipah virus—Malaysia and Singapore, 1999. MMWR Morb Mortal Wkly Rep 1999b; 48: 335–337.

Anon. Emerging Disease Futures: Identifying Risks, Exploring Solutions, Vol. 2005. Bio Economic Research Associates 2004a.

Anon. Nipah encephalitis outbreak over wide area of Western Bangladesh, 2004. Health Sci Bull 2004b; 2: 7–11.

Anon. Nipah virus outbreak(s) in Bangladesh, January–April 2004. Wkly Epidemiol Rec 2004c; 79: 168–171.

Anon. Person-to-person transmission of Nipah virus during outbreak in Faridpur District, 2004. Health Sci Bull 2004d; 2: 5–9.

Bellini WJ, Rota P, Parashar UD. Zoonotic paramyxoviruses. In: Clinical Virology (Richman DD, Whitley RJ, Hayden FG, editors). 2nd ed. Washington, DC: ASM Press; 2002; pp. 845–855.

Bowden TR, Boyle DB. Completion of the full-length genome sequence of Menangle virus: characterisation of the polymerase gene and genomic 5′ trailer region. Arch Virol 2005; 150: 2125–2137.

Breed A, Field H, Plowright R. Volant viruses: a concern to bats, humans and other animals. Microbiol Aust 2005; 26: 59–63.

Chadha MS, Comer JA, Lowe L, Rota P, Rollin PE, Bellini WJ, Ksiazek T, Mishra AC. Nipah virus-associated encephalitis outbreak, Siliguri, India. Emerg Infect Dis 2006; 12: 235–240.

Chan KP, Rollin PE, Ksiazek TG, Leo YS, Goh KT, Paton NI, Sng EH, Ling AE. A survey of Nipah virus infection among various risk groups in Singapore. Epidemiol Infect 2002; 128: 93–98.

Chant K, Chan R, Smith M, Dwyer DE, Kirkland P. Probable human infection with a newly described virus in the family *Paramyxoviridae*. Emerg Infect Dis 1998; 4: 273–275.

Chong HT, Kamarulzaman A, Tan CT, Goh KJ, Thayaparan T, Kunjapan SR, Chew NK, Chua KB, Lam SK. Treatment of acute Nipah encephalitis with ribavirin. Ann Neurol 2001; 49: 810–813.

Chong HT, Kunjapan SR, Thayaparan T, Tong J, Petharunam V, Jusoh MR, Tan CT. Nipah encephalitis outbreak in Malaysia, clinical features in patients from Seremban. Neurol J Southeast Asia 2000; 5: 61–67.

Chua KB. Nipah virus outbreak in Malaysia. J Clin Virol 2003; 26: 265–275.

Chua KB, Bellini WJ, Rota PA, Harcourt BH, Tamin A, Lam SK, Ksiazek TG, Rollin PE, Zaki SR, Shieh W, Goldsmith CS, Gubler DJ, Roehrig JT, Eaton B, Gould AR, Olson J, Field H, Daniels P, Ling AE, Peters CJ, Anderson LJ, Mahy BW. Nipah virus: a recently emergent deadly paramyxovirus. Science 2000a; 288: 1432–1435.

Chua KB, Goh KJ, Wong KT, Kamarulzaman A, Tan PS, Ksiazek TG, Zaki SR, Paul G, Lam SK, Tan CT. Fatal encephalitis due to Nipah virus among pig-farmers in Malaysia. Lancet 1999; 354: 1257–1259.

Chua KB, Koh CL, Hooi PS, Wee KF, Khong JH, Chua BH, Chan YP, Lim ME, Lam SK. Isolation of Nipah virus from Malaysian Island flying-foxes. Microbes Infect 2002; 4: 145–151.

Chua KB, Lam SK, Goh KJ, Hooi PS, Ksiazek TG, Kamarulzaman A, Olson J, Tan CT. The presence of Nipah virus in respiratory secretions and urine of patients during an outbreak of Nipah virus encephalitis in Malaysia. J Infect 2001; 42: 40–43.

Chua KB, Lam SK, Tan CT, Hooi PS, Goh KJ, Chew NK, Tan KS, Kamarulzaman A, Wong KT. High mortality in Nipah encephalitis is associated with presence of virus in cerebrospinal fluid. Ann Neurol 2000b; 48: 802–805.

Daniels P, Ksiazek T, Eaton BT. Laboratory diagnosis of Nipah and Hendra virus infections. Microbes Infect 2001; 3: 289–295.

Daszak P, Tabor GM, Kilpatrick AM, Epstein J, Plowright R. Conservation medicine and a new agenda for emerging diseases. Ann N Y Acad Sci 2004; 1026: 1–11.

Field H, Young P, Yob JM, Mills J, Hall L, Mackenzie J. The natural history of Hendra and Nipah viruses. Microbes Infect 2001; 3: 307–314.

Field HE, Barratt PC, Hughes RJ, Shield J, Sullivan ND. A fatal case of Hendra virus infection in a horse in north Queensland: clinical and epidemiological features. Aust Vet J 2000; 78: 279–280.

Goh KJ, Tan CT, Chew NK, Tan PS, Kamarulzaman A, Sarji SA, Wong KT, Abdullah BJ, Chua KB, Lam SK. Clinical features of Nipah virus encephalitis among pig farmers in Malaysia. N Engl J Med 2000; 342: 1229–1235.

Guillaume V, Contamin H, Loth P, Georges-Courbot MC, Lefeuvre A, Marianneau P, Chua KB, Lam SK, Buckland R, Deubel V, Wild TF. Nipah virus: vaccination and passive protection studies in a hamster model. J Virol 2004; 78: 834–840.

Halpin K, Young PL, Field HE, Mackenzie JS. Isolation of Hendra virus from pteropid bats: a natural reservoir of Hendra virus. J Gen Virol 2000; 81: 1927–1932.

Harcourt BH. Genetic characterization of nipah virus, Bangladesh, 2004. Emerg Infect Dis 2005; 11: 1594–1597.

Harcourt BH, Tamin A, Halpin K, Ksiazek TG, Rollin PE, Bellini WJ, Rota PA. Molecular characterization of the polymerase gene and genomic termini of Nipah virus. Virology 2001; 287: 192–201.

Harcourt BH, Tamin A, Ksiazek TG, Rollin PE, Anderson LJ, Bellini WJ, Rota PA. Molecular characterization of Nipah virus, a newly emergent paramyxovirus. Virology 2000; 271: 334–349.

Hooper PT, Gould AR, Hyatt AD, Braun MA, Kattenbelt JA, Hengstberger SG, Westbury HA. Identification and molecular characterization of Hendra virus in a horse in Queensland. Aust Vet J 2000; 78: 281–282.

Hooper PT, Williamson MM. Hendra and Nipah virus infections. Vet Clin North Am Equine Pract 2000; 16: 597–603 xi.

Hsu VP, Hossain MJ, Parashar UD, Ali MM, Ksiazek TG, Kuzmin I, Niezgoda M, Rupprecht C, Bresee J, Breiman RF. Nipah virus encephalitis reemergence, Bangladesh. Emerg Infect Dis 2004; 10: 2082–2087.

Hyatt AD, Zaki SR, Goldsmith CS, Wise TG, Hengstberger SG. Ultrastructure of Hendra virus and Nipah virus within cultured cells and host animals. Microbes Infect 2001; 3: 297–306.

Koopman KF. O1_MRKO1_MRKOrder Chiroptera. In: Mammal Species of the World: A Taxonomy and Geographic Reference (Wilson DE, Reeder DM, editors). Washington, DC: Smithsonian Institution Press; 1992; pp. 137–241.

Lee KE, Umapathi T, Tan CB, Tjia HT, Chua TS, Oh HM, Fock KM, Kurup A, Das A, Tan AK, Lee WL. The neurological manifestations of Nipah virus encephalitis, a novel paramyxovirus. Ann Neurol 1999; 46: 428–432.

Lim CC, Lee KE, Lee WL, Tambyah PA, Lee CC, Sitoh YY, Auchus AP, Lin BK, Hui F. Nipah virus encephalitis: serial MR study of an emerging disease. Radiology 2002; 222: 219–226.

Lim CC, Lee WL, Leo YS, Lee KE, Chan KP, Ling AE, Oh H, Auchus AP, Paton NI, Hui F, Tambyah PA. Late clinical and magnetic resonance imaging follow up of Nipah virus infection. J Neurol Neurosurg Psychiatry 2003; 74: 131–133.

Mayo MA. A summary of taxonomic changes recently approved by ICTV. Arch Virol 2002; 147: 1655–1663.

McCormack JG. Hendra and Nipah viruses: new zoonotically-acquired human pathogens. Respir Care Clin N Am 2005; 11: 59–66.

McCormack JG, Allworth AM, Selvey LA, Selleck PW. Transmissibility from horses to humans of a novel paramyxovirus, equine morbillivirus (EMV). J Infect 1999; 38: 22–23.

Middleton DJ, Westbury HA, Morrissy CJ, van der Heide BM, Russell GM, Braun MA, Hyatt AD. Experimental Nipah virus infection in pigs and cats. J Comp Pathol 2002; 126: 124–136.

Mohd Nor MN, Gan CH, Ong BL. Nipah virus infection of pigs in peninsular Malaysia. Rev Sci Tech 2000; 19: 160–165.

Moll M, Diederich S, Klenk HD, Czub M, Maisner A. Ubiquitous activation of the Nipah virus fusion protein does not require a basic amino acid at the cleavage site. J Virol 2004; 78: 9705–9712.

Morse SS. Factors in the emergence of infectious diseases. Emerg Infect Dis 1995; 1: 7–15.

Mounts AW, Kaur H, Parashar UD, Ksiazek TG, Cannon D, Arokiasamy JT, Anderson LJ, Lye MS. A cohort study of health care workers to assess nosocomial transmissibility of Nipah virus, Malaysia, 1999. J Infect Dis 2001; 183: 810–813.

Murray K, Rogers R, Selvey L, Selleck P, Hyatt A, Gould A, Gleeson L, Hooper P, Westbury H. A novel morbillivirus pneumonia of horses and its transmission to humans. Emerg Infect Dis 1995a; 1: 31–33.

Murray K, Selleck P, Hooper P, Hyatt A, Gould A, Gleeson L, Westbury H, Hiley L, Selvey L, Rodwell B, et al. A morbillivirus that caused fatal disease in horses and humans. Science 1995b; 268: 94–97.

Ng BY, Lim CC, Yeoh A, Lee WL. Neuropsychiatric sequelae of Nipah virus encephalitis. J Neuropsychiatry Clin Neurosci 2004; 16: 500–504.

O'Sullivan JD, Allworth AM, Paterson DL, Snow TM, Boots R, Gleeson LJ, Gould AR, Hyatt AD, Bradfield J. Fatal encephalitis due to novel paramyxovirus transmitted from horses. Lancet 1997; 349: 93–95.

Parashar UD, Sunn LM, Ong F, Mounts AW, Arif MT, Ksiazek TG, Kamaluddin MA, Mustafa AN, Kaur H, Ding LM, Othman G, Radzi HM, Kitsutani PT, Stockton PC, Arokiasamy J, Gary Jr. HE, Anderson LJ. Case–control study of risk factors for human infection with a new zoonotic paramyxovirus, Nipah virus, during a 1998–1999 outbreak of severe encephalitis in Malaysia. J Infect Dis 2000; 181: 1755–1759.

Park MS, Shaw ML, Munoz-Jordan J, Cros JF, Nakaya T, Bouvier N, Palese P, Garcia-Sastre A, Basler CF. Newcastle disease virus (NDV)-based assay demonstrates interferon-antagonist activity for the NDV V protein and the Nipah virus V, W, and C proteins. J Virol 2003; 77: 1501–1511.

Paterson DL, Murray PK, McCormack JG. Zoonotic disease in Australia caused by a novel member of the *paramyxoviridae*. Clin Infect Dis 1998; 27: 112–118.

Paton NI, Leo YS, Zaki SR, Auchus AP, Lee KE, Ling AE, Chew SK, Ang B, Rollin PE, Umapathi T, Sng I, Lee CC, Lim E, Ksiazek TG. Outbreak of Nipah-virus infection among abattoir workers in Singapore. Lancet 1999; 354: 1253–1256.

Philbey AW, Kirkland PD, Ross AD, Davis RJ, Gleeson AB, Love RJ, Daniels PW, Gould AR, Hyatt AD. An apparently new virus (family *Paramyxoviridae*) infectious for pigs, humans, and fruit bats. Emerg Infect Dis 1998; 4: 269–271.

Ramasundrum V, Chong TT, Chua KB, Chong HT, Goh KJ, Chew NK, Tan KS, Thayaparan T, Kunjapan SR, Petharunam V, Loh YL, Ksiazek TG, Lam SK. Kinetics of IgM and IgG seroconversion in Nipah virus infection. Neurol J Southeast Asia 2000; 5: 23–28.

Ramasundrum V, Tan CT, Chong HT, Goh KJ, Chew NK, Lam SK, Ksiazek T. Presence of CSF IgM do not have a protective effective in Nipah encephalitis. Neurol J Southeast Asia 1999; 4: 73–76.

Reynes JM, Counor D, Ong S, Faure C, Seng V, Molia S, Walston J, Georges-Courbot MC, Deubel V, Sarthou JL. Nipah virus in Lyle's flying foxes, Cambodia. Emerg Infect Dis 2005; 11: 1042–1047.

Rogers RJ, Douglas IC, Baldock FC, Glanville RJ, Seppanen KT, Gleeson LJ, Selleck PN, Dunn KJ. Investigation of a second focus of equine morbillivirus infection in coastal Queensland. Aust Vet J 1996; 74: 243–244.

Selvey LA, Wells RM, McCormack JG, Ansford AJ, Murray K, Rogers RJ, Lavercombe PS, Selleck P, Sheridan JW. Infection of humans and horses by a newly described morbillivirus. Med J Aust 1995; 162: 642–645.

Tan CT, Goh KJ, Wong KT, Sarji SA, Chua KB, Chew NK, Murugasu P, Loh YL, Chong HT, Tan KS, Thayaparan T, Kumar S, Jusoh MR. Relapsed and late-onset Nipah encephalitis. Ann Neurol 2002; 51: 703–708.

Tan KS, Tan CT, Goh KJ. Epidemiological aspects of Nipah virus infection. Neurol J Southeast Asia 1999; 4: 77–81.

Wacharapluesadee S, Lumlertdacha B, Boongird K, Wanghongsa S, Chanhome L, Rollin PE, Stockton P, Rupprecht CE, Ksiazek TG, Hemachudha T. Bat Nipah virus, Thailand. Emerg Infect Dis 2005; 11: 1949–1951.

Wang L, Harcourt BH, Yu M, Tamin A, Rota PA, Bellini WJ, Eaton BT. Molecular biology of Hendra and Nipah viruses. Microbes Infect 2001; 3: 279–287.

Wang LF, Yu M, Hansson E, Pritchard LI, Shiell B, Michalski WP, Eaton BT. The exceptionally large genome of Hendra virus: support for creation of a new genus within the family *Paramyxoviridae*. J Virol 2000; 74: 9972–9979.

Ward MP, Black PF, Childs AJ, Baldock FC, Webster WR, Rodwell BJ, Brouwer SL. Negative findings from serological studies of equine morbillivirus in the Queensland horse population. Aust Vet J 1996; 74: 241–243.

Weingartl H, Czub S, Copps J, Berhane Y, Middleton D, Marszal P, Gren J, Smith G, Ganske S, Manning L, Czub M. Invasion of the central nervous system in a porcine host by Nipah virus. J Virol 2005; 79: 7528–7534.

Westbury HA, Hooper PT, Brouwer SL, Selleck PW. Susceptibility of cats to equine morbillivirus. Aust Vet J 1996; 74: 132–134.

Williamson MM, Hooper PT, Selleck PW, Gleeson LJ, Daniels PW, Westbury HA, Murray PK. Transmission studies of Hendra virus (equine morbillivirus) in fruit bats, horses and cats. Aust Vet J 1998; 76: 813–818.

Williamson MM, Hooper PT, Selleck PW, Westbury HA, Slocombe RF. Experimental Hendra virus infection in pregnant guinea pigs and fruit bats (*Pteropus poliocephalus*). J Comp Pathol 2000; 122: 201–207.

Williamson MM, Hooper PT, Selleck PW, Westbury HA, Slocombe RF. A guinea-pig model of Hendra virus encephalitis. J Comp Pathol 2001; 124: 273–279.

Wong KT, Grosjean I, Brisson C, Blanquier B, Fevre-Montange M, Bernard A, Loth P, Georges-Courbot MC, Chevallier M, Akaoka H, Marianneau P, Lam SK, Wild TF, Deubel V. A golden hamster model for human acute Nipah virus infection. Am J Pathol 2003; 163: 2127–2137.

Wong KT, Shieh WJ, Kumar S, Norain K, Abdullah W, Guarner J, Goldsmith CS, Chua KB, Lam SK, Tan CT, Goh KJ, Chong HT, Jusoh R, Rollin PE, Ksiazek TG, Zaki SR. Nipah virus infection: pathology and pathogenesis of an emerging paramyxoviral zoonosis. Am J Pathol 2002; 161: 2153–2167.

Wong SC, Ooi MH, Wong MN, Tio PH, Solomon T, Cardosa MJ. Late presentation of Nipah virus encephalitis and kinetics of the humoral immune response. J Neurol Neurosurg Psychiatry 2001; 71: 552–554.

Wright PJ, Crameri G, Eaton BT. RNA synthesis during infection by Hendra virus: an examination by quantitative real-time PCR of RNA accumulation, the effect of ribavirin and the attenuation of transcription. Arch Virol 2005; 150: 521–532.

Yob JM, Field H, Rashdi AM, Morrissy C, van der Heide B, Rota P, bin Adzhar A, White J, Daniels P, Jamaluddin A, Ksiazek T. Nipah virus infection in bats (order Chiroptera) in peninsular Malaysia. Emerg Infect Dis 2001; 7: 439–441.

Young PL, Halpin K, Selleck PW, Field H, Gravel JL, Kelly MA, Mackenzie JS. Serologic evidence for the presence in *Pteropus* bats of a paramyxovirus related to equine morbillivirus. Emerg Infect Dis 1996; 2: 239–240.

Yu M, Hansson E, Langedijk JP, Eaton BT, Wang LF. The attachment protein of Hendra virus has high structural similarity but limited primary sequence homology compared with viruses in the genus *Paramyxovirus*. Virology 1998; 251: 227–233.

Emerging Viruses in Human Populations
Edward Tabor (Editor)
DOI 10.1016/S0168-7069(06)16010-3

Japanese Encephalitis Virus: The Geographic Distribution, Incidence, and Spread of a Virus with a Propensity to Emerge in New Areas

John S. Mackenzie[a], David T. Williams[a], David W. Smith[b]

[a]*Australian Biosecurity Cooperative Research Centre for Emerging Infectious Diseases, Curtin University of Technology, GPO Box U1987, Perth, WA6845, Australia*
[b]*Division of Microbiology and Infectious Diseases, PathWest, Locked Bag 2009, Nedlands, WA6909, Australia*

Introduction

Japanese encephalitis (JE) virus (JEV) is the major mosquito-borne encephalitic flavivirus of rural eastern, southeastern and southern Asia. It is believed to be responsible for more than 40,000 cases of encephalitis annually, with at least 10,000 deaths, but these figures are generally regarded as a significant underestimate, and it has been suggested that the true disease burden might be closer to 175,000 cases annually (Tsai, 2000). Indeed, with the near eradication of poliomyelitis, JE is now the leading cause of childhood viral neurological infection and disability in Asia (Halstead and Jacobson, 2003). In 2002, the global burden was estimated to be 709,000 disability adjusted life years (WHO, 2004). The lack of a more accurate indication of the disease burden is due to the absence of good surveillance (surveillance is incomplete or even non-existent in some affected countries) and by the paucity of diagnostic laboratories in a number of affected countries. It has been calculated that about 2 billion people live in rural JE-prone areas of the world, the majority in China and India, with 700 million children under the age of 15 at risk of infection (Tsai, 2000; Keiser et al., 2005). Over the past 60 years, it has been estimated that JEV has infected more than 10 million people, of whom 3 million died and 4 million suffered long-term disabilities.

Historically, epidemics of encephalitis suggestive of JE had been recorded in Japan since 1871, but the first large outbreak to be described occurred in 1924 with

> 6000 cases and a fatality rate of 60%. The disease was termed "Type B" epidemic encephalitis initially to distinguish it from epidemic encephalitis lethargica, "Type A", but the use of the designation "Type B" has now been dropped from the name. Observations of the 1924 epidemic and subsequent epidemics suggested that JE had a seasonal occurrence and was therefore probably transmitted by mosquito vectors. The virus was first isolated from the brain of a fatal case in Japan in 1934 (T. Miatamura et al., 1936, cited by Burke and Leake, 1988; Monath, 1988) and characterised as the prototype strain (Nakayama strain). It was subsequently isolated from *Culex tritaeniorhynchus* mosquitoes (T. Mitamura et al., 1938, cited by Burke and Leake, 1988). Much of our knowledge of the animal–vector–human transmission cycles between viraemic pigs and birds through the vector, *Cx. tritaeniorhynchus*, and to humans as incidental hosts, was later elucidated in a series of excellent studies in Japan by Scherer, Buescher, and their colleagues (Buescher and Scherer, 1959; Buescher et al., 1959a,b; Scherer, 1959).

JEV was shown to be antigenically related to St Louis encephalitis virus (SLEV) and West Nile virus (WNV) by Smithburn (1942). Subsequently Casals and Brown (1954) grouped these viruses as the "Group B arboviruses", together with yellow fever, dengue, and other similar viruses on the basis of serological cross-reactions detected by haemagglutination inhibition. More recently, these viruses were classified as members of the family *Flaviviridae* based on a number of similar features and properties (Westaway et al., 1985), and subsequently in the genus *Flaviviruses*, within that family. While all flaviviruses share group-reactive epitopes, cross-neutralisation tests have been shown to further discriminate most members of the genus into eight serological groups or serocomplexes, the JE serological group being one of these complexes (Madrid and Porterfield, 1974; Calisher et al., 1989). Phylogenetic studies have generally supported and extended these earlier serological relationships and have given some indication of the possible evolutionary origins of these viruses (Kuno et al., 1998; Gould et al., 2001).

Japanese encephalitis virus

The JE serological group of viruses

The JE serological group comprises eight antigenically related virus species and two strains or subtypes, with members found on all continents except Antarctica. The virus species are Cacipacore virus (CPCV), JEV, Koutango virus (KOUV), Murray Valley encephalitis virus (MVEV), SLEV, Usutu virus (USUV), WNV, and Yaounde virus (YAOV), with Alfuy virus (ALFV) and Kunjin virus (KUNV) being subtypes of MVEV and WNV, respectively (Mackenzie et al., 2002a; Thiel et al., 2005). Of the latter two viruses, there is increasing genetic evidence to indicate that ALFV should be re-classified as a separate species in the group (May et al., 2006), and KUNV is generally recognised to be a clade within WNV lineage 1 viruses (Lanciotti et al., 1999; Scherret et al., 2001, 2002), and is referred to here as WNV (KUNV clade). In addition to these recognised members, there have been reports of other potential species or subtypes from central Europe and the Volga delta of Russia that appear to be closely related to WNV (Lvov et al., 2004; Bakonyi et al., 2005). SLEV, MVEV, and WNV are major causes of human disease: SLEV in North, Central, and South America; MVEV in Australia and Papua New Guinea; and WNV in Africa, southern Europe, western Asia, Australasia (as KUNV clade), and most recently in North America. KOUV and USUV cause occasional human infections in Africa. The other three viruses, ALFV in Australia, CPCV in South America, and YAOV in Africa, have not been associated with human infection or disease. The phylogenetic relationships between putative members of the serological group, based on molecular biology studies, have been described by a several groups (Poidinger et al., 1996; Kuno et al., 1998; Gould et al., 2001) and in general are consistent with the serological grouping, with the exception that SLEV clusters more closely with Rocio and Ilheus viruses in the Ntaya virus serological group than with members of the JE serological group. The evolution and divergence of the members is more complex and difficult to determine, but it is likely that a precursor to JEV emerged from Africa and gave rise to the current genetically recognisable form of the virus within the past few centuries (Uchil and Satchidanandam, 2001; Gould, 2002; Solomon et al., 2003a).

The JE serological group members have demonstrated a strong propensity to spread into new areas. This has been clearly demonstrated over the past few years with the spread of WNV into North America (Briese et al., 1999; Lanciotti et al., 1999), USUV into the avifauna of Austria (Weissenbock et al., 2002), and JEV into Pakistan (Igarashi et al., 1994) and Australasia (Hanna et al., 1996b; Mackenzie et al., 2002b). Indeed it is this propensity to spread together with the geographic range that forms the major focus of this chapter.

Properties of the virus

JEV is a positive-sense single-stranded RNA virus, approximately 11 kb long and capped at its 5′ end but, unlike cellular mRNAs, is not 3′-polyadenylated (Burke and Monath, 2001; Lindenbach and Rice, 2003). It contains a single open reading frame (ORF) encoding a polyprotein, which is cleaved co- and post-translationally. The 5′ quarter of the ORF encodes three structural proteins (capsid (C), membrane (M) that is formed from its precursor (prM), and envelope (E)), and the remaining 3′ end of the genome encodes seven non-structural proteins (NS1, NS2a, NS2b, NS3, NS4a, NS4b, and NS5). The ORF is flanked by a 5′ untranslated region (UTR) of approximately 95 nucleotides, and a polymorphic 3′ UTR, 560–585 nucleotides in length (Poidinger et al., 1996; Nam et al., 2002).

JE virions contain the surface proteins E and prM/M, and the nucleocapsid C protein that encapsulates the viral RNA (Lindenbach and Rice, 2003). The E protein forms an icosahedral protein shell and is responsible for cellular attachment and fusion of the virus envelope with the plasma membrane (Heinz et al., 2004). The prM protein facilitates the intracellular maturation and transport of E protein during virus particle morphogenesis (Heinz and Allison, 2003). Shortly before virus egress, prM undergoes proteolytic cleavage—an event required to produce fully infectious virus leaving the M protein in the mature viral envelope (Elshuber et al., 2003; Heinz and Allison, 2003). The main functions of the non-structural proteins are viral RNA replication, involving NS1, NS2A, NS3, NS4A, and NS5, and translation and polyprotein processing, mediated by NS2B, NS3, NS4, and NS5 (Westaway et al., 2002; Lindenbach and Rice, 2003). Conserved elements and secondary structures located in the 5′ and 3′ UTRs are also involved in viral RNA replication and translation (Markoff, 2003).

Antigenic and genomic variation

Antigenic variation

JEV exists as a single serotype, but antigenic variation has been recognised using polyclonal and monoclonal antibodies. Two major immunotypes were differentiated using polyclonal sera and represented by the prototype strain, Nakayama, and the Beijing-1 strain (Okuno et al., 1968), which are also the strains used in inactivated mouse brain-derived JE vaccines. Monoclonal antibody analyses have demonstrated at least five antigenic subgroups (Kobayashi et al., 1984; Kedarnath et al., 1986); the Nakayama virus strain isolated in 1934, the Beijing-1 virus strain which had been isolated in 1949, the Kamiyama strain isolated in 1966, the 691004 strain isolated in 1969 in Sri Lanka, and the Muar strain isolated in 1952 in Singapore. Further putative subtypes were subsequently identified from 5 viruses isolated in Thailand, China Taiwan, and India, of which four had some antigenic similarities to the Kamiyama subtype and one, the Thai KE093 strain, was very different (Satake et al., 1994; Hasegawa et al., 1995). Interestingly, most of the currently circulating strains fall into the Kamiyama subtype (Satake et al., 1994; Hasegawa et al., 1995), but the data also suggest that there is antigenic drift from the Kamiyama subtype, and that additional antigenic subtypes may be circulating in other geographic areas.

Genomic variation

Genetic variation among JEV strains isolated from widely different time periods and geographical regions has been demonstrated and investigated in several studies (Chen et al., 1990, 1992; Ali and Igarashi, 1997; Williams et al., 2000; Uchil and Satchidanandam, 2001; Solomon et al., 2003a). Sequence information from the highly variable prM gene was used to define four genotypes (Chen et al., 1990, 1992). These genotypes were subsequently confirmed by phylogenetic studies using the E gene and full-length genomic sequences (Williams et al., 2000; Uchil and Satchidanandam, 2001; Solomon et al., 2003a). Genotype 1 was found to comprise strains from Cambodia, Korea, northern Thailand, Vietnam, Japan, and Australia; genotype 2 comprised strains from Indonesia, Malaysia, southern Thailand, and Australia; genotype 3 contained viruses isolated from the known geographic range of JEV—with the exception of the Australasian region—and included strains from Japan, China, Taiwan, the Philippines, and Southeast Asia; and genotype 4 comprised isolates found only in Indonesia. Interestingly, all isolates from Indian subcontinent belong to genotype 3, and no other genotype has been found in India, Nepal, or Sri Lanka. Genotype 4 is the most divergent clade in phylogenetic analyses and is therefore thought to represent the oldest lineage of JEV (Solomon et al., 2003a). Based on E gene phylogeny, the Muar strain from Singapore has been proposed as a fifth genotype (Uchil and Satchidanandam, 2001; Solomon et al., 2003a), but this isolate clusters with genotype 3 strains in prM gene phylogeny (Chen et al., 1990, 1992; Williams et al., 2000) and it has been suggested that sequencing errors introduced into an otherwise conserved region of the Muar E gene sequence may have confounded phylogenetic analyses (Gould et al., 2004). In the absence of confirmatory sequences for the Muar strain or the isolation of additional strains belonging to this proposed genotype, the fifth genotype remains uncertain. The phylogenetic relationship between the different genotypes is shown in Fig. 1.

The genetic variation observed in flaviviruses was thought to arise predominantly through the accumulation of mutational changes (clonal evolution). Recently, however, evidence for recombination has been found for flaviviruses including JEV, providing an alternative and more dramatic means by which JEV may evolve (Twiddy and Holmes, 2003; Gould et al., 2004). Recombination events may lead to evolution of novel viruses with altered tissue tropism, pathogenesis, and disease associations. In terms of molecular epidemiological investigations, the presence of recombination in a given genome may lead to its misclassification in single gene analysis. This may be avoided by using either full-length genomes or different regions of the same genome in phylogenetic analyses.

A correlation between genetic variation and JEV activity has been observed, with isolates from northern temperate areas where JE occurs as summer epidemics predominantly caused by genotypes 1 and 3, whereas endemic strains found in tropical equatorial regions have been associated with genotypes 2 and 4 (Chen et al., 1990, 1992). However, several exceptions to this pattern have now been demonstrated, with the so-called epidemic genotypes found in endemic areas, and vice versa. One such example can be found in India where epidemic virus activity occurs in the north of the country and endemic, year-round activity is found in the south (Reuben and Gajanana, 1997). Thus far, all Indian isolates belong to genotype 3 (Uchil and Satchidanandam, 2001), which includes strains from countries of epidemic virus activity. Hence, genotype not only correlates with virus activity, but also with place of isolation, suggesting that the epidemic potential of a virus may depend more on environmental factors (viz., climate, availability of suitable mosquito vectors/vertebrate hosts and immune status of the host population) than viral genetic determinants (Williams et al., 2000). Despite this, genetic analysis of genotype 4 strains identified unique residues in the E gene predicted to be involved in cellular entry (Solomon et al., 2003a). It was hypothesized that these differences resulted in altered viral tropism that restricted

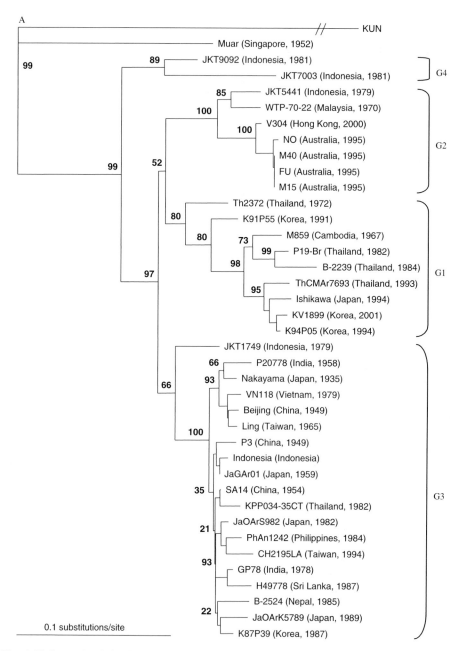

Fig. 1 Phylogenetic relationships of Japanese encephalitis virus strains predicted from E gene sequence information. Phylogenetic groupings corresponding to the genotype classification of Chen et al. (1990, 1992) and Williams et al. (2000) are indicated (G1–G4). The tree was constructed using the neighbour-joining method in ClustalX (Thompson et al., 1997), with percentage bootstrap values indicated at branch nodes. The scale at the bottom of the trees indicates the number of nucleotide substitutions per site. Horizontal branch lengths are proportional to genetic distance while vertical branch lengths have no significance. The tree was rooted using cognate sequence information from the genome of West Nile Kunjin (KUN) clade. Adapted from Lam et al. (2005b).

vector and/or host range of genotype 4 viruses and confined their circulation to an ecological niche within Indonesia; conversely, changes in this region of the E protein might have resulted in enhanced viral tropism, allowing the expanded transmission and spread observed for the recent genotypes (Solomon et al., 2003a). Further investigation will be required to fully delineate the relationship between genetic variation and virus transmission and spread.

In the last decade, the phenomenon of genotypic shift or genotypic replacement in circulating JEV has been increasingly reported (Nam et al., 1996; Pyke et al., 2001; Ma et al., 2003; Nga et al., 2004). A shift from genotype 3 to 1 was reported to have occurred in Korea in the early 1990s, and in Japan and Vietnam in the mid-to-late 1990s (Nam et al., 1996; Ma et al., 2003; Nga et al., 2004; Yang et al., 2004). A similar phenomenon took place in the Australasian region; since the year 2000, only genotype 1 strains of JEV have been isolated following a history of genotype 2 virus activity (Pyke et al., 2001; Johansen et al., 2004). The Indonesia–Malaysia region was implicated as the most likely source of these genotype 1 incursions (Pyke et al., 2001; Nga et al., 2004).

Clinical description and disease associations

Encephalitis is a common manifestation of a number of flavivirus infections, including JEV, MVEV, WNV (including WNV KUNV clade), SLEV, and tick-borne encephalitis virus. Despite some variation in clinical manifestations and severity of illness, the pathogenesis, disease states and outcomes are similar for most of these. JE is the most common of the human flavivirus encephalitides, though we still know relatively little about the disease process and its effective treatment.

Apart from rare instances of laboratory-acquired infection, human JEV infection and disease are always the result of the bite of an infected mosquito. The initial infection event is thought to be uptake of virus into the dendritic cells (Langerhans' cells) in the skin. These antigen-processing cells carry the virus to peripheral lymph nodes, and viral replication occurs within the macrophages and other cells of the peripheral lymphatic system. This is followed by a short-lived viraemia, usually <1 week, which precedes the entry of the virus into the central nervous system. In the vast majority of patients, the infection resolves at this stage; nervous system involvement sufficient to produce clinical disease occurs in only 1 : 200–1 : 1000 cases. When it does occur, it is likely that it occurs via penetration of the blood–brain barrier through the vascular endothelium. Although a mouse model has been used to show direct entry via the olfactory bulb with retrograde spread along the olfactory nerve, there is no direct evidence that this occurs in humans.

The virus invades neuronal cells and later also can be found in phagocytic cells within the nervous system. The major effects are seen within the central cerebral structures including the hippocampus, thalamus, substantia nigra, and brainstem. The temporal lobes may also be involved, as well as the cerebellum and upper spinal cord, particularly the anterior horn cells of the latter. The affected areas show an inflammatory infiltrate and oedema, with a predominance of activated T cells, macrophages, and B cells. The inflammatory response is important in causing cerebral disease, though there are also other probable mechanisms of neuronal damage, such as apoptosis.

In endemic areas, JEV mainly causes disease in children, as the majority of adults are immune. However, disease occurs at all ages in new residents or travellers who have come from non-endemic areas, or when outbreaks occur outside the endemic areas. The very young and the elderly are more likely to develop encephalitis and to have a poor outcome of infection, a particularly common feature of flavivirus encephalitis resulting from WNV and MVEV infections.

There are three major categories of clinical illness: non-encephalitic disease, encephalitis or related neurological disease, and late-onset illness. The vast majority of infected individuals have a self-limiting illness that is either asymptomatic or is a non-specific febrile illness, with or without headache. This mild, non-encephalitic illness due to JEV infection is probably underdiagnosed; it may not be considered in the diagnosis and it may clinically and serologically resemble other infections, including other flavivirus infections (Watt and Jongsakul, 2003).

The JEV encephalitic illness classically is preceded by fever, headache, and gastrointestinal symptoms, followed by deteriorating consciousness. JE has an incubation period that is usually < 1 week, but may be up to 16 days. Neck stiffness is present in about half of cases. Sudden onset with fever and convulsions may occur in children and occasionally in adults, and it is generally a bad prognostic feature. Cranial nerve palsies are common and patients may demonstrate either flaccid or spastic paralysis. Cerebrospinal fluid (CSF) typically shows lympho-cytosis (> 100×10^9 cells per litre), but the CSF cell count may be normal in some cases. Protein levels are normal or mildly elevated. Magnetic resonance imaging commonly shows lesions in the thalamus and/or adjacent structures in patients with severe encephalitis and is substantially more sensitive than CT scan (Kalita and Misra, 2000).

In the worst cases, patients progress to coma with respiratory failure requiring ventilatory support. Tremor, cogwheel rigidity, cerebellar ataxia, and upper limb weakness are seen in some cases. Approximately 25% die even within the most sophisticated medical settings, while about half the survivors have residual neurological disease. In those who survive, recovery begins after about 1 week, though it may take weeks or months for neurological deficits to resolve. In up to 50% of patients, there will be residual long-term deficits including cranial nerve palsies, peripheral nerve palsies, epilepsy, blindness, parkinsonism, and movement disorders. In children, residual long-term behavioural and psychiatric disturbances are very common, including memory impairment, emotional lability, and aggressiveness (Hoke et al., 1988).

At present we have a limited understanding of the factors that influence the outcome of flavivirus encephalitides, including JE. Those with more severe disease at presentation and older patients have a poorer outcome, as do young children

(Libraty et al., 2002; Tiroumourougane et al., 2002). Other factors, such as co-existent neurocysticercosis, are associated with more severe disease (Tiroumour-ougane et al., 2002). Also, the presence in the CSF of JEV-IgM and JEV neutralising antibody are both indicators of a better outcome (Libraty et al., 2002; Potula et al., 2003).

There has been considerable discussion about the potential protective role of pre-existing antibody to dengue virus. The early epidemiological data, reviewed by Grossman et al. (1974), concluded, with some significant reservations, that prior dengue did offer some protection against JEV encephalitis. A follow-up at 1 year of the surviving JEV encephalitis cases (Edelman et al., 1975) also found that neurological outcomes were better in children who had previous dengue infection. A later study of paediatric cases in Thailand also found prior flavivirus infection, presumed to be dengue, was an independent predictor of lower risk of severe disease or death, presumably because there was a more rapid anamnestic protective flavivirus immune response in those children (Libraty et al., 2002). Currently, the protective role of past infection with dengue virus or other flaviviruses has not been proven, but it remains an interesting possibility.

JEV neurological disease may also present without overt signs of encephalitis. JEV is a common cause of polio-like acute flaccid paralysis in children in endemic areas (Solomon et al., 1998), and it may also present as acute psychosis or as benign aseptic meningitis (Kuwayama et al., 2005).

JEV infection in pregnancy is rare, but it has been described in a small number of women, resulting in intrauterine foetal infection and death in 2/5 cases (Chaturvedi et al., 1980).

There is no proven beneficial specific therapy for JEV encephalitis, and the available treatment is supportive. Access to respiratory support is important in the survival of severe cases. Neither corticosteroids (Hoke et al., 1992) nor alpha-interferon (Solomon et al., 2003b) appear to be effective. Dehydroepiandrosterone (DHEA) has been shown to reduce the severity of encephalitis in the mouse model, but there are no data available yet for humans (Chang et al., 2005) Intravenous immunoglobulin has had very limited use for treatment of WNV encephalitis (Haley et al., 2003).

Laboratory diagnosis

Viraemia lasts only a few days; the virus can rarely be cultured from either blood or CSF. Nucleic acid detection tests, with a number of methods available for PCR-based detection of JEV and other flaviviruses appear to have been successful in experimental evaluations. In a recent Indian study, the sensitivity of PCR for detection of JEV in the CSF was 65% (Kabilan et al., 2004b). Where possible, early blood samples and CSF samples should be tested for viral RNA to confirm the diagnosis and provide material for molecular characterisation. Antigen detection methods have also been used, usually for tissue samples.

Diagnosis is usually reliant upon detection of antibodies in serum and CSF, most commonly using either an enzyme immunoassay (EIA) or haemagglutination inhibition assays (HIA), though immunofluorescent antibody assays have also been used. Rapid immunochromatographic antibody tests have also been developed for JEV infection (Cuzzubbo et al., 2000). During the acute illness, detection of IgM in serum and CSF is the most commonly used methods for diagnosing suspected JEV infection. IgM is present in serum of 75–90% of cases within a few days of onset of illness and in nearly all by 10 days after the onset. Previous studies in Asia have detected IgM to JEV in CSF in 30–67% of cases, with negative results more likely in very early samples (Lowry et al., 1998). A recent study of samples from Thai patients showed that IgM detection in CSF was more sensitive than serum IgM (Chanama et al., 2005) for the early diagnosis of JEV encephalitis. Using an IgM capture EIA, IgM was found in 60% of serum samples and 90% of CSF samples collected 1–4 days after the onset of illness. All CSF samples were positve by day 7 while 100% of serum samples are not positive until day 13.

As IgM will cross-react with other flavivirus antigens, a positive IgM to JEV may be obtained following infection with other flaviviruses, including WNV, MVEV, SLEV, and the dengue viruses. Therefore, detection of IgM antibodies to JEV is not in itself sufficient to definitively diagnose JEV infection. It is more reliable if there are no other possible infecting flaviviruses, which is unusual in JEV endemic areas, or where it can be demonstrated that there is only IgM to JEV and not to other flaviviruses. IgM also persists for many months following infection so that detection of IgM does not, of itself, prove that a current illness is a JEV infection. Rising titres of IgG between acute and convalescent serum samples are required to demonstrate recent infection. However, IgG is even more broadly cross-reactive than IgM and identifying the virus-specific antibody is challenging and requires more specific tests. Classically this is done using neutralising antibody titres, but these are technically difficult and may not always yield clear results. An epitope-blocking EIA using a JEV-specific monoclonal antibody has been developed that can identify IgG antibodies to JEV (Spicer et al., 1999), though antibodies to very closely related flaviviruses such as MVEV may still cross-react. Tests for antibodies directed to the premembrane protein may show better specificity (Cardosa et al., 2002).

The co-circulating flaviviruses that might lead to heterotypic responses are discussed under individual countries below, but it should be recognised that dengue viruses co-circulate with JEV in much of tropical and subtropical countries of Asia.

Ecology: vertebrate hosts and vectors

JEV is a zoonotic virus that is maintained in nature by transmission cycles involving *Culex* sp. mosquitoes and certain species of wild and domestic birds and pigs as the vertebrate hosts. Humans become infected when they are bitten by an infected mosquito, but they are incidental, dead-end hosts. Much of our basic knowledge of the ecology of JEV has come from studies carried out in Japan by

Scherer and Buescher and their colleagues (Scherer, 1959). They established the role of pigs as amplifiers of the disease, the involvement of ardeid birds such as Black-crowned night herons (*Nycticorax nycticorax*), Little egrets (*Egretta garzetta*), and other ardeid species as maintenance hosts, and the importance of *Cx. tritaeniorhynchus* mosquitoes as the major vector between vertebrate hosts and humans, as incidental hosts. Work by a number of other groups, notably in India, Japan, and Thailand, have confirmed and extended these earlier observations. Of particular importance in the ecology is the interplay between rice cultivation, vector densities, and pig rearing in close proximity to human habitation (Mishra et al., 1984; Geevarghese et al., 1994; Gajanana et al., 1997; Kanojia et al., 2003; Phukan et al., 2004). The ecology and epidemiology of JEV have been extensively reviewed by Endy and Nisalak (2002).

Vertebrate hosts

Pigs are the principle amplification hosts of JEV, especially in epidemic areas, and are maintenance hosts in endemic areas. The importance of pigs in the maintenance and amplification of JEV was demonstrated by the seminal studies carried out by Scherer and Buescher and their colleagues in Japan (Gresser et al., 1958; Scherer, 1959). They found that there was a high JEV seroprevalence rate among pigs, that pigs developed a high and prolonged viraemia following natural infection with JEV which lasted 2–4 days and was capable of infecting *Cx. tritaeniorhynchus* mosquitoes, that *Cx. tritaeniorhynchus* mosquitoes were able to transmit JEV between pigs in a laboratory setting, and that large numbers of susceptible young pigs were bred for commercial purposes and thus available for amplification of JEV each year. A number of other investigations have confirmed the importance of pigs as amplifying hosts, and extended these early observations, including Hurlbut (1964), Konno et al. (1966), Carey et al. (1968), Sazawa (1968), Yamada et al. (1971), Johnsen et al. (1974), Fukumi et al. (1975), Van Peenen et al. (1975b), Burke et al. (1985a,b), Gingrich et al. (1987, 1992), and Peiris et al. (1993). In serological surveys, pigs consistently display higher geometric mean titres than other domestic or wild animals. They are particularly attractive to the major mosquito vectors as the source of blood meals, providing a sensitive indicator of virus transmission in endemic areas (Burke et al., 1985a). Despite their potential danger to humans if raised in open pens near human habitation, have been used in this way as sentinel animals to monitor for virus activity as an early warning system in Japan (Maeda et al., 1978), Taiwan (Detels et al., 1976), Thailand (Johnsen et al., 1974; Burke et al., 1985b), India (Geevarghese et al., 1987, 1991), Sri Lanka (Peiris et al., 1993), Indonesia (Van Peenen, 1974b), and Australia (Shield et al., 1996). Adult pigs do not show any overt signs of infection. Infected pregnant sows, however, can produce mummified foetuses or give birth to stillborn or weak piglets, and JEV may be associated with infertility in boars. Young piglets may occasionally show signs of disease, including hydrocephalus (Joo and Chu, 1999; Daniels et al., 2002).

Porcine vaccination has been undertaken in Japan (Igarashi, 2002), Taiwan, and Nepal (Daniels, 2003).

Horses can be infected by JEV and may develop severe encephalitis, although inapparent infections are more common than recognisable cases (Ellis et al., 2000). The clinical disease in horses is similar to that in humans. A number of countries require vaccination of thoroughbred racehorses, including Japan, Hong Kong (China), Macau, Malaysia, and Singapore. Horses are dead-end hosts for JE, although experimental transmission by *Cx. tritaeniorhynchus* has been reported from horses to birds and from horses to horses (Gould et al., 1964).

Cattle, buffaloes, and goats are also dead-end hosts (Carey et al., 1969a), but because they are particularly attractive to a number of the major vector species, especially *Cx. tritaeniorhynchus*, they make good potential hosts for surveillance and may act as "dampers" in an outbreak situation (Carey et al., 1969a; Johnsen et al., 1974; Ilkal et al., 1988; Peiris et al., 1993; Gajanana et al., 1995; Reuben and Gajanana, 1997; Rajendran et al., 2003). This was further demonstrated in a study of JEV in the Thanjavur district of India, a rice-growing area with a very low incidence of JEV, which was explained by the high cattle to pig ratio (400:1) (Vijayarani and Gajanana, 2000). Indeed, JEV seroprevalence in cattle and goats was found to be a better predictor of human infection risk than was porcine seroprevalence in Sri Lanka (Peiris et al., 1993). Other animals may have relatively high seroprevalence rates, such as sheep and dogs, but viraemia levels are believed to be too low to infect mosquitoes (Johnsen et al., 1974; Banerjee et al., 1979). Rodents do not appear to be involved in JEV transmission. JEV has been isolated from a number of bats belonging to the Orders *Microchiroptera* and *Megachiroptera*, but most studies of their potential role in maintenance and transmission have been carried out in *Microchiroptera* (much of this work has been done by Sulkin and colleagues; reviewed in Sulkin and Allen, 1974). The viraemia in bats lasts as long as 25–30 days at a level high enough to infect mosquitoes; transplacental transmission also occurs. Experimental transmission of JEV has also been demonstrated in fruit bats of the order *Megachiroptera*, suggesting that they may be good candidates for virus maintenance and also possibly for geographic movement of the virus (Banerjee et al., 1979, 1984).

Birds, particularly ardeid species, are believed to be important maintenance hosts of JEV, and may act as amplifiers in epidemics where pigs are present in insignificant numbers or absent. Early work by Hammon et al. (1951) and Scherer and colleagues (Buescher et al., 1959a) clearly showed that wild birds may be important to the natural transmission cycle, with several ardeid species having antibodies to JEV, and indeed a number of JEV isolates were obtained from three species, the Black-crowned night heron (*Nycticorax nycticorax*), Plumed egrets (*Egretta intermedia*), and Little egrets (*Egretta garzetta*). While antibodies to JEV have been described in many avian species, these findings do not necessarily indicate an involvement in natural transmission cycles. Experimental infection and transmission of JEV in Pond herons (*Ardeola grayii*), Cattle egrets (*Bubulcus ibis*), Little egrets, and Little cormorants (*Phalacrocorax niger*) was successfully undertaken by Soman et al (1977), and experimental infection leading to viraemia in Nankeen night herons (*Nycticorax caledonicus*) and an Intermediate egret (*Egretta intermedia*) in Australia (Boyle et al., 1983). Experimental transmission has also been reported with sparrows (*Passer domestica*) (Hammon et al., 1951), Japanese tree sparrows (*Passer montanus saturatus*) (Hasegawa et al., 1975), pigeons (Banerjee et al., 1979), and between ducks and from ducks to chickens (Dhanda et al., 1977), but the relevance of these latter studies is questionable. Ducks have been suggested as possible epidemic hosts in the absence of pigs, and indeed duck antibodies to JEV have been reported from a number of countries. Chickens appear to be only rarely infected and may have a limited role in either transmission or surveillance. Nevertheless, a number of mosquito transmission studies have employed chickens successfully, either as a host of origin or as a recipient host. Wild birds have been implicated as the source of virus in outbreaks where pigs are uncommon (Soman et al., 1977; Rosen, 1986; Phanthumachinda, 1995), and as a means by which JEV can spread to colonise new areas (Scott, 1988; Hoke and Gingrich, 1994; Hanna et al., 1996b; Solomon et al., 2003a). In support of the role of ardeid birds in transmission cycles to humans, a study demonstrated that in villages with rice fields but which did not have herons in close proximity to the villages, seroconversion rates in children aged 0–5 and 6–15 years were 0% and 5%, respectively, whereas in villages with a similar ecology but where herons were found nearby, the corresponding rates were 50% and 56%, respectively (Mani et al., 1991).

Vectors

JEV has been isolated from a wide range of mosquito species, but not all are believed to be able or competent to transmit the virus to new hosts. There is a general concensus that *Cx. tritaeniorhynchus* is the major vector throughout most of Asia, but other species may be locally important, such as *Cx. gelidus*, *Cx. vishnui*, *Cx. fuscocephala*, *Cx. pseudovishnui*, *Cx. whitmorei*, *Cx. annulus*, *Cx. bitaenior-hynchus*, *Cx. annulirostris*, *Cx. quinquefasciatus*, *Anopheles subpictus*, *Aedes togoi*, *Ochlerotatus japonicus*, and *Mansonia uniformis* (Rosen, 1986; Burke and Leake, 1988; Sucharit et al., 1989; Vaughn and Hoke, 1992; van den Hurk et al., 2001a, 2003a; Mackenzie et al., 2002b). JEV has been isolated from several other species of mosquito as well as single isolates from midges and ticks, but the importance of these other species in transmission cycles is unknown, and it is probable that in most instances they are not involved in transmission either on epidemiological grounds or because they are not competent to transmit. The major *Culex* vectors of JEV are rice field-breeding species that bite during the night, particularly in the period shortly after sunset and in the early morning between midnight and about 4 am (Wada et al., 1970; Gould et al., 1974), and are zoophilic, preferring animals to humans for obtaining blood meals. A number of studies have demonstrated that *Cx. tritaeniorhynchus* feed preferentially on bovine species (reviewed by Colless, 1959; Mitchell et al., 1973; Gould et al., 1974; Rodrigues, 1988; Thein et al., 1988;

Reuben et al., 1992), even when pigs are equally available. However, in a study carried out in Assam, northern India, a high percentage of *Cx. tritaeniorhynchus* (40%) and *Cx. vishnui* (35%) were found to have fed on pigs rather than other species that were prevalent in the area, whereas *Cx. pseudovishnui* were not attracted to pigs (0.4%) (Bhattacharyya et al., 1994). In southern India, *Cx. pseudovishnui* and *Cx. vishnui* were also found to have fed preferentially on bovine species rather than pigs (Reuben et al., 1992). *Cx. fuscocephala* also appear to have a preference for bovine species rather than pigs (Mitchell et al., 1973; Gould et al., 1974), whereas *Cx. gelidus* appear to feed equally freely on pigs and bovine species in some studies (Colless, 1959; Macdonald et al., 1967), but with a preference for bovine species in another study (Gould et al., 1974). None of these mosquito species have a preference for humans, with feeding levels usually <1%. In traps baited with animals, pigs attracted and were bitten by many more *Cx. tritaeniorhynchus* than were black-crowned night herons or participating humans, but traps baited with black-crowned night herons were 3–15 times more attractive to *Cx. tritaeniorhynchus* than traps containing egrets or chickens (Scherer, 1959). In Australasia, where members of the *Cx. sitiens* subgroup, and particularly *Cx. annulirostris*, are major vectors of MVEV and JEV, *Cx annulirostris* feed preferentially on mammals, especially bovine species (Kay et al., 1979) and marsupials such as the agile wallaby in the Cape York area (van den Hurk et al., 2003b), although they will readily feed on other hosts depending on availability, including pigs, birds, and humans (Kay et al., 1979).

Overwintering

There has been much speculation about how JEV survives the winter months in its northern range. There are four major hypotheses: (1) that the virus spends winters in mosquito eggs after vertical transmission; (2) that the virus survives in hibernating mosquitoes; (3) that the virus survives in hibernating animals such as cold-blooded animals or bats; or (4) that the virus is re-introduced each year by migratory birds or even by mosquitoes blown by prevailing wind patterns from endemic areas. The answer may well be that each of the four methods contributes to overwintering in different situations. Vertical transmission has been shown to occur in *Ae. togoi*, *Ae. albopictus*, *Ae. esoensis*, and possibly *Cx. tritaeniorhynchus* in nature, and in a number of species under laboratory conditions including *Cx. tritaeniorhynchus*, *Cx. vishnui*, *Cx. pipiens*, *Cx. quinquefasciatus*, and *Oc. japonicus* (reviewed by Rosen, 1986; Rosen et al., 1989). The evidence for overwintering in dormant or hibernating mosquitoes is questionable and it would appear that this may not be an effective strategy for maintaining the virus in the environment (Min and Xue, 1996). Survival of virus in hibernating poikilothermic animals or bats is a possible method for overwintering, and several species of reptiles can be infected with JEV (Shortridge et al., 1974, 1977; Doi et al., 1983). However, bats perhaps have the best potential as a mechanism for maintenance through winter months, as the virus can remain viable in brown fat during hibernation, a second round of viraemia can initiate after hibernation is finished, and the virus can also cross the placenta to infect the young (Sulkin and Allen, 1974). Finally, migrating birds and mosquitoes may also re-introduce virus into the environment. Migratory patterns of herons coincide with seasonal transmission of JEV in Japan (Ogata et al., 1970, cited by Endy and Nisalak, 2002). With respect to migrating mosquitoes, *Cx. tritaeniorhynchus* mosquitoes may use wind as a means of migration each year in China, flying north in the spring and returning south in the autumn (Ming et al., 1993; Min and Xue, 1996). Both of these possible migratory methods are discussed more fully in the Section on "Mechanisms of spread and changing epidemiological patterns".

Geographic range, incidence, and seasonality

Epidemics of JEV have been reported in Japan, maritime Siberia, China, Taiwan, Korea, northern Vietnam, Guam, Saipan, Cambodia, Laos, northern Thailand, northern India, and Nepal, whereas sporadic cases of JE, probably resulting from endemic activity, have been reported from the Philippines, southern Vietnam, southern Thailand, Malaysia, Singapore, Indonesia, Myanmar, Bangladesh, southern India, and Sri Lanka (Umenai et al., 1985; Burke and Leake, 1988; Vaughn and Hoke, 1992; Solomon et al., 2000; Endy and Nisalak, 2002; Halstead and Jacobson, 2003). JEV has spread into Pakistan in the west (Igarashi et al.,

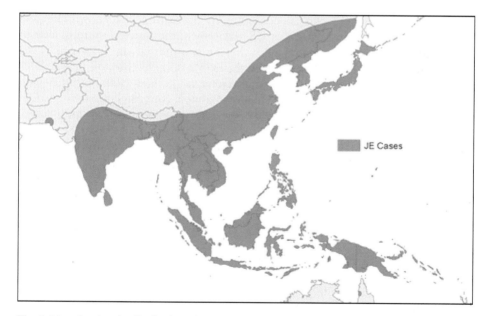

Fig. 2 Map showing the distribution of JE cases (modified from CDC, Atlanta). (For colour version: see Colour Section on page 353).

1994) and Australasia in the east (Hanna et al., 1996b; Mackenzie et al., 2002b). The geographic range of the virus is shown in Fig. 2.

In general, two epidemiological patterns of JEV have now been recognised: tropical, where the disease is endemic with sporadic cases throughout the year and there is no seasonal pattern, although a peak number of cases may occur after the start of the rainy season; and temperate or northern tropical, where the disease is epidemic with outbreaks in summer or early autumn (from about June to September), after the rainy season. Further south, this period may be longer and extend from March to November, or even year round. The reasons for this difference in patterns are unclear. While rainfall is obviously an important factor for vector breeding, temperature may be a more defining factor, certainly in some locations (Solomon et al., 2000). The two patterns of endemic and epidemic transmission also blur in subtropical areas such as northern Thailand and Vietnam where epidemic activity may be superimposed on low-level endemic or year-round transmission.

JE is mostly a disease of children and young adults, with the most important age group being from 3 to 9 years of age, possibly reflecting behavioural patterns, and it is found slightly more often in males than females, but when epidemics first occur at new locations, all age groups may be infected (Umenai et al., 1985). In endemic areas, there is a 100% seropositivity rate by the time children reach adulthood. Most infections, however, are asymptomatic or result in a non-specific flu-like illness (Solomon et al., 2000). The ratio of symptomatic to asymptomatic infection varies in different populations, but is commonly between 1 : 50 and 1 : 300, although the reasons why clinical disease rarely develops is not known (Vaughn and Hoke, 1992). In non-indigenous US servicemen, the ratio of symptomatic to asymptomatic cases have been higher, variously reported as 1 : 25 and 1 : 63 (Halstead and Grosz, 1962; Benenson et al., 1975).

The introduction of vaccination programmes in the late 1960s, together with widespread use of pesticides in the rice paddies, almost completely eliminated JE in the economically affluent Asian countries such as Japan, Korea, Taiwan (Okuno, 1978; Igarashi, 1992; Igarashi, 2002), and in Singapore. In addition, the disease burden of JEV infection in China has been significantly reduced by vaccination (Halstead and Jacobson, 2003). However, despite these successes, there has been an apparent increase in geographic spread and disease incidence in much of southeast and southern Asia (Lowry et al., 1998; Halstead and Jacobson, 2003; Kabilan et al., 2004a). Part of the reason for this has been the development of new areas of irrigated agriculture and the introduction of new crops.

One of the pressing needs is a better understanding of the disease burden in countries of this region, both those with endemic and epidemic disease, to better assess the need and potential effectiveness of introducing JEV immunisation programmes into the various national EPIs. This is currently a major project of the Program for the Appropriate Technology in Health (PATH), with its partners including WHO and UNICEF, and funded by the Bill and Melinda Gates Foundation. Surveillance and laboratory diagnostic facilities are lacking in many

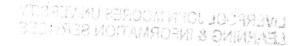

affected countries, which makes the disease burden in those countries difficult to determine. Indeed available information is very limited from Bangladesh, Bhutan, Laos and North Korea, and poor for countries such as Myanmar, Cambodia, Papua New Guinea, and Timor-Leste. With more than 700 million children believed to be at risk of JE, the programme of PATH to introduce JEV vaccination to those countries with a substantial JE burden becomes all the more important. The following sections provide a brief overview of JE in each country in which epidemic or endemic JEV infections occur. [Bhutan is not included because there is only anecdotal information about the incidence of JE there. Nevertheless, ecological conditions are suitable, the major vectors are present, and JE is a serious problem in bordering areas of India, the states of West Bengal and Assam (Brantly et al., 2004). Brunei Darussalam is also not included, but it is assumed that the pattern of JEV endemicity there is similar to that of East Malaysia (Sarawak).]

Japan

As reported above, epidemics of encephalitis believed to have been due to JEV have been recorded in Japan since 1871. The large epidemic of 1924, which resulted in 6125 cases and 3797 deaths (W.C. Rappleye, 1939, cited by Burke and Leake, 1988), brought recognition of the public health importance of JE. Regular epidemics of varying severity occurred until the mid-1960s, with several thousand cases annually. The more severe epidemics were in 1935 and 1948. No epidemics have been reported in Japan since 1968, due largely to the widespread use of pesticides on rice paddies and to mass vaccination, although sporadic cases continue to occur (Igarashi, 1992, 2002). JE has become a disease of the older age groups in Japan, the case-fatality rates being highest in the elderly, and there is growing concern that a gradual decrease in herd immunity may create the potential for future outbreaks (Umenai et al., 1985). Thus, it is interesting that recent discussions have queried the need to continue vaccination programmes due to concern about the neurological side effects of inactivated JE vaccine (Fukuda et al., 1997; Plesner et al., 1998). Nevertheless, serological studies to detect antibodies to NS1, which are indicative of natural exposure to the virus, have indicated that significant levels of JEV continue to circulate in central Japan in both humans and racehorses (Konishi et al., 2006). Circulation of JEV also probably continues in pigs, especially in southeastern Japan and in foci on Hokkaido. The Japanese government, however, elected to suspend routine JE immunisation on 30 May 2005, with continued vaccination only in high-risk areas and for travellers to endemic countries outside Japan.

Maritime Siberia, Russia

JEV infections are found in maritime Siberia (I.V. Dandurov, 1968, cited by Burke and Leake, 1988; Vaughn and Hoke, 1992; Halstead and Jacobson, 2003), but although it was first reported in 1938 (Solomon et al., 2000), little is known of the incidence. Certain mosquito species have been implicated in transmission to humans there, including *Cx. pipiens, Cx. quinquefasciatus, Ae. esoensis, Oc. japonicus, Ae. koreicus,* and *Ae. togoi*; in addition, it is transmitted by *Cx. bitaeniorhynchus,* which is believed to be a vector of JEV transmission to animals but not to humans (K.P. Chagin and P.Y. Kondratev, 1943, and P.A. Petrishcheva, 1948, cited by Rosen, 1986). The first reports of human cases in 30 years have appeared recently (CDC Traveller's Health, Yellow Book, Japanese encephalitis).

China

The ecology and epidemiology of JEV in China have been reviewed by Huang (1982) and Yu (1995). Clinical cases of JE were first recognised in China in 1940 (Chu et al., 1940), and the virus first isolated in China in 1940 by Yen (Huang, 1982). Further JEV isolations of importance were obtained in 1949 (Beijing and P3 strains). The disease has been most prevalent in the central and eastern parts of China where surface water is abundant and the average temperature in July exceeds 20°C (Chu, 1982). In the 1960s and 1970s, the disease tended to extend northwards and involve older age groups (Chu, 1982), and new epidemic areas have appeared in several provinces (Yu, 1995). Indeed, clinical cases of JE have been reported from all provinces except Xinjiang (Sinkiang) and Xizang (Tibet) (Chu, 1982; Umenai et al., 1985; Yu, 1995).

JE was not regarded as a public health problem in China until the mid-1960s. During the mid-1970s, JEV was responsible for an average of 100,000 cases annually in China (Halstead and Jacobson, 2003), and although this number has decreased significantly since the introduction of vaccination, China still accounts for the majority of cases reported from the Western Pacific region, with 10,000–20,000 cases annually. In 1998, 11,891 cases were reported from 1303 counties, with high incidences of cases in 10 provinces: Sichuan (2133); Guizhou (1390); Sshanxi (1222); Henan (1192); Chongqing (783); Hubei (694); Yunnan (670); Anhui (582); Shanxi (548); and Hunan (547) (Su and Liang, 2002). In 2003, only 7900 suspected JE cases were reported, an incidence of 0.6 per 100,000 population (W. Lixia, personal communication to Petersen and Marfin, 2005), although the incidence in children younger than 15 years of age may exceed 10 per 100,000 in remote areas. China has been using a live-attenuated vaccine, SA-14-14-2, and over 200 million children have now received this vaccine, which has been found to be safe, immunogenic, and efficacious. The vaccination programme has resulted in a decrease in the incidence of clinically recognised JEV infection from about 2.5/100,000 to 0.5/100,000.

In Hong Kong, sporadic cases have been recognised; in the period 1992–2004, 11 cases were reported, of which 7 were locally acquired and 4 were imported cases, with 5 of the locally acquired cases occurring in 2004 (ProMED Posting, 2004; Lam et al., 2005a). In a subsequent serological survey of people living near these 5 cases, 2.4% were found to have antibodies to JEV, but most were over the age of 40 (A.A. Fu cited by Lam et al., 2005a). Serosurveillance in 6-month-old pigs in Hong Kong between 1999 and 2000 found that between 11% and 91% of animals were seropositive depending on the season (T.M. Ellis, personal communication to Lam et al., 2005b), demonstrating that JEV circulates regularly in Hong Kong. In addition, a fatal case of JEV infection in a thoroughbred racehorse in Hong Kong in 2000 was reported by Lam et al. (2005b). As has been the requirement since 1972 for all racehorses in training in Hong Kong, this horse had been vaccinated against JE earlier that year. As a direct consequence of this case, a 6-month booster vaccination programme for JE was introduced in 2001 for all horses in Hong Kong (Lam et al., 2005b).

Taiwan

JE in Taiwan was first studied in detail by Grayston and colleagues (Chu and Grayston, 1962; Grayston et al., 1962; Hsu and Grayston, 1962; Wang and Grayston, 1962; Wang et al., 1962a,b). Their observations, together with those of a number of authors of subsequent studies (Okuno et al., 1975a,b; Detels et al., 1976; Wu et al., 1999), described the pattern of outbreaks, the importance of pigs as amplifiers of disease, and the involvement of the major mosquito species, especially *Cx. tritaeniorhynchus* and *Cx. annulus*. The involvement of pigs remains unchanged over the past 40 years, and human cases follow virus amplification in the pigs. The introduction of childhood vaccination in 1968 reduced the incidence significantly, from 2.05 per 100,000 in 1967 to 0.03 per 100,000 in 1999. JE continues to occur sporadically in all parts of Taiwan, but the cases have changed from being a childhood disease (largely in 2–7 year olds) to being a disease of adults. In addition, the peak number of cases previously was in August, but is now in June. JEV continues to circulate in mosquitoes (Weng et al., 1999, 2005), and infected domestic pigs are found to be infected throughout the year (Chang, 2002) with prevalence rates between 49% and 70% in different regions of the island. Chang (2002) also indicated that JEV propagation may be active in winter as well as in other seasons of the year, sporadic cases occurring between December and April.

Korea

Although regular epidemics of summer encephalitis had been recognised in Korea in the 1930s, the first isolation of JEV was made in 1946 from an American soldier stationed in Korea (Sabin et al., 1947). An extensive serological survey was then carried out in four areas of South Korea and the results showed that JEV was widely disseminated there (Deuel et al., 1950). The first major epidemic in South Korea occurred in 1949 with at least 5548 cases and 2429 deaths, the highest incidence being in Seoul and Kyonggi Province (Hullinghorst et al., 1951; Pond and Smadel, 1954; Umenai et al., 1985). Epidemics continued to occur every 2 or 3 years with several thousand cases annually until the mid-1960s, with more cases in the southwestern provinces than in the northeastern provinces. Most cases occurred in August and September, particularly in children below 15 years of age. The largest recorded epidemic was in 1958 involving 6897 cases (Chang, 1959). After 1968, the number of cases dropped significantly with the introduction of limited vaccination and the increased use of pesticides in rice paddies (Igarashi, 1992; Vaughn and Hoke, 1992). Despite an estimated 80% vaccination coverage among school children, an unexpected epidemic occurred in 1982 in the rice-growing area of southwest Korea (Umenai et al., 1985). A national immunisation programme was initiated after the 1982 outbreak. The total number of cases and deaths reported in the Republic of Korea (South Korea) annually between 1956 and 1975 were listed by Okuno (1978), and between 1973 and 1990 were described by Igarashi (1992). The average annual number of cases between 1973 and 1983 was 500, and this dropped to an average of one case per year between 1985 and 1990. In the period 1985–1998, only 21 cases were serologically confirmed, with more cases in adults than in children (Sohn, 2000). An epidemic forecast programme, which was started in 1975 and based on various factors including virus isolation from *Cx. tritaeniorhynchus* mosquitoes, vector densities, and porcine seroconversions from animals in the slaughterhouse, provides an early warning of the potential for increased virus activity (Sohn, 2000).

Philippines

Serological surveys and sporadic clinical cases had indicated that JEV is active in rice-growing areas of the Philippines (Hammon et al., 1958a; Venzon et al., 1972; Cross et al., 1977; Barzaga, 1989). Most cases occur in the 1–10 year age group, and the fatality rate is 7–30%. Virus isolation was first reported in 1980 from *Cx. tritaeniorhynchus, Cx. bitaeniorhynchus, Cx. vishnui,* and *An. annularis* mosquitoes collected at various sites in central Luzon (Ksiazek et al., 1980; Trosper et al., 1980). A more detailed study carried out in 1984–1985 found 83 cases of JEV infection from 1000 specimens submitted from hospitals in Manila and the surrounding area. Cases occurred throughout the year, with higher numbers during the rainy season between August and December. Most cases were in children between 1 and 10 years of age in rural areas in central Luzon, with a fatality rate of 11% (O'Rourke et al., 1986). A few cases were also reported from Mindanao and Romblon. While most human cases and sentinel pig seroconversions occurred during the rainy season, a significant number of human cases and pig seroconversions surprisingly occurred in the second year of the study at the end of the hot, dry season. The authors suggested that environmental factors such as the onset of irrigation practices may have been important in the initiation of JEV transmission activity. This was supported in a later study in Luzon in which mosquito abundance was observed several months after the onset of both the rainy season and the irrigation period (Shultz and Hayes, 1993). In recent years, JE cases have been reported from Bataan, Bulacan, Nueva Ecija, Pampanga, Tarlac and Zambales Provinces in Central Luzon region, and from Luguna and Quezon Provinces in Calabarzon region.

Western Pacific: Guam and Saipan

An outbreak of 49 cases of JE was reported in Guam from December 1947 to March 1948 (Hammon et al., 1958b). The vector implicated in the outbreak was *Cx. annulirostris mariani* (Reeves and Rudnick, 1951), which was shown to transmit JEV experimentally (Hurlbut and Thomas, 1949). The second outbreak in the Pacific occurred on the island of Saipan, Commonwealth of the Northern Mariana Islands in 1990 (Paul et al., 1993). Ten cases were reported during the outbreak. The antibody prevalence in residents after the outbreak was 4.2%, but antibody was not detected in any of 288 sera stored prior to the outbreak, suggesting that the virus had recently been introduced onto the island. The antibody prevalence in pigs was 96%, and it was suggested that the outbreak ended because of the exhaustion of the supply of susceptible amplifier hosts. A subsequent mosquito survey found that *Cx. tritaeniorhynchus* was the predominant species in the southern half of Saipan where human cases had occurred, and was therefore implicated as the probable vector species (Mitchell et al., 1993).

Vietnam

The first recorded outbreak of JE in northern Vietnam occurred in 1965. The pattern of JE in Vietnam is epidemic in the subtropical north, with an epidemic season between May and August, and is endemic in the tropical south, with disease reported all year round but with a slight peak in July (Ketel and Ognibene, 1971; Igarashi, 1992). Several thousand cases occur annually, with most cases coming from the heavily populated delta regions of the Red River in the north and the Mekong River in the south (Nguyen and Nguyen, 1995), although some JEV activity occurs in most parts of the country, with 62 of 64 provinces reporting cases in 2004 (data from Japanese encephalitis Prevention Network [JEPN], http://www.jepn.org). Virus isolates have been obtained from patients, pigs, mosquitoes, and wild birds (Thi-Kim-Thoa et al., 1974; Le, 1986; Igarashi, 1992). Most cases of JE in north Vietnam occur in young children in the 2–7 year age group (Le, 1986), and this vulnerability of young children to JE was clearly consistent with a subsequent study of hospitalised cases of encephalitis in Hanoi, in which 67% of encephalitis cases in children were due to JE compared with only 6% of adults (Lowry et al., 1998). The median age of the children with JE was 6 years of age. These results were later reflected in a seroprevalence study in southern Vietnam in which antibody positivity was associated with increasing age in children (Bartley et al., 2002).

In 1989, the WHO country office in Vietnam, and the WHO Western Pacific Regional Office in collaboration with the Japanese Biken Institute, assisted the National Institute of Hygiene and Epidemiology (NIHE) to establish the production of Nakayama strain inactivated mouse brain vaccine, with Phase III clinical trials conducted in 1993–1997. Prior to 1993, JEV control in Vietnam focused on vector control. After 1993, vaccine use began with the introduction of vaccine into the at-risk population focusing on 1–15 year olds. In 1997, free vaccination against JEV was introduced into the Expanded Program of Immunization (EPI) for children 1–5 years old in the first year, and then for 1 year olds, in selected high-risk districts. There are now plans to expand vaccination to other areas, because the area of JEV transmission has extended over the past few years. Vaccine production has been increased with capacity reported to be 4.5 million doses in 2004. Budget constraints are the main limiting factor for providing vaccine through the EPI (Nguyen, 2002).

Cambodia

JEV was isolated in 1965 for the first time in Phnom Penh, from *Cx. tritaeniorhynchus* mosquitoes (Chastel and Rageau, 1966, cited by Chanthap, 2002). Little information is available about the epidemiology and ecology of JEV in Cambodia (Sunnara and Touch, 1995). On clinical grounds, epidemic activity appeared to occur between October and December, and it occurred principally in the 0–4 year age group, with a mortality rate of > 50%. More recently, confirmed cases of JE have been reported from the National Pediatric Hospital in Phnom Penh (Chhour et al., 2002) and from the Takao Provincial Hospital (Srey et al., 2002), accounting for 18% of children with clinical encephalitis in the former, and 31% of children with encephalitis in the latter. In 2004, 578 cases of confirmed JE were reported from 3 hospitals, Kantha Bopha I and II in Phnom Penh and Jayavarman VII in Siem Reap Province (JEPN website, www.jepn.org), with most cases occurring in children under 5 years of age in the rainy season between June and August.

Laos

As with Cambodia, little information is available about the incidence of JE in Laos (Okuno, 1978; Vongxay, 1995). A serological survey has suggested that 28% of the inhabitants of Vientiane have neutralising antibody to JEV (Kanamitsu M and Ogata T, personal communication to Okuno, 1978). There were 54 cases of encephalitis with 14 deaths in 1974 and 6 cases with 5 deaths in 1975. Most cases occurred during August. Confirmed cases of JE were reported between 1989 and 1991 (Vongxay, 1995). The prevalence of antibody was relatively low, from none to 25% in children <5 years of age, increasing with age to approximately 75% of adults over 30 years of age.

Thailand

Clinical JE has been recognised in Thailand since the mid-to-late 1950s (Thongcharoen, 1985; Endy and Nisalak, 2002). The first serological evidence was found in horses in Chonburi Province north of Bangkok (Thongcharoen, 1985). JEV was subsequently isolated from *Cx. tritaeniorhynchus* and *Cx. gelidus* mosquitoes in the same area in 1962 (Simasathien et al., 1972), from clinical cases in Phitsanuloke Hospital in central Thailand in 1964, and from paediatric cases in Sukhothai Province in northern Thailand in 1965 (Thongcharoen, 1985). Sporadic confirmed cases were recorded between 1964 and 1966 in Sukhothai, Phitsanulok and Korat Provinces (Bunnag et al., 1976; Sangkawibha, 1982). The first major outbreak of JE occurred in the Chiang Mai valley in northern Thailand between May and August, 1969, peaking in July (Yamada et al., 1971; Bunnag et al., 1976; Sangkawibha et al., 1982). The incidence rate was 20.3/100,000 (Yamada et al., 1971). The epidemic was mainly in the young, between 1 and 19 years of age, with a peak in 10 year olds. A second epidemic occurred the following year with 83 cases occurring between May and July, and a further 17 cases between August and December, with a total of 20 deaths, and an overall incidence rate of 14.7/100,000 (Grossman et al., 1973a).

Studies by Yamada et al. (1971) in 1969 and Grossman and colleagues in 1970–1971 of human infections (Grossman et al., 1972, 1973a,b,c), animal infections (Johnsen et al., 1974), and vectors (Gould et al., 1974) have been central to our understanding of the epidemiology and ecology of JEV in northern Thailand and with important lessons for JEV elsewhere. The Chiang Mai Valley has been one of the most intensively studied areas of JEV activity, and various studies have clearly demonstrated that JE is primarily a childhood disease there, with the peak in the 5—9 year age group. All children there have antibodies to JEV by the time they reach adulthood, and the lifetime risk of JEV infection is 100%. Inapparent infection was relatively common, with a ratio of inapparent to apparent JEV infection of 300 : 1. The major amplifying vertebrate hosts are pigs and the major vector species are *Cx. tritaeniorhynchus*, *Cx. gelidus* and *Cx. fusocephala* mosquitoes.

After the 1969 and 1970 epidemics in Thailand, the epidemic area of JEV expanded, with the number of cases of encephalitis increasing to 1500–2500 annually by the 1980s, for a case incidence rate of 3–5/100,000 and case-fatality rate of 20–35% (Chunsuttiwat, 1989). The incidence has been highest in the northern provinces and lowest in the central provinces. The spatial and temporal case of encephalitis by province in Thailand have been described (Endy and Nisalak, 2002). Thus, during the late 1970s and early 1980s, the northeastern provinces began reporting JE disease, and the southern provinces did so subsequently. The north and northeastern provinces have a seasonal occurrence of JEV activity with transmission occurring in the rainy season between May and September. The central region is less affected than the other regions, and there is more continuous transmission of JEV, similar to the year-round transmission found in the tropical/ endemic southern provinces. During the period 1994–2004, all 76 provinces of Thailand reported cases of JE (JEPN website, www.jepn.org).

The control of JEV in Thailand was initially based on vector-borne disease control beginning in 1973, but after a series of vaccine efficacy studies, the Ministry of Health introduced JEV vaccination as part of the EPI in 1990 for eight northern provinces. A year later vaccination was introduced into all 17 northern provinces, and then into all 36 provinces with encephalitis incidences of more than 1/100,000 (S. Chunsuttiwat, 1998, cited by Endy and Nisalak, 2002). Average case rates per 100,000 during the period 1989–1993 in the northern, southern, north-eastern, and central regions were 3.5, 2.4, 1.43, and 1.21, respectively (Chunsuttiwat and Warachit, 1995), but these have continued to fall during the late 1990s (Endy and Nisalak, 2002). Currently, the vaccine programme is part of the EPI throughout Thailand, and Thailand has an excellent national surveillance programme.

Malaysia

The possible occurrence of JEV in Malaysia was first suggested in a report of illness among British prisoners of war during World War II (Cruickshank, 1951). It was subsequently recognised in the Malaysian peninsula in the early 1950s, with virus isolation, serological evidence of human and equine infections, and cases of encephalitis (Paterson et al., 1952; Hale and Witherington, 1954; Pond et al., 1954; Hale and Lee, 1955). However, like other tropical endemic areas, clinical cases of JE have been sporadic, and from figures maintained at the Institute of Medical Research in Kuala Lumpur, the incidence is low and fairly evenly distributed throughout the year. Thus, it was not considered a major public health problem in Malaysia (Fang et al., 1980; Sinniah, 1989). However, 172 cases were reported between 1989 and 1993, most of which were in children, with a case-fatality rate of 7% (Tan, 1995). In addition, serological investigations and clinical case studies of paediatric patients with encephalitis in Perak and Penang suggested that there is probably more JE in Malaysia than the national figures reflect (Cardosa et al., 1991, 1995). A serological survey of animal sera from all parts of Malaysia indicated that antibodies to JEV are relatively common, with high titres in pigs, cattle, and buffalo (Oda et al., 1996), and JEV has been isolated from several species of mosquitoes in Selangor in recent years, including *Cx. tritaeniorhynchus*, *Cx. vishnui*, *Cx. bitaeniorhynchus*, and *Cx. sitiens* (Vythilingam et al., 1994, 1995, 1997). Thus, there is good evidence for widespread endemic activity in the Malaysian peninsula. Interestingly, the 1999 outbreak of Nipah virus was first thought to have been due to JEV, and indeed there were some confirmed cases of JE at the start of the Nipah outbreak, leading to a local programme of vector control and JE vaccination, but the occurrence of cases of encephalitis in vaccinated individuals and the death of significant numbers of pigs indicated that another agent was responsible, later shown to be Nipah virus.

Studies of JEV in East Malaysia in the 1970s clearly demonstrated that JEV was the principal cause of encephalitis in Sarawak, with an incidence rate of 5–10% per year (Smith et al., 1974). JEV was isolated from *Cx. tritaeniorhynchus* and *Cx. gelidus* mosquitoes, and ecological studies demonstrated that JEV was maintained throughout the year mainly by a cycle involving pigs and *Cx. gelidus*. During rice planting and harvesting, the numbers of infected *Cx. tritaeniorhynchus* increased, with a concomitant risk of human infections (Simpson et al., 1970a,b, 1974). Interestingly, two isolates of WNV were identified in Sarawak in the late 1960s, the first as WNV and the second as KUNV (Bowen et al., 1970; Karabatsos, 1985), which, if still enzootic in the region, may present problems in serological diagnoses because of potential heterotypic responses. A recent 5-year study at Sibu hospital in central Sarawak, which covers a referral population of 600,000, found 101 cases of JE at an annual incidence of 20 cases, with a mortality rate of 9% (Ooi, 2002). Sporadic cases of JE continue to occur in Sarawak, indicative of endemic activity, with an average of greater than 40 recognised cases occurring throughout the year, with a peak in the period October to December (M.J. Cardosa, personal communication). JEV continues to be a public health problem in Sarawak, and, it is assumed, in Sabah and Brunei.

The true incidence of JE in Malaysia is unknown and almost certainly underestimated (Tan, 1995).

Singapore

Prior to 1980, sporadic cases of JE occurred in Singapore, with a biannual increase in cases around both April and October, and with the highest morbidity rate being in children in the 5–14 year age group (Wo, 1963; Doraisingham, 1982). Infection was reported to be widespread, with neutralising antibodies found in about 70% of the population over 12 years of age (Hale and Lee, 1955). Antibody was also found to be widespread in horses (Hale and Witherington, 1954) and pigs (A.C. Lim, personal communication to Doraisingham, 1982) and the virus was isolated from *Cx. tritaeniorhynchus* mosquitoes (Hale et al., 1957). Most cases were in rural areas of Singapore in association with *Culex* breeding sites (Doraisingham, 1982). In the early 1980s, pig farming was phased out in Singapore, a process that was completed in 1992. The incidence of indigenous cases dropped from 101 during the period 1977–1984 to 15 cases for the period 1985–1993, with the last fatal case occurring in 1984 (Anon., 1993, 1994). Thus JEV transmission appeared to cease, with only very occasional cases occurring thereafter. Between 1991 and 2000, only 3 cases were reported (Anon., 2003), but in the light of these occasional cases further investigations were undertaken and it was found that wild boars on an offshore island (See et al., 2002) and various animals and birds in Singapore (Anon., 2003; Ting et al., 2004) have neutralising antibodies, suggesting that JEV transmission is continuing in peripheral parts of Singapore. An indigenous case of JE occurred in 2005 (Koh et al., 2006), which suggested that regular surveillance be initiated in these areas to further elucidate the activity of JEV in Singapore.

Myanmar

JE was first recognised in Myanmar in 1974 in Shan State, which borders Chiang Mai Province of Thailand, and cases have been reported each year thereafter (Ming et al., 1977; Umenai et al., 1985). A seroepidemiological study carried out in the north-western Myanmar in 1976 near the border with India suggested that JEV was present in some areas (Swe et al., 1979). An outbreak of encephalitis in horses occurred in 1977, and JEV was isolated from horses at autopsy (Than Swe, Khin Khin Soe, Than Aung, unpublished data, cited by Khin, 1982). A prospective study of JE in Rangoon in 1982 found serological evidence of JEV infection in 52% of pigs, but concurrent human infection could not be detected (Thein et al., 1988).

Bangladesh

Very little is known about the incidence of JEV infection in Bangladesh. JE was reported for the first time on clinical grounds in 1977 without serological confirmation. In the 1977 outbreak in the Modhupur Forest area, in Tangail District, 22 patients were reported to have been infected, of whom 7 died, and serological evidence of probable JEV infection was obtained, but the authors were unable to isolate JEV from mosquitoes (Khan et al., 1981). Serological surveys have suggested a moderate prevalence of JEV antibodies in northeast (Sylhet) and southwest (Kushtia) Bangladesh, and a low incidence in Chittagong (Islam et al., 1982). Most recently, a prospective study of encephalitis in Bangladesh in 2003–2004 enrolled every fourth encephalitis patient admitted to Dhaka, Mymensingh, and Rajshahi Medical College Hospitals (ICDDR, 2004). A total of 176 patients were tested for JEV, of whom 10 (6%) were found to have antibodies to JEV, including 7/63 from Rajshahi Hospital and the other cases from Mymensingh Hospital. The mean age of patients was 18 years; 40% were male. Four JE patients resided in Chapai Nawabganj District (Rajshahi Division in northwest Bangladesh), two were from Kishoreganj District (Dhaka Division in the north), and four patients were from Naogaon (Rajshahi Division), Pabna (Rajshahi Division), Rajshahi (Rajshahi Division), and Mymensingh (Dhaka Division) Districts, respectively. Thus, all were from the north of the country, but this may reflect the catchment areas of the participating hospitals.

India

JEV in India has been reviewed (Banerjee, 1975; Kumar and Misra, 1988; Reuben and Gajanana, 1997; Sehgal and Dutta, 2003; Jacobson and Sivalenka, 2004; Kabilan et al., 2004a). JE was first recognised in India in 1955 during an outbreak in and around Vellore, Tamil Nadu, and the neighbouring areas of Andhra Pradesh (Webb and Pereira, 1956; Work and Shah, 1956; Carey et al., 1969b; Jacobson and Sivalenka, 2004). Further cases were observed every year thereafter in various districts in the states of Tamil Nadu and Andhra Pradesh in south India, almost all in children, and presenting in the latter half of the year during the rainy season (Carey et al., 1969b). Serological surveys carried out between 1955 and 1972 showed that JEV infections occurred in widely scattered areas in eight states, comprising Gujarat, Maharashtra, Orissa, Assam, Arunachal Pradesh, Tamil Nadu, Andhra Pradesh, and Karnataka (F.M. Rodrigues, cited by Reuben and Gajanana, 1997). JEV was first isolated from mosquitoes of the Cx. vishnui subgroup in 1956, and from the brain of a fatal case of encephalitis in 1958.

JEV was not recognised as a major public health problem in India until 1973, when the first major epidemic occurred in the Bankura and Burdwan districts of West Bengal (Arora and Singh, 1974; Chakravarti et al., 1975). Since then, epidemics of various size have been reported from a number of states and union territories, including Karnataka in 1977–1978, Bihar in 1978, Uttar Pradesh in 1978, Tamil Nadu in 1978, Maharashtra in 1979, Assam in 1980, Pondicherry in 1981, Manipur in 1982, Goa in 1982, Nagaland in 1985, Orissa in 1989, Haryana in 1990, and Kerala in 1996. The major outbreaks have usually coincided with heavy rainfall and/or flooding. Examples of these and other JEV epidemics are shown in Table 1, and a map depicting the location of JEV virus activity in India can be viewed at the website

Table 1

Examples of epidemics of JEV in India

Year	State	References
1973	West Bengal	Arora and Singh (1974); Chakraveri et al. (1975)
1977–1978	Karnataka	Prasad et al. (1982)
1978	Bihar	Mohan Rao et al. (1980)
	West Bengal	Mohan Rao et al. (1980)
	Uttar Pradesh	Mathur et al. (1982)
	Tamil Nadu	Rao et al. (1982)
1979	Maharashtra	Rodrigues et al. (1980)
1980	Assam	Chakraborty et al. (1987)
	Bihar	Loach et al. (1983)
1981	Pondicherry	Rao et al. (1988)
1982	Manipur	Chakraborty et al. (1984)
	Goa	Mohan Rao et al. (1983); Choudhury et al (1983)
1985	Nagaland	Angami et al. (1989); Mukherjee et al. (1991)
1987	Nagaland	Mukherjee et al. (1991)
1988	Nagaland	Mukherjee et al. (1991)
	Uttar Pradesh	Rathi et al. (1993)
1989	Assam	Vajpayee et al. (1992)
	Orissa	Vajpayee et al. (1991)
1990	Haryana	Sharma and Panwar (1991); Prasad et al. (1993)
1996	Kerala	Dhanda et al. (1997)
1997	Maharashtra	Thakare et al. (1999)
1998	Uttar Pradesh	http://www.nicd.org
1999	Uttar Pradesh	http://www.nicd.org
1999	Karnataka	http://www.nicd.org
1999	Andhra Pradesh	Rao et al. (2000), http://www.nicd.org
2000	Assam	Kaur et al. (2002); Phukan et al. (2004)
2000	Uttar Pradesh	http://www.nicd.org
2001	Assam	Phukan et al. (2004)
2002	Assam	Phukan et al. (2004)
2005	Uttar Pradesh	Kumar et al. (2006); http://w3.whosea/org/en/Section1226/Section2073.asp

of the Vector Control Research Centre in Pondicherry http://www.pon.nic.in/fil-free/
vrcc/jel.html, or the website of the National Vector Borne Disease Control
Programme at http://www.namp.gov.in/je.html. The most recent outbreak in Uttar
Pradesh in 2005, with a spillover of cases in Bihar, may have been one of the largest
recorded epidemics of JEV (Mudur, 2005; Kumar et al., 2006; WHO, SEARO,
website http://w3.whosea.org/en/Section1226/Section2073.asp). In all, JEV activity
has been reported from at least 25 states and union territories of India. While a few
states have not reported JEV activity, transmission is widespread and endemic in
some states with high infection rates, such as in Andhra Pradesh, Tamil Nadu and
some parts of Karnataka, Uttar Pradesh, Assam, and West Bengal, and other states
may have occasional but limited, focal transmission, such as in Punjab (Ratho et al.,
1999), Madhya Pradesh (Mathur et al., 1981), and Arunachal Pradesh (Chattopadhyay, 2001).

Thus, it appears that JEV probably became established first in southeast India.
It may then have subsequently spread out from this endemic area to cause epidemic
activity in the north in 1978 (Uttar Pradesh and Bihar), reaching the north-east
(Assam, Manipur, and Nagaland) between 1980 and 1985, and the west coast
(Goa) and north-west (Haryana) in 1982 and 1990 respectively, and eventually into
the southwest in 1996 (Kerala). Alternatively, it may have been re-introduced a
second time into India to cause the first epidemic in West Bengal, and then have
spread to other areas from this new introduction. Indeed, this latter possibility
seems more likely from phylogenetic data, which suggest that there have been
multiple introductions of JEV into India, notably into West Bengal in 1973 and
into Assam in 1978, the former introduction spreading to other states of India,
including Goa, and subsequently to Sri Lanka, and from Sri Lanka to Nepal (Uchil
and Satchidanandam, 2001). Despite genomic differences, all JEV strains from the
Indian subcontinent have belonged to genotype 3.

The epidemiology of JEV outbreaks varies considerably between states and
between districts within states. This latter aspect is clearly shown in Andhra
Pradesh where 98% of all JE cases were reported from 10 of the 23 districts in the
state (Jacobson and Sivalenka, 2004). JE is primarily a rural disease in India, with
scattered cases over a wide area, and there are rarely more than a handful of cases
in any one village. Most cases of JE occur in areas of endemic activity and
outbreaks occur in children below the age of 14; but in areas where JEV infection is
uncommon or in areas that are experiencing JEV activity for the first time, all age
groups are affected. Morbidity rates of between 0.30 and 1.5/100,000 have been
estimated (Reuben and Gajanana, 1997). The number of cases reported annually
over the 10-year period 1992–2001 ranged from 1172 to 3395, with case-fatality
rates varying from 19 to 51.5 (National Institute of Communicable Diseases, Delhi,
website http://www.nicd.org, and reproduced in Kabilan et al., 2004a). Indeed,
case-fatality rates in excess of 50% are not uncommon in some outbreaks (eg.
Mathur et al., 1981; Vajpayee et al., 1992; Chattopadhyay, 2001), although in most
outbreaks the case-fatality rates were usually between 15% and 30%. There is
growing awareness that the incidences of JE and related deaths have been

increasing over recent years, and that JEV is spreading into previously unaffected areas (Kabilan et al., 2004a). However, the burden of disease in India is still not known with any accuracy, and until there are enough laboratories capable of diagnosing JEV and an improved national surveillance system, it is unlikely that the real burden of JE will be known.

The major mosquito vectors in India vary from region to region, depending on ecological factors. JEV has been isolated from 16 species of mosquito and the most important vector species are members of the *Cx. vishnui* subgroup especially *Cx. tritaeniorhynchus*, *Cx. vishnui*, and *Cx. pseudovishnui*, which are rice paddy breeders, but other mosquito species are important locally (Samuel et al., 2000; National Vector Borne Disease Control Programme website at http://www.namp.gov.in/je.html).

Two other mosquito-borne arboviral encephalitides occur in India, WNV and Chandipura virus, and have implications for clinical and laboratory diagnosis of JEV infection. WNV was first detected in India by serology in the early 1950s (Smithburn et al., 1954), and cases of both febrile disease and encephalitis due to WNV were reported from the Udaipur area of Rajastan, and from Buldhanam, Marathwada, and Khandesh districts of Maharashtra (Banerjee, 1996). The virus has been isolated from sporadic human infections, both classical febrile cases (Paul et al., 1970) and encephalitis cases (George et al., 1984; Kedarnath et al., 1984; George et al., 1987), and from mosquitoes (Pavri and Singh, 1965; Dandawate et al., 1969; Rodrigues et al., 1980). Cases of febrile disease with arthralgia and encephalitis due to WNV have been reported; 7 cases of WNV encephalitis were identified by detection of IgM in the CSF in Goa, Maharashtra, Orissa and Rajasthan (Thakare et al., 2002). Neutralising antibodies were detected in human sera collected from Tamil Nadu, Karataka, Andhra Pradesh, Gujarat, Maharashtra, Madhya Pradesh, Orissa, and Rajastan (R.G. Damle, cited by Paramasivan et al., 2003). Thus, although WNV has not been responsible for epidemic activity, it is relatively widespread in India. Of concern, is the potential for both WNV and JEV to co-circulate, as described in an outbreak of JEV in Karnataka when a few cases of WNV infection were detected by brain biopsy (George et al., 1987). While it is probable that immunity gained from subclinical infection with either virus will give some level of protection against the other, there is no field evidence to support this. Experimental studies in domestic pigs have shown that prior exposure to JEV prevented the development of viraemia on subsequent exposure to WNV, but HI antibodies were induced to both viruses. Interestingly, WNV challenge did not significantly boost the antibodies to JEV. However, in the converse experiments, prior exposure to WNV did not prevent the occurrence of a low viraemia on subsequent infection with JEV, although the viraemia was probably too low to infect mosquitoes, but there was a boosting effect on the already existing WNV antibodies (Ilkal et al., 1994). These results were consistent with earlier observations in bonnet macaques (*Macaca radiata*), in which immunisation with WNV reduced the severity of disease due to JEV without prevention of infection, whereas immunisation with JEV protected the animals against WNV (Goverdhan et al., 1992). It is interesting, however, that both viruses appear to be able to co-circulate in a region despite having similar ecologies.

A second virus, Chandipura virus, a Rhabdovirus transmitted by phlebotomus flies (sandflies) and mosquitoes, has recently been associated with highly fatal epidemics of encephalitis and may cause difficulties with JEV diagnosis. It was first isolated from two adult cases of febrile illness in the Chandipura (Nagpur) region in Maharashtra (Bhatt and Rodrigues, 1967), and from a child with encephalitis in Raipur in Chhattirgarh (formerly part of Madhya Pradesh) (Rodrigues et al., 1983). Most recently it has been associated with two outbreaks of encephalitis with high mortality. The first was in children in Andhra Pradesh in 2003 (Rao et al., 2004), which had a case-fatality rate of 55.6%, and the second occurred in eastern districts of Gujarat and included patients of all ages (Chadha et al., 2005).

India's first commercially available JEV vaccine, Nakavac (Kabilan, 2004), is available but is not widely used. An improved immunisation programme was initiated by the Andhra Pradesh State Government in collaboration with PATH and has successfully reduced JE there by 90% in its first year (Cooley, 2004). It is hoped that this will serve as a model for a wider and more concerted attempt to reduce the JEV infections in India.

Nepal

An epidemic of JEV occurred for the first time in Nepal in 1978 in the lowland (Terai) region, a rice-growing area bordering Uttar Pradesh and where about half of the population of Nepal live, including 12.5 million children <15 years old. A total of 422 cases were reported with 119 deaths (Umenai et al., 1985; Joshi, 1986, 1995; Parajuli, 1989). Sporadic cases of JE had been reported even earlier than 1978, however, from all hospitals in the Terai areas (Joshi, 1995). During the next few years, the disease fluctuated between 50 and 800 cases annually, with a case-fatality rate between 30% and 50% (Igarashi, 1992). Most cases occurred between July and November, peaking in August to October after the monsoon season (Igarashi, 1992; Endy and Nisalak, 2002). Outbreaks in 1985 and 1986 in the Terai region resulted in 595 and 1299 cases, respectively, in all age groups, with mortality rates of 26.5% and 27.5%, respectively (Joshi, 1987). Interestingly, outbreaks in two districts, Kailali and Kanchanpur, occurred despite the absence of pigs or ducks as reservoir hosts. Analysis of epidemiological data collected during the 1986 epidemic in the Koshi Zone in the Terai region in southeastern Nepal suggested that the virus had only been recently introduced. Children accounted for most of the hospital admissions but had a markedly lower fatality rate than adults, the overall fatality rate being 15% (McCallum, 1991). From 1993 to 1997, the total number of cases of JE within the 25 districts of the Terai increased from 446 cases in 1993 to 2953 cases in 1997 (Bista et al., 1999). JEV spread from the Terai to the Kathmandu Valley in September and October 1995 to cause an outbreak with a mortality of 53% (Zimmerman et al., 1997). Annual epidemics continue to occur in the Terai region, often associated with epidemic activity across the border in Uttar

Pradesh. In 2004, 24 of 75 districts reported cases of JE (JEPN website, www.jepn.org). The number of suspect cases was 2824, of which 316 died, and a further 33 suspect cases were recorded in the first 6 weeks of 2006 (WHO SEARO website: http://w3.whosea.org/en/Section1226/Section2073.asp). JE vaccination has been undertaken in high-risk districts of the Terai using inactivated vaccine, although a highly successful trial using a single dose of the Chinese SA-14-14-2 live vaccine in 1999 has made this a more plausible tool for use in the future (Bista et al., 2001; Ohrr et al., 2005).

Pakistan

Serological studies carried out in Karachi, Pakistan between 1983 and 1985 provided evidence suggesting that some cases of central nervous system disease may have been due to JEV, although most cases were caused by WNV (Ishii et al., 1988; Sugamata et al., 1988). These results were subsequently confirmed and extended in 1992 when JEV genome sequences were found by RT-PCR in the CSF from a patient with encephalitis (Igarashi et al., 1994). WNV was found in CSFs from an additional eight cases, indicating that a significant proportion of encephalitis cases in Karachi were caused by WNV, while JEV was a minor cause in some cases.

Sri Lanka

JEV was first isolated in Sri Lanka in 1968 (Hermon and Anandarajah, 1974). From 1971 to 1981, 1030 hospital admissions of sporadic cases of encephalitis were reported, with a case-fatality rate of 25–45%, of which about 43% of admissions for encephalitis may have been due to JEV (Vitarana, 1982; Vitarana et al., 1988). The first major outbreak of JEV occurred between November 1985 and February 1986 in the North-Central (dry-zone rice cultivation area) and Western provinces of the country, with 406 cases and 76 deaths in Anuradhapura district in the North-Central province and 106 cases and 18 deaths in Chilaw (Puttalum) district in the Western province coastal belt (Vitarana et al., 1988). The Anuradhapura outbreak appeared to start in a major new irrigation system, the giant Mahaweli Irrigation Scheme; 73% were adult cases with a peak incidence in the 20–40 year age group, whereas the Chilaw outbreak had the more usual endemic pattern with most cases in children (Vitarana et al., 1988). The authors concluded that the new irrigation scheme contributed to the Anuradhapura outbreak with higher vector densities and a 10-fold increase in domestic pigs. This conclusion was supported by the increased numbers of nocturnally active mosquitoes able to transmit JEV, especially *Cx. tritaeniorhynchus, Cx. quinquefasciatus*, and *Mansonia uniformis*, and to a lesser extent, *Cx. fuscocephala* (Amerasinghe and Ariyasena, 1991). A second, larger outbreak occurred in November to December 1987 in North-Central province at Anuradhapura, with 744 cases diagnosed on clinical grounds, of whom 361 were confirmed by laboratory studies (Peiris et al., 1992). The epidemic was preceded 2–3

weeks earlier by seroconversions in sentinel pigs. The major vectors identified were
Cx. tritaeniorhynchus, *Cx. gelidus*, and to a lesser extent, *Cx. fuscocephala*, *Cx. whitmorei*, and *Ma. uniformis*. Comparing the epidemic period in 1987 with the same period in the following year when no epidemic occurred, the major differences were a lower vector biomass and a lower JEV carriage rate in the vectors. Peiris et al. (1993) also investigated the ecology of JEV in different climatological areas of Sri Lanka in relation to the abundance of mosquito vectors, infection in domestic livestock, and human infection and disease. Little or no virus activity was documented above 1200 m in elevation. Interestingly, JEV seroprevalence in cattle and goats were better predictors of human infection risk than was porcine seroprevalence, especially in epidemic regions. The dry-zone area around Anuradhapura was classified as an epidemic area for JEV, whereas the wet zone in the Western Province was classified as endemic for the virus. Vaccination of children between 1 and 10 years of age was begun in 1988 in the Anuradhapura and Puttalam districts, and was then extended to high prevalence areas in the Kurunegala, Polunnaruwa, and Gampaha districts. The incidence of JE dropped significantly in the immunised age group thereafter (Vitarana, 1995). Other control procedures used were porcine immunisation using a live vaccine, water management in irrigation schemes, and spraying of pigpens with malathion (Vitarana, 1995). JE cases continue to occur throughout the year with a peak between October and February, and 21 districts out of 26 reported cases between 1994 and 2003 (JEPN website, www.jepn.org). The vaccination programme is run only in high-risk districts and uses an inactivated vaccine.

Indonesia

The ecology of JEV in Indonesia is complicated to some extent by the zoogeographic separation of the country by the hypothetical Wallace and Weber lines, both purporting to provide a demarcation between the Oriental and Australasian zoogeographic regions (Kanamitsu et al., 1979; Marshall, 1988; Mackenzie et al., 1997a, 2002b), and by the large number of flaviviruses endemic to the region (Mackenzie, 2000; Mackenzie et al., 2002b). The latter fact may make serological surveys difficult to interpret because of heterotypic immune responses. Of particular concern are various members of the JEV serological group, WNV and WNV (KUNV clade), which have been found on Borneo (albeit in Sarawak) (Bowen et al., 1970; Karabatsos, 1985), and MVEV, WNV (KUNV clade), and ALFV, which can be found in some parts of the eastern archipelago. In addition to these members of the JEV serological group, dengue viruses are found widely throughout the region, Zika and Tembusu viruses are of concern in the western archipelago, and Edge Hill, Kokobera, Sepik, Zika and Tembusu viruses may be found in parts of the eastern archipelago. Early seroepidemiological studies had suggested that JEV was present in various parts of Indonesia (Hotta et al., 1967, 1970a,b), but because of the problems associated with antigenic cross-reactivities in the HI tests, the results were inconclusive. For ease of discussion, the data from the Western archipelago (Sumatra, Java, Bali, and Kalimantan) will be described first.

Java, Sumatra, Kalimantan, and Bali

The first report of clinical illness attributed to JEV was from a clinical case in 1971 in Jakarta (L.K. Kho, cited by Van Peenen et al., 1975b). Studies carried out in a major pig raising area at Bogor, near Jakarta, showed that a pig–mosquito transmission cycle of JEV was present, implicating *Cx. tritaeniorhynchus* mosquitoes through vector numbers and virus isolation (Atmosoedjono et al., 1973; Van Peenen et al., 1974a), and the demonstration of antibody-positive pigs (Van Peenen et al., 1974b). Further isolations of JEV were made from pig sera and from *Cx. tritaeniorhynchus*, *Cx. gelidus*, and *Cx. fuscocephala* mosquitoes trapped in the pig-raising areas (Van Peenen et al., 1975a,b). These studies suggested that there was a correlation with agricultural practices rather than climate and rainfall, although the mosquitoes were trapped in the rainy season. The association between vector density dynamics and JEV activity was shown in a study carried out in Kapuk, a suburb of Jakarta (Olson et al., 1985b), in which JEV was isolated from *Cx. tritaeniorhynchus*, *Cx. fuscocephala*, *Cx. gelidus*, and *Cx. vishnui*. In central Java where pigs are less common, JEV was isolated from seven species of mosquitoes trapped in cattle shelters, suggesting that cattle may be involved in some natural transmission cycles in Indonesia (Tan et al., 1993). In a survey of encephalitis cases in hospitals throughout Indonesia between 1979 and 1986, there was an average of 1586 cases reported each year with case-fatality rates ranging from 28% to 45%, with most cases in children. Hospitals from East Java, West Java, and Bali reported the highest incidence of cases (Sumarmo et al., 1995). After a case of JE was found in a 10-year-old female tourist from Australia visiting Denpasar in 1989 (Macdonald et al., 1989), a prospective study in Bali of children hospitalised for encephalitis between 1990 and 1992 found 19 of 47 cases of encephalitis that could be serologically confirmed as JE (Jennings and colleagues, unpublished results cited by Sumarmo et al., 1995). Further studies in Bali of another 77 suspected cases of JE found that 44 of them had JEV antibodies in their CSF (T. Soroso, S. Ganefa, B. Widarso, personal communication cited by Mackenzie et al., 2002b). In addition, Yoshida et al. (1999) recently reported serologically confirmed cases of JE in Bali, and in a prospective study, 40–50% of hospitalised encephalitis cases, mostly children, were shown to be caused by JEV (Xu, personal communication to Halstead and Jacobson, 2003). More recent data from the current project run jointly by the Ministry of Health and PATH is described below. JEV has been isolated from mosquitoes in Bali (R. Graham, personal communication cited in Mackenzie et al., 2002b), and several vector species have been found in significant numbers, including *Cx. tritaeniorhynchus*, *Cx. gelidus*, *Cx. fuscocephala*, and *Cx. vishnui* (Lee et al., 1983). A small number of tourists have become infected with JEV while visiting Bali (Macdonald et al., 1989; Wittesjo et al., 1995; Buhl et al., 1996; Ostlund et al., 2004).

West Nusa Tenggara (including Lombok and Sumbawa), East Nusa Tenggara (including Flores, West Timor, Komodo and Sumba), Sulawesi, Moluccas and West Papua

A serological survey carried out by Kanamitsu et al. (1979) found neutralising antibodies to JEV at various locations in Wallacea (the area between the Wallace and Weber lines, and comprising Lombok, Flores, Timor, and Sulawesi) and also in West Papua. However, most of the sera reacted with more than one of the flaviviruses, and only a few sera from Lombok were believed to be positive for JEV. Olson et al. (1983) also found heterotypic responses in human sera, but subsequently isolated JEV from three species of mosquitoes, *Cx. tritaeniorhynchus, An. vagus*, and *An. anularis*, in Lombok (Olson et al., 1985a) and from *Cx. tritaeniorhynchus* in Flores (J.G. Olson, unpublished results, cited by Mackenzie et al., 2002b). A single case of JE was reported from Timika, West Papua, in 1997 (Spicer, 1997), and subsequent serological investigations demonstrated that five indigenous people from the Timika region had serological evidence of past infection with JEV (Spicer et al., 1999). However, it should be recalled that other members of the JE serological group, especially MVEV, are endemic in West Papua, and MVEV has been responsible for at least one reported case of encephalitis (Essed and Van Tongeran, 1965). Porcine sera from various parts of the Eastern archipelago including West Timor (P.W. Daniels and I. Sandow, personal communication to Mackenzie et al., 2002b), Sulawesi, East Nusa Tenggara, and West Nusa Tenggara (T. Soroso, S. Ganefa, B. Widarso, personal communication to Mackenzie et al., 2002b) have also been found to have HI antibodies to JEV.

The JE project of PATH has initiated a surveillance system for JE at various sites throughout Indonesia in collaboration with the Indonesian Ministry of Health to determine the burden of disease so that more informed decisions can be made concerning childhood immunisation. Starting in Janury 2005, the surveillance is hospital based and incorporates 15 hospitals in 6 provinces. In the first 6 months of the project, 19 cases of JE were found from 397 encephalitis cases, with confirmed cases in West Sumatra, West Kalimantan, East Java, West Nusa Tenggara (Lombok), and East Nusa Tenggara (West Timor). No cases were found in that period in West Papua.

Timor-Leste

Two serologically confirmed cases of JEV infection were reported from the Viqueque district of Timor-Leste in 2000, one of which was fatal (Hueston et al., 2001).

Papua New Guinea

JEV was first found in Papua New Guinea during an investigation into the source of an outbreak in the Torres Strait of northern Australia (see below). Serological surveys found strong evidence of JEV in human sera collected from various sites in Western, Gulf, and Southern Highlands Provinces between 1989 and 1995 (Johansen et al., 1997), and in porcine sera from Western Province (J. Shield and R. Lunt, unpublished data cited by Mackenzie et al., 2002b). Three isolates of JEV were obtained from Lake Murray and Balimo in Western Province in 1997 and 1998, respectively from *Cx. annulirostris* and *Cx. palpalis* (Johansen et al., 2000), and four cases of JE were recognised at a mission hospital near Kiunga (J. Oakley. S. Flew, C.A. Johansen, R.A. Hall, D. Phillips, J.S. Mackenzie, unpublished results cited in Mackenzie et al., 2002b). In addition, two outbreaks of JEV have been reported, one on Normanby Island in Milne Bay Province in eastern Papua New Guinea, and the other at Alotau, capital of Milne Bay Province, although both outbreaks remain unconfirmed. Finally, a case of JEV infection was recently reported from the Port Moresby area (Hanson et al., 2004).

A number of flaviviruses are endemic in Papua New Guinea, thus making the interpretation of some serological surveys problematical. MVEV has been isolated from mosquitoes in East Sepik Province in the north of Papua New Guinea (Marshall, 1988) and from Western Province in the south (Johansen et al., 2000), and been responsible for a case of fatal encephalitis in Papua (French et al., 1957). Antibodies to WNV (KUNV clade) have been detected in sera collected in East Sepik Province (R.A. Hawkes unpublished data, cited by Marshall, 1988); and two other flaviviruses have been isolated in Papua New Guinea, Sepik, and Kokobera viruses (Marshall, 1988; Johansen et al., 2000). Thus it is perhaps not surprising that in an earlier seroepidemiological study in 1956–1957, some sera, particularly from the Aramia River near Balimo in Western Province, had shown higher neutralising antibody titres to JEV than to MVEV, which was explained by the authors as heterotypic responses (Anderson et al., 1960). As found in India with WNV, JEV appears to co-circulate with MVEV and WNV (KUNV clade), and indeed JEV, MVEV, and Sepik virus were isolated from mosquitoes during a single night of trapping at Balimo in Western Province (Johansen et al., 2000).

Australia

JE was first reported in the Torres Strait of northern Australia in March to April 1995. Three cases, two of which were fatal, occurred on Badu, an island in the central Torres Strait (Hanna et al., 1996b). A further 55 people from islands in the central and northern Torres Strait were found to have evidence of subclinical infection, and a large number of domestic pigs on nine islands were found to have seroconverted. Ten isolates of JEV were obtained, two from subclinical human sera, and eight from *Cx. annulirostris* mosquitoes (Hanna et al., 1996b; Ritchie et al., 1997). In response to the outbreak, all inhabitants of the Torres Strait were offered inactivated JEV vaccine (Hanna et al., 1996a). In addition, a sentinel pig surveillance programme was initiated (Shield et al., 1996; Ellis et al., 2000). Two more cases of JE occurred in 1998, one in an unvaccinated child on Badu and the other in an individual on the Australian mainland at the mouth of the Mitchell River in southwest Cape York (Hanna et al., 1999). The latter was the first human case on the Australian mainland. These two cases were accompanied by pig seroconversions from the northern Torres Strait islands to Cape York, and JEV was isolated from *Cx. annulirostris* and *Oc. vigilax* mosquitoes in Badu and from pig sera in Cape York (Hanna et al., 1999; Johansen et al., 2001). Genetic sequencing of the 1995 and 1998 virus isolates showed they were genotype 2, similar to strains from Java, and were closely related to each other and to the 1997 and 1998 isolates from Papua New Guinea, indicating that Papua New Guinea was the probable source of the incursions of JEV into Australia. It was hypothesised that JEV reached Australasia by island hopping across the eastern Indonesia archipelago, spread by birds, establishing the bird–mosquito and pig–mosquito transmission cycles on each island as it moved (Mackenzie et al., 2002b).

In further JEV infections in the Torres Strait in 2000, the virus was isolated from pig sera and *Cx. gelidus* mosquitoes on Badu and from *Cx. sitiens* mosquitoes on Saibai, an island in the north of the Torres Strait a few kilometres from the Papua New Guinea coast (Mackenzie et al., 2001; Pyke et al., 2001; van den Hurk et al., 2001a; Johansen et al., 2004). Interestingly, the virus isolates in this outbreak were genetically different from those of the previous outbreak, belonging instead to genotype 1, indicating a second introduction of JEV into the Torres Strait region of Australia (Pyke et al., 2001). The finding of JEV in *Cx. gelidus* mosquitoes was unexpected as this species was not known to be in the Torres Strait, although it had been found on the Australian mainland for the first time the previous year (Muller et al., 2001), and its range was later found to extend across northern Australia (Whelan et al., 2000). JEV was detected on the Australian mainland for the second time in 2004 and isolated from *Cx. sitiens* subgroup mosquitoes in Cape York (van den Hurk et al., 2006; G.A. Smith, A.T. Pyke, P. Daniels, unpublished data). This was the first isolate from a mosquito trapped on mainland Australia. Over the period 1995–2005, JEV infections occurred every year in the Torres Strait except 1999, and on the Australian mainland in 1998 and 2004 (Mackenzie, 2005; G.A. Smith, S.A. Ritchie, J. Lee, P.W.Daniels, unpublished observations).

It was hypothesised that the outbreak in 1998 in the Torres Strait and mainland Australia resulted from wind-borne virus blown southwards from Western Province of Papua New Guinea during cyclonic weather patterns (Ritchie and Rochester, 2001), and it was suggested that this may have been the route also taken by the virus in other years, although wild birds have also been suggested, as noted above (Hanna et al., 1996b). Despite JEV occurring on mainland Australia in at least two locations in 1998 and again in 2004, there is no evidence at this time that the virus has become established there, although mosquito species able to transmit JEV are present (van den Hurk et al., 2003a), and large numbers of ardeid birds and feral pigs are present that could serve as potential vertebrate hosts (Mackenzie et al., 2002b). Of the ardeid birds, it is believed that the Nankeen night heron (*Nycticorax caledonicus*), which is closely related to the Black-crowned night heron of Asia, may be the most important, as it is also thought to be the major host of MVEV (Marshall, 1988; Mackenzie et al., 1994). The Nankeen night heron is found widely across Australia, and vagrant birds can travel substantial distances, including moving between the Australian mainland and Papua New Guinea.

A number of other flaviviruses circulate in northern Australia and the Torres Strait, including the three other viruses in the JEV serological group, MVEV, ALFV, and WNV (KUNV clade), and four additional mosquito-borne flaviviruses, Kokobera, Stratford, New Mapoon, and Edge Hill viruses (Mackenzie et al., 1994; van den Hurk et al., 2001b; Johansen et al., 2003, 2004; Nisbet et al., 2005). Serological surveys are therefore often difficult to interpret, since a person or animal may have been infected with more than one flavivirus. The three JEV serological group viruses appear to co-circulate. While it is not known at this time whether JEV will also co-circulate, should it become established in northern Australia, mice passively immunised with antisera generated by JEV infection are immune to subsequent infection with MVEV, and mice passively immunised with antisera generated by MVEV infection are immune to subsequent infection with JEV (Broom et al., 2000). However, passive immunisation with antibody generated by infection with WNV (KUNV clade) did not protect against MVEV infection. Thus while JEV and WNV are able to co-circulate in India, JEV and MVEV are closer antigenically and it is less clear whether they will also be able co-exist, although it is unclear whether JEV and MVEV will be able co-co-circulate in Australia, data from Papua New Guinea (above) suggest that they have the potential to do so. This is an important question in assessing the risk of JEV establishment in northern Australia.

Virus spread

Possible spread of JEV from Japan

There is little doubt that over the past five decades JEV has spread into new areas and is an increasing threat to large numbers of children in southern and southeastern Asia. The method and direction of spread, however, is not clear. It must also be remembered that epidemic activity is much more recognisable than endemic activity, where occasional, sporadic and unconnected cases occur and which, if the virus is not known to be present, JEV may remain undiagnosed or misdiagnosed.

Although it is possible that summer epidemics of encephalitis in Japan in 1871 may have been caused by JEV, the virus itself was not isolated and identified until the mid-1930s. The possible spread of the virus thereafter is perceived within a time frame which incorporates information based on epidemic activity or virus isolations, and this may not always fit comfortably with information from other geographic areas. While it appears to be relatively simple to trace the possible movement of the virus as it spread from Japan into Siberia around 1938, and into China and Korea around 1940 (although summer epidemics of encephalitis had been recognised in Korea since the early 1930s), and then into northern Thailand and Vietnam possibly in the late 1950s or early 1960s (Solomon, 2003), these dates are not necessarily consistent with the apparent presence of the virus a decade or more earlier in tropical, endemic areas further south and west (Fig. 3). Indeed there is evidence from prisoner-of-war records that the virus may have been in Malaya in the mid-to-late 1940s, or shortly thereafter, and that the virus was in southern India in the early 1950s. More localised spread in the Indian subcontinent is easier to recognise with the virus spreading south to Sri Lanka around 1968. However, genetic evidence suggests that multiple incursions of JEV have occurred into India, one of which caused the first epidemic in West Bengal in 1973 and then spread across the country to Goa, and another of which spread into Assam and Nepal (Uchil and Satchidanandam, 2001). Even the spread south to Sri Lanka may not be as straight forward, and there is genetic evidence to indicate that both the 1955 epidemic JEV strain and the later West Bengal epidemic strain may have spread to Sri Lanka. Thus, one major question raised by this apparent sequential spread is

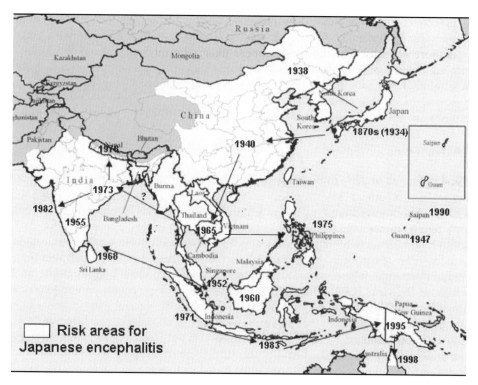

Fig. 3 Map showing the temporal spread of JEV from the initial isolation in Japan. Modified from Solomon (2000). (For colour version: see Colour Section on page 354).

why the virus was present in Malaysia and India before northern Thailand and northern Vietnam. Possible explanations could be that it was introduced to the Indo-Malay peninsula by Japanese troops during the World War II, or that it was introduced into tropical ecosystems by migratory birds (see below).

Evidence for evolution and spread of JEV from molecular and phylogenetic studies

Genomic studies provide an alternative explanation for the direction of JEV dispersal, suggesting that JEV might have actually originated in southeast Asia, and then spread north and west as different genotypes. Exhaustive analyses of sequence data for JEV reveal that the Indonesia–Malaysia region supports the circulation of all JEV genotypes and is the only region where the oldest and most divergent genotype (genotype 4) has been found (Solomon et al., 2003a). It was therefore suggested that JEV originated in this region from an ancestral virus, from which genotype 4 diverged, followed later by genotypes 1, 2, and 3 (Fig. 4). When these newer genotypes spread across Asia and Australasia, genotype 4 remained in the Indonesia–Malaysia region (Solomon et al., 2003a). The timing of such movment is difficult to determine, particularly given the epidemic activity in Japan, and the apparently recent arrival of JEV in Australasia.

Was JE in tropical areas slow to be recognised, perhaps being misdiagnosed as smear-negative cerebral malaria, whereas the epidemic activity in temperate areas was more obvious? This does not appear likely, although misdiagnosis can be a problem in the absence of laboratory support, as seen in Papua New Guinea. The divergence of genotype 4 JEV from the common ancestor has been estimated to have occurred ~300 years ago, whereas genotypes 1, 2, and 3 diverged ~130 years ago (Uchil and Satchidanandam, 2001; Solomon et al., 2003a).

Mechanisms of spread and changing epidemiological patterns

Genotype 1 strains of JEV have recently spread and replaced genotype 3 in Japan, Korea, and northern Vietnam (see Section on "Genomic variation" above). The mechanisms for this genomic spread and displacement are unknown; however, it has been suggested that genotype 1 strains may have acquired increased virulence for avian hosts, enabling its spread via bird migration along the "East Asian-Australasian flyway" (Nga et al., 2004), Migrating ardeid birds, such as the Blackcrowned night heron, have been suggested as a means of virus movement and dispersal. Indeed it has been suggested that viraemic birds may be responsible for spreading JEV to new areas and for reintroducing JEV into epidemic areas each season (Ogata et al., 1970). Migratory patterns of herons from China, Taiwan, Philippines, and Java, to Japan at the beginning of the summer coincide with the seasonal transmission of JEV in Japan (Ogata et al., 1970).

Another ardeid species, the Asiatic cattle egret (*Bubulcus ibis coromandus*) is an important host in the dispersal of the virus to new geographic areas (Solomon et al., 2003a), in part due to its greatly expanded range across Asia following

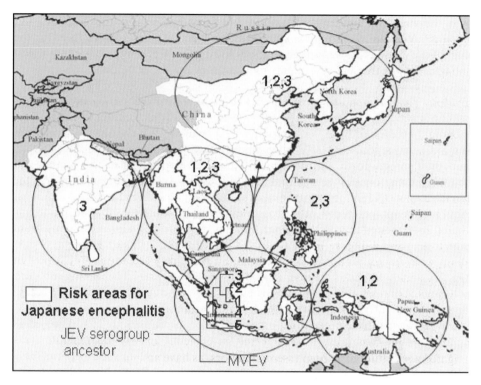

Fig. 4 Map showing the possible origin and distribution of JEV, showing the geographic distribution of the genotypes. The ancestral virus is hypothesized to have given rise to genotype 4, and then to the other genotypes. A possible genotype 5, based on the Muar strain, would have been the earliest genotype if its sequence is confirmed. From Solomon and Winter (2004) and Solomon et al. (2003a). (For colour version: see Colour Section on page 355).

changes in agricultural practices, which also coincided with the evolution and spread of the more recent genotypes of JEV.

Wind is central to insect dispersal, often over long distances, and thus virus movement, providing it is sufficiently warm and moist for flight. There is a substantial literature concerned with the role of wind in the genesis of epidemic activity of arboviruses through the movement of infected mosquitoes (e.g. Garrett-Jones, 1962; Sellers,1989; Sellers and Maarouf, 1990,1993; Ming et al., 1993; Min and Mei, 1996; Reynolds et al., 1996; Mackenzie et al., 2000). Flights of 5–100 km have been recorded for *Cx. taeniorhynchus* (a vector of Venezuelan equine encephalitis virus) and 175 km for *Ae. sollicitans* (a vector of Venezuelan and Eastern equine encephalitis viruses) (Sellers, 1980). These flights were completed at temperatures of 15–35°C at heights of up to 1.5 km (Sellers, 1980). Most studies, however, have tended to capture mosquitoes at lower heights, and most commonly below about 500 m (e.g. Ming et al., 1993; C.G. Johnson, cited by Sellers, 1980).

Wind has also been suggested as a means by which *Cx. tritaeniorhynchus* mosquitoes migrate or are assisted in migrating each year in China, where they fly north in the spring and return south in the autumn (Ming et al., 1993; Min et al., 1996).

The accidental transportation of exotic mosquito species around the world when they have bred in pools of water trapped in deck cargo, or when they travel as stowaways on aircraft (Lounibos, 2002; Mackenzie et al., 2004; Larish and Savage, 2005), may also assist in the establishment of JEV in new geographic areas. Aircraft disinfection is not a widespread practice everywhere, including some countries in Asia. Some mosquito species known to transmit JEV have spread to other continents; for instance *Oc. japonicus* reached the continental US (Peyton et al., 1999), where it has spread widely in both East and West Coasts as well as to Hawaii (Larish and Savage, 2005) and to Europe (Medlock et al., 2005). *Oc. japonicus* mosquitoes are probably most important as transmitters of JEV in temperate areas of eastern Asia (Vaughn and Hoke, 1992). They have been shown to transmit JEV experimentally, including by vertical transmission (Takashima and Rosen, 1989). They also have been shown to transmit both WNV (Turell et al., 2002) and SLEV in the USA (Sardelis et al., 2003).

There are many other factors associated with the spread and establishment of JEV, although their interplay is not well understood. Changes in land use and agricultural practices have been particularly important; increases in rice fields and irrigated agriculture have been essential factors, as have an increase in pig breeding with the promotion of pigs as a food source (Umenai et al., 1985; Tsai, 1997; Keiser et al., 2005). Deforestation with indiscriminate clear-felling, in which small streams become blocked to form swamps, can provide ideal conditions for mosquitoes to breed.

Prevention

Vector reduction, animal host control, and personal protection

Pesticide usage on rice fields had a substantial effect in northern temperate areas of JEV activity prior to vaccination programmes, but insecticide use has generally been of very limited value. It is expensive, and even when mosquito numbers drop, new populations of mosquitoes will fly in from nearby rice fields (Vaughn and Hoke, 1992).

Various other methods of mosquito vector reduction have been investigated, including the use of larvicidal bacteria such as *Bacillus sphaericus* and *B. thuringiensis*, the use of nematode parasites of mosquitoes such as *Romanomermis culicivorax*, the use of invertebrate predators, the use of larvivorous fish such as *Gambusia affinis*, and the use of certain fungi to destroy larvae, but none have been effective for more than a short period, and most are expensive and time consuming to deploy (reviewed by Lacey and Lacey, 1990; Keiser et al., 2005). One environmental method, alternate wet and dry irrigation, however, does warrant further experimental investigation (Reuben and Gajanana, 1997; Keiser et al., 2005). The most effective means of reducing the numbers of infected mosquitoes around human habitation is to ensure that pigsties and cattle pens are a distance from houses. The removal of pigs from around human habitation to communal pig pens located 3 km away was suggested as a reason for the absence of human cases in Badu in 2000 (J.N. Hanna, S.A. Ritchie, personal communication; Mackenzie et al., 2002b), despite the isolation of JEV from sentinel pigs and *Cx. gelidus* mosquitoes on the island (Pyke et al., 2001; van den Hurk et al., 2001a). It is also essential to take effective personal precautions against mosquito bites including the use of bednets, minimising outdoor exposure at dusk and dawn, wearing long-sleeved shirts and trousers, using personal insect repellants with at least 30% DEET (*N,N*-diethyl-meta-tolumide) on exposed skin, maintaining insect screens on all windows and doors, and sleeping under mosquito netting.

Vaccines

Currently, three human vaccines are available for prevention of JE (Monath, 2002a; Chang et al., 2004; Halstead and Tsai, 2004). A formalin inactivated mouse brain-derived vaccine is manufactured in China, Japan, North Korea, South Korea, Taiwan, and in limited quantities in India, Thailand, and Vietnam. It is given in childhood vaccination programs in Japan, South Korea, and Taiwan, nearly eliminating the disease in these countries (Hoke et al., 1988; Wu et al., 1999; Sohn, 2000). This vaccine has also become a part of the Expanded Program of Immunization in Thailand; elsewhere, it is administered at a regional level to those at risk in various countries including in Vietnam, Sri Lanka, and Nepal (Halstead and Tsai, 2004; Hombach et al., 2005).

Mouse brain-derived vaccine manufactured and exported from Japan by the Biken Institute is the only commercial JE vaccine available internationally and it is indicated for travellers to JEV endemic countries (Shlim and Solomon, 2002). Although the vaccine has relatively high efficacy (91% after two doses; Hoke et al., 1988), its use is limited by high production costs (US$3–5 per dose), poor induction of long-term immunity, requirement for multiple boosters, and the incidence of vaccine-induced adverse reactions (Poland et al., 1990; Plesner et al., 2000; Takahashi et al., 2000; Halstead and Tsai, 2004). The mouse brain vaccine is derived from a genotype 3, virus strain but there is no evidence that its efficacy is affected by the antigenic variation that has been reported within and between genotypes of JEV (Wills et al., 1992; Ali and Igarashi, 1997). This vaccine has been effective in regions where heterologous genotypes circulate, indicating that it results in high levels of cross-protection.

In China, a formalin-inactivated, cell culture-derived vaccine (derived from P3 strain, grown in primary hamster kidney [PHK] cells) is produced and reported to have similar efficacy to the mouse brain-derived vaccine (84–95%) after two doses (Monath, 2002a; Halstead and Tsai, 2004). However, the P3 inactivated vaccine suffers from the same shortcomings as the mouse brain-derived vaccine and is gradually being replaced by a live-attenuated virus vaccine (SA14-14-2 strain), also produced in PHK cells (Halstead and Tsai, 2004). The SA14-14-2 vaccine is administered in three doses in annual childhood vaccination campaigns and, in contrast to inactivated vaccines, is inexpensive to make (~US$0.05 per dose) and is relatively safe (Yu et al., 1988; Liu et al., 1997; Halstead and Tsai, 2004). This vaccine has also been shown to be immunogenic and effective, with a protective efficacy of 96–98% following two doses in children (Hennessy et al., 1996; Sohn et al., 1999) and comparable efficacy with a single dose (Bista et al., 2001; Ohrr et al., 2005). A single-dose immunisation schedule would reduce vaccination costs even further and would extend vaccine supply. However, the SA14-14-2 vaccine has yet to be accepted outside of China, with the exception of South Korea, because of concerns about compliance with international regulatory standards and about its safety in specific recipients such as immunocompromised patients (Monath, 2002a; Halstead and Tsai, 2004; WHO, 2005). Implementation of childhood vaccination programs for JEV, using inactivated mouse brain vaccine in Thailand or P3 and SA14-14-2 vaccines in China, has been shown to be cost efficient, suggesting that their inclusion in immunisation programmes of other JEV endemic countries may also be economically feasible. (Siraprapasiri et al., 1997; Ding et al., 2003).

The economic benefits of veterinary vaccines for JEV are also well recognised. Since JEV infection can lead to abortion in pigs and encephalitis in horses, inactivated mouse brain-derived or live-attenuated virus veterinary vaccines have been used throughout East Asia (Barrett, 1997; Daniels et al., 2002; Igarashi, 2002).

Given the limitations of existing vaccines, the WHO has highlighted the need for a safe, low cost, and efficacious vaccine that meets international regulatory standards and is suitable for large-scale public health use (Hombach et al., 2005). The advancement of such a vaccine and its integration into immunisation schemes are among the objectives of the newly established JE program funded by the Bill and Melinda Gates Foundation and developed by PATH through the Children's Vaccine Program (with partners in the Global Alliance for Vaccines and Immunization (GAVI), including various national ministries of health, UNICEF, and WHO) (http://www.childrensvaccine.com/html/jep.htm; Hombach et al., 2005). Second-generation vaccine development is focused on both improving current vaccines and developing new ones. To avoid possible safety risks associated with the mouse brain vaccine and to reduce production costs, attempts have been made to switch to making the vaccine in Vero cells (certified for vaccine manufacture). In clinical evaluations, candidate second-generation vaccines displayed comparable or higher levels of immuno-genicity than the mouse brain-derived vaccine (Kuzuhara et al., 2003; Chang et al., 2004; Hombach et al., 2005).

Efforts to gain approval for the attenuated SA14-14-2 vaccine are also underway. China's largest producer of the vaccine, the ChengDu Institute, has upgraded its facilities to WHO Good Manufacturing Practices standards and has established a pathogen-free facility to provide controlled primary hamster kidney cell substrate (Hombach et al., 2005).

The most promising new vaccine candidate, the ChimeriVax™-JE vaccine, is a recombinant live-attenuated vaccine based on the Yellow Fever 17D vaccine strain, in which the structural genes (prM/E) have been replaced by the cognate genes of the SA14-14-2 vaccine strain (Monath, 2002a; Jones, 2004). Early clinical trials have shown safety and protective efficacy after only one dose of the ChimeriVax vaccine (Monath et al., 2002b, 2003). Passive transfer of antibody raised to the new vaccine provides protection against all four genotypes of JEV in a murine model system (Beasley et al., 2004).

Future spread of JEV

JEV, like WNV, has the propensity to spread and colonise new areas. Over the past 15 years it has spread into naive districts in various states of India as well as into the states of Haryana and Kerala to cause epidemics in 1990 and 1996 respectively, and now it threatens to expand into the Thar desert irrigation areas of Rajasthan, the Indus valley of Pakistan, with the potential to become entrenched in southern Pakistan, and most recently into the eastern Indonesian archipelago, Papua New Guinea, the Torres Strait of northern Australia, and northern mainland Australia. The apparent ease of spread into West Papua, Papua New Guinea, and the Torres Strait, despite the absence of rice growing in those areas, is of concern. The reasons for the ability of JEV and WNV to spread so readily and establish in new areas so effectively may be because of their similar ecologies, and especially their use of avian hosts and to the wide range of mosquito vectors which are competent under a variety of ecological conditions (Mackenzie et al., 2004). JEV has the additional advantage of employing pigs as amplifying hosts, which can have a major effect on the number of infected mosquitoes in the environment.

The lack of many reported cases from Pakistan since JEV was first detected there some 15 years ago may suggest limited access due to the dearth of pig farming in a Muslim country. In northern Australia, JEV has been detected on the mainland in at least two of the past 10 years with infected pigs and mosquitoes yielding virus isolates and a single human case, but there is not yet any evidence to indicate that the virus has established local transmission cycles, although ardeid birds and feral pigs exist there as potential vertebrate hosts, and several mosquito species are excellent vectors. There is some evidence to indicate that the mosquito vectors preferentially bite certain marsupial species rather than feral pigs, and that some of the marsupials may function as dead-end hosts for JEV due to the development of low levels of viraemia (P.W. Daniels, D. Middleton, D. Boyle, K.Newberry, D.Williams, R.Lunt, unpublished results, cited in Mackenzie et al., 2002b; van den Hurk et al., 2003b). If so, the marsupials may play a dampening role, rather as cattle have been hypothesized to do in Asia, but conversely, the similar ecosystems found in Western Province of PNG and Cape York would indicate that the Cape York area should be receptive to JEV establishment. The general belief is that JEV will eventually establish enzootic cycles in northern Australia, but it is difficult to predict a time frame in which this will happen.

The ease and speed with which JEV appears to have emerged and established in Papua New Guinea serves notice to other island territories and nations, many of which have all the necessary ingredients including competent mosquito vectors, pigs, and ardeid birds. The islands most at risk are Bougainville, the Solomon Islands, New Caledonia, Vanuatu, and possibly Fiji, although the risks diminish significantly with greater distances from endemic and epidemic areas (Mackenzie et al., 2002b). The spread of JEV to Guam, Saipan, and the eastern Indonesian archipelago, suggests that JEV could spread to some of these other islands by means of vagrant, infected birds also, or mosquitoes and birds could be blown in prevailing winds.

Spread of JEV further afield is less likely, but it is probable that most new destinations will have competent mosquito vectors, pigs, and ardeid birds. The ability of WNV to jump the Atlantic Ocean suggests that JEV could potentially find its way east to Hawaii and the continental US, or to Europe. The most likely mechanisms would be through aircraft stowaways or birds and/or mosquitoes blown long distances by major storm fronts. The importance of international aircraft disinfection, therefore, cannot be over-emphasised. Although the risks are small, they are finite and therefore cannot be discounted. JEV, like other viruses of the genus Flavivirus, has often surprised us, and could well do so again in the future.

Acknowledgements

The generous help given by Mrs Debra Gendle in the preparation of this manuscript is gratefully acknowledged.

References

Ali A, Igarashi A. Antigenic and genetic variations among Japanese encephalitis virus strains belonging to genotype 1. Microbiol Immunol 1997; 41: 241.

Amerasinghe FP, Ariyasena TG. Survey of adult mosquitoes (Diptera: *Culicidae*) during irrigation development in the Mahaweli Project, Sri Lanka. J Med Entomol 1991; 28: 387.

Anderson SG, Price AVG, Nanadai-Koia, Slater K. Murray Valley encephalitis in Papua and New Guinea. II. Serological survey. Med J Aust 1960; 2: 410.

Angami K, Chakravarty SK, Das MS, Chakraborty MS, Mukherjee KK. Seroepidemiological study of Japanese encephalitis in Dimapur, Nagaland. J Commun Dis 1989; 21: 87.

Anon. Epidemiology of Japanese encephalitis in Singapore. Epidemiol News Bull (Sing) 1993; 19: 40.

Anon. Prevalence of Japanese encephalitis virus infection in Singapore. Epidemiol News Bull (Sing) 1994; 20: 25.

Anon. Seroepidemiology of Japanese encephalitis virus infection in Singapore. Epidemiol News Bull (Sing) 2003; 29(8): 49.

Arora RR, Singh NN. Epidemiological study of an epidemic of Japanese encephalitis in Bankura district of West Bengal during 1973. J Commun Dis 1974; 6: 310.

Atmosoedjono S, Van Peenen PF, Joseph SW, Saoso JS, See R. Observations on possible Culex arbovirus vectors in Djakarta, Indonesia. Southeast Asian J Trop Med Public Health 1973; 4: 108.

Bakonyi T, Hubalek Z, Rudolf I, Nowotny N. Novel flavivirus or new lineage of West Nile virus, central Europe. Emerg Infect Dis 2005; 11: 225.

Banerjee K. Japanese encephalitis in India. Ann Indian Acad Med Sci 1975; 11: 51.

Banerjee K. Emerging viral infections with special reference to India. Indian J Med Res 1996; 103: 177.

Banerjee K, Ilkal MA, Bhat HR, Sreenivasan MA. Experimental viraemia with Japanese encephalitis virus in certain domestic and peridomestic vertebrates. Indian J Med Res 1979; 70: 364.

Banerjee K, Ilkal MA, Deshmukh PK. Susceptibility of *Cynopterus sphinx* (frugivorous bat) and *Suncus murinus* (house shrew) to Japanese encephalitis virus. Indian J Med Res 1984; 79: 8.

Barrett AD. Japanese encephalitis and dengue vaccines. Biologicals 1997; 25: 27.

Bartley LM, Carabin H, Vinh Chau N, Ho V, Luxemburger C, Hien TT, Garnett GP, Farrar J. Assessment of the factors associated with flavivirus seroprevalence in a population in southern Vietnam. Epidemiol Infect 2002; 128: 213.

Barzaga NG. A review of Japanese encephalitis cases in the Philippines. Southeast Asian J Trop Med Public Health 1989; 20: 587.

Beasley DW, Li L, Suderman MT, Guirakhoo F, Trent DW, Monath TP, Shope RE, Barrett AD. Protection against Japanese encephalitis virus strains representing four genotypes by passive transfer of sera raised against ChimeriVax-JE experimental vaccine. Vaccine 2004; 22: 3722.

Benenson MW, Top FH, Gresso W, Ames CW, Altstatt LB. The virulence to man of Japanese encephalitis virus in Thailand. Am J Trop Med Hyg 1975; 24: 974.

Bhatt PN, Rodrigues FM. Chandipura virus: a new arbovirus isolated in India from patients with a febrile illness. Indian J Med Res 1967; 55: 1295.

Bhattacharyya DR, Handique R, Dutta LP, Doloi P, Goswami BK, Sharma CK, Mahanta J. Host feeding patterns of *Culex vishnui* subgroup of mosquitoes in Dibrugarh district of Assam. J Commun Dis 1994; 26: 133.

Bista M, Bastola S, Shrestha S, Gautam P. Japanese encephalitis in Nepal (1993–1997): epidemiological analysis and review of the literature. Epidemiology and Disease Control Division, Department of Health Services, Ministry of Health and the World Health Organization, Kathmandu, Nepal; 1999; pp. 1–46.

Bista MB, Banerjee MK, Shin SH, Tandan JB, Kim MH, Sohn YM, Ohrr HC, Tang JL, Halstead SB. Efficacy of a single dose SA 14-14-2 vaccine against Japanese encephalitis: a case–control study. Lancet 2001; 358: 791.

Bowen ETW, Simpson DIH, Platt GS, Way HJ, Smith CEG, Ching CY, Casals J. Arbovirus infections in Sarawak: the isolation of Kunjin virus from mosquitoes of the *Culex pseudovishnui* group. Ann Trop Med Parasitol 1970; 64: 263.

Boyle DB, Dickerman RW, Marshall ID. Primary viraemia responses of herons to experimental infection with Murray Valley encephalitis, Kunjin and Japanese encephalitis viruses. Aust J Exp Biol Med Sci 1983; 61: 655.

Brantly E, Wijeyaratne P, Singh D, Pandey S. Environmental Health Project. Activity Report 136. Interccountry Collaboration for Improving Surveillance and Control of Vector-borne Diseases. Final Report on EHP support for Bangladesh, Bhutan, India and

Nepal. Office of Health, Infectious Diseases and Nutrition, Bureau for Global Health, U.S. Agency for International Development, Washington, USA; 2004.

Briese T, Jia XY, Huang C, Grady LJ, Lipkin WI. Identification of a Kunjin/West Nile-like virus in brains of patients with New York encephalitis. Lancet 1999; 354: 1261.

Broom AK, Wallace MJ, Mackenzie JS, Smith DW, Hall RA. Immunisation with gamma globulin to Murray Valley encephalitis virus and with an inactivated Japanese encephalitis virus vaccine as a prophylaxis against Australian encephalitis: evaluation in a mouse model. J Med Virol 2000; 61: 259.

Buescher EL, Scherer WF. Ecologic studies of Japanese encephalitis virus in Japan. IX. Epidemiologic correlations and conclusions. Am J Trop Med Hyg 1959; 8: 719.

Buescher EL, Scherer WF, McClure HE, Moyer JT, Rosenberg MZ, Yoshi M, Okada Y. Ecologic studies of Japanese encephalitis virus in Japan. IV. Avian infection. Am J Trop Med Hyg 1959a; 8: 678.

Buescher EL, Scherer WF, Rosenberg MZ, Gresser I, Hardy JL, Bullock HR. Ecologic studies of Japanese encephalitis virus in Japan. II. Mosquito infection. Am J Trop Med Hyg 1959b; 8: 651.

Buhl MR, Black FT, Andersen PL, Laursen A. Fatal Japanese encephalitis in a Danish tourist visiting Bali for 12d. Scand J Infect Dis 1996; 28: 189.

Bunnag T, Singharaj P, Sindhusen S, Punyagupta S. Japanese encephalitis in Nakorn Rajsima. J Med Assoc Thai 1976; 50: 590.

Burke DS, Leake CJ. Japanese encephalitis. In: The Arboviruses: Epidemiology and Ecology (Monath TP, editor). vol. III. Boca Raton: CRC Press; 1988; p. 63.

Burke DS, Monath TP. Flaviviruses. In: Fields Virology (Knipe DM, Howley PM, Griffin DE, Lamb RA, Martin MA, Roizman B, Straus SE, editors). 3rd ed. Philadelphia: Lippincott Williams & Wilkins; 2001; p. 1043.

Burke DS, Tingpalapong M, Ward GS, Andre R, Leake CJ. Intense transmission of Japanese encephalitis virus to pigs in a region free of epidemic encephalitis. Southeast Asian J Trop Med Public Health 1985a; 16: 199.

Burke DS, Ussery MA, Elwell MR, Nisalak A, Leake CJ, Laorakpongse T. Isolation of Japanese encephalitis virus strains from sentinel pigs in North Thailand, 1982. Trans R Soc Trop Med Hyg 1985b; 79: 420.

Calisher CH, Karabatsos N, Dalrymple JM, Shope RE, Porterfield JS, Westaway EG, Brandt WE. Antigenic relationships between flaviviruses as determined by cross-neutralization tests with polyclonal antisera. J Gen Virol 1989; 70: 37.

Cardosa MJ, Choo BH, Zuraini I. A serological study of Japanese encephalitis virus infections in northern Peninsula Malaysia. Southeast Asian J Trop Med Public Health 1991; 22: 341.

Cardosa MJ, Hooi TP, Kaaur P. Japanese encephalitis virus is an important cause of encephalitis among children in Penang. Southeast Asian J Trop Med Public Health 1995; 26: 272.

Cardosa MJ, Wang SM, Sum MS. Antibodies against prM protein distinguish between previous infection with dengue and Japanese encephalitis viruses. BMC Microbiol 2002; 2: 9.

Carey DE, Myers RM, Reuben R, Webb JKG. Japanese encephalitis in south India. A summary of recent knowledge. J Indian Med Assoc 1969b; 52: 10.

Carey DE, Reuben R, Myers RM. Japanese encephalitis studies in Vellore. South India. V. Experimental infection and transmission. Indian J Med Res 1969a; 57: 283.

Carey DE, Reuben R, Myers RM, George S. Japanese encephalitis studies in Vellore, South India. Part IV. Search for virological and serological evidence of infection in animals other than man. Indian J Med Res 1968; 56: 1340.

Casals J, Brown LV. Hemagglutination with arthropod-borne viruses. J Exp Med 1954; 99: 429.

Chadha MS, Arankalle VA, Jadi RS, Joshi MV, Thakare JP, Mahadev PVM, Mishra AC. An outbreak of Chandipura virus encephalitis in the eastern districts of Gujarat State, India. Am J Trop Med Hyg 2005; 73: 566.

Chakraborty AK, Chakravarti SK, Chakravarty MS. Outbreak of Japanese encephalitis in two districts of Assam during 1980. Some serological features. Indian J Public Health 1987; 31: 5.

Chakraborty AK, Chakraborty SK, Chakraborty MS, Singh NC. Outbreak of Japanese encephalitis in Manipur during 1982—some epidemiological features. J Commun Dis 1984; 16: 227.

Chakravarti SK, Sarkar JK, Chakravarty MS, Mukherjee MK, Mukherjee KK, Das BC, Hati AK. The first epidemic of Japanese encephalitis studied in India. Indian J Med Res 1975; 63: 77.

Chanama S, Sukprasert W, Sa-ngasang A, A-nuegoonpipat A, Sangkitporn S, Kurane I, Anantapreecha S. Detection of Japanese encephalitis (JE) virus-specifc IgM in cerebrospinal fluid and serum samples from JE patients. Jpn J Infect Dis 2005; 58: 294.

Chang CC, Ou YC, Raung SL, Chen CJ. Antiviral effect of dehydroepiandrosterone on Japanese encephalitis virus infection. J Gen Virol 2005; 86: 2513.

Chang G-JJ, Kuno G, Purdy DE, Davis BS. Recent advancement in flavivirus vaccine development. Expert Rev Vaccines 2004; 3: 199.

Chang IJ. Epidemiology of Japanese encephalitis in Korea. Korean Med J 1959; 4: 35.

Chang KJ. Seasonal prevalence of anti-Japanese encephalitis virus antibody in pigs in different regions of Taiwan. J Microbiol Immunol Infect 2002; 35: 12.

Chanthap L. JE in Cambodia. In: Personal Communication, presented to the Joint Japanese Encephalitis Meeting of the Global Alliance for Vaccines and Immunization (GAVI) South-East Asia & Western Pacific Regional Working Groups. Setting the Global Agenda on Public Health Solutions and National Needs, June 18–19 2002, Bangkok.

Chattopadhyay UK. A study on the status of Japanese encephalitis in Arunachal Pradesh. J Commun Dis 2001; 33: 261.

Chaturvedi UC, Mathur A, Chandra A, Das SK, Tandon HO, Singh UK. Transplacental infection with Japanese encephalitis virus. J Infect Dis 1980; 141: 712.

Chen WR, Rico-Hesse R, Tesh RB. A new genotype of Japanese encephalitis virus from Indonesia. Am J Trop Med Hyg 1992; 47: 61.

Chen WR, Tesh RB, Rico-Hesse R. Genetic variation of Japanese encephalitis virus in nature. J Gen Virol 1990; 71: 2915.

Chhour YM, Ruble G, Hong R, Minn. K, Kdan Y, Sok T, Nisalak A, Myint KS, Vaughn DW, Endy TP. Hospital-based diagnosis of hemorrhagic fever, encephalitis, and hepatitis in Cambodian children. Emerg Infect Dis 2002; 8: 485.

Choudhury N, Saxena NBL, Dwivedi SR, Khamre JS. Study of the outbreak of Japanese encephalitis in Goa. J Commun Dis 1983; 15: 111.

Chu CM. Viral diseases in China. In: Viral Diseases in South-East Asia and the Western Pacific (Mackenzie JS, editor). Sydney: Academic Press; 1982; p. 243.

Chu FT, Wu JP, Teng CH. Acute encephalitis in children; clinical and serologic study of ten epidemic cases. Chin Med J 1940; 58: 68.

Chu IH, Grayston JT. Encephalitis on Taiwan. VI. Infections in American servicemen on Taiwan and Okinawa. Am J Trop Med Hyg 1962; 11: 159.

Chunsuttiwat S. Japanese encephalitis in Thailand. Southeast Asian J Trop Med Public Health 1989; 20: 593.

Chunsuttiwat S, Warachit P. Japanese encephalitis in Thailand. Southeast Asian J Trop Med Public Health 1995; 26(Suppl 3): 43.

Colless DH. Notes on the culicine mosquitoes of Singapore. VII. Host preferences in relation to the transmission of disease. Ann Trop Med Parasitol 1959; 53: 259.

Cooley L. Andhra Pradesh builds a model immunization system Indian state protects millions and shows what new vaccines and technologies can do. Indian J Public Health 2004; 48: 67.

Cross JH, Banzon T, Wheeling CH, Cometa H, Lien JC, Clake R, Petersen H, Sevilla J, Basaca-Sevilla V. Biomedical survey in North Samar Province, Philippine Islands. Southeast Asian J Trop Med Public Health 1977; 8: 464.

Cruickshank EK. Acute encephalitis in Malaya. Trans R SocTrop Med 1951; 45: 113.

Cuzzubbo AJ, Vaughn DW, Nisalak A, Solomon T, Kalayanarooj S, Aaaskov J, Dung NM, Devine PL. Comparison of PanBio dengue duo IgM and IgG capture ELISA and venture technologies dengue IgM and IgG dot blot. J Clin Virol 2000; 16: 135.

Dandawate CN, Rajagopalan PK, Pavri KM, Work TH. Virus isolation from mosquitoes collected in North Arcot District, Madras State, and Chittoor District, Andhra Pradesh between November 1955 and October 1957. Indian J Med Res 1969; 57: 1420.

Daniels PW. Arboviruses of veterinary significance in the Asia-Pacific region, such as Japanese encephalitis. In: Compendium of Technical Items Presented to the International Committee or to Regional Commissions, 2001–2002. Paris: OIE; 2003; p. 167.

Daniels PW, Williams DT, Mackenzie JS. Japanese encephalitis virus. In: Trends in Emerging Viral Infections of Swine (Morilla A, Yoon K-J, Zimmermen JJ, editors). Ames: Iowa State University Press; 2002; p. 249.

Detels R, Cross JH, Huang WC, Lien JC, Chen S. Japanese encephalitis virus in Northern Taiwan, 1969–1973. Am J Trop Med Hyg 1976; 25: 477.

Deuel RE, Bawell MB, Matsumoto M, Sabin AB. Status and significance of inapparent infection with virus of Japanese B encephalitis in Korea and Okinawa in 1946. Am J Hyg 1950; 51: 13.

Dhanda V, Banerjee K, Deshmukh PK, Ilkal MA. Experimental viraemia and transmission of Japanese encephalitis virus by mosquitoes in domestic ducks. Indian J Med Res 1977; 66: 881.

Dhanda V, Thenmozhi V, Hiriyan J, Arunachalam N, Batasubramanian A, Ilango A, Gajanana A. Virus isolation from wild-caught mosquitoes during a Japanese encephalitis outbreak in Kerala in 1996. Indian J Med Res 1997; 106: 4.

Ding D, Kilgore PE, Clemens JD, Liu W, Xu Z-Y. Cost-effectiveness of routine immunization to control Japanese encephalitis in Shanghai, China. Bull World Health Organ 2003; 81: 334.

Doi R, Oya A, Shirasaka A, Yabe S, Sasa M. Studies on Japanese encephalitis virus infection of reptiles. II. Role of lizards on hibernation of Japanese encephalitis virus. Jpn J Exp Med 1983; 53: 125.

Doraisingham S. Viral diseases in Singapore—a national overview. In: Viral Diseases in South-East Asia and the Western Pacific (Mackenzie JS, editor). Sydney: Academic Press; 1982; p. 229.

Edelman R, Schneider RJ, Chieowanich P, Pompibul R, Voodhikul P. The effect of dengue virus infection on the clinical sequelae of Japanese encephalitis: a one year follow-up study in Thailand. Southeast Asian J Trop Med Public Health. 1975; 6: 308.

Ellis P, Daniels PW, Banks DJ. Emerging infectious diseases: Japanese encephalitis. Vet Clinics North America: Equine Pract 2000; 16: 565.

Elshuber S, Allison SL, Heinz FX, Mandl CW. Cleavage of protein prM is necessary for infecton of BHK-21 cells by tick-borne encephalitis virus. J Gen Virol 2003; 84: 183.

Endy TP, Nisalak A. Japanese encephalitis virus: ecology and epidemiology. Curr Top Microbiol Immunol 2002; 267: 11.

Essed WCAH, Van Tongeran HAE. Arthropod-borne virus infections in Western New Guinea. I. Report of a case of Murray Valley encephalitis in a Papuan woman. Trop Geogr Med 1965; 1: 52.

Fang R, Hsu DR, Lim TW. Investigation of a suspected outbreak of Japanese encephalitis in Pulau, Langkawi. Malaysian J Pathol 1980; 3: 23.

French EL, Anderson SG, Price AVG, Rhodes FA. Murray Valley encephalitis in New Guinea. I. Isolation of Murray Valley encephalitis virus from the brain of a fatal case of encephalitis occurring in a Papuan native. Am J Trop Med Hyg 1957; 6: 827.

Fukuda H, Umehara F, Kawahigashi N, Suehara M, Osame M. Acute disseminated myelitis after Japanese B encephalitis vaccination. J Neurol Sci 1997; 148: 113.

Fukumi H, Hayashi K, Mifune K, Schichijo A, Matsuo S. Ecology of Japanese encephalitis virus in Japan. I. Mosquito and pig infection with the virus in relation to human incidences. Trop Med 1975; 17: 97.

Gajanana A, Rajendran R, Samuel PP, Thenmozhi V, Tsai TF, Kimura-Kuroda J, Reuben R. Japanese encephalitis in south Arcot district, Tamil Nadu, India: a three-year longitudinal study of vector abundance and infection frequency. J Med Entomol 1997; 34: 651.

Gajanana A, Thenmozhi V, Samuel PP, Reuben R. Community-based study of subclinical flavivirus infections in children in an area of Tamil Nadu, India, where Japanese encephalitis is endemic. Bull World Health Organ 1995; 73: 237.

Garrett-Jones C. The possibility of active long distance migration of *Anopheles pharoensis*. Bull World Health Organ 1962; 27: 299.

Geevarghese G, George S, Bhat HR, Prasanna Y, Pavri KM. Isolation of Japanese encephalitis virus from a sentinel domestic pig from Kolar district in Karnataka. Indian J Med Res 1987; 86: 273.

Geevarghese G, Mishra AC, Jacob PG, Bhat HR. Studies on the mosquito vectors of Japanese encephalitis virus in Mandya District, Karnataka, India. Southeast Asian J Trop Med Public Health. 1994; 25: 378.

Geevarghese G, Shaikh BH, Jacog PG, Bhat HR. Monitoring Japanese encephalitis virus activity using domestic sentinel pigs in Mandya district, Karnataka State (India). Indian J Med Res 1991; 93: 140.

George S, Gourie-Devi M, Rao JA, Prasard SR, Pavri KM. Isolation of West Nile virus from the brains of children who had died of encephalitis. Bull World Health Organ 1984; 62: 879.

George S, Prasad SR, Rao JA, Yergolkr PN, Setty CVS. Isolation of Japanese encephalitis and West Nile viruses from fatal cases of encephalitis in Kolar district of Karanataka. Indian J Med Res 1987; 86: 131.

Gingrich JB, Nisalak A, Latendresse JR, Pomsdhit J, Paisansilp S, Hoke CH, Chantalakana C, Satayaphantha C, Uechiewcharnkit K. A longitudinal study of Japanese encephalitis in suburban Bangkok, Thailand. Southeast Asian J Trop Med Public Health 1987; 18: 558.

Gingrich JB, Nisalak A, Latendresse JR, Sattabongkot J, Hoke CH, Pomsdhit J, Chantalakana C, Satayaphanta C, Uechiewcharnkit K, Innis BL. Japanese encephalitis virus in Bangkok: factors influencing vector infections in three suburban communities. J Med Entomol 1992; 29: 436.

Gould DJ, Byrne RD, Hayes DE. Experimental infection of horses with Japanese encephalitis virus by mosquito bite. Am J Trop Med Hyg 1964; 13: 742.

Gould DJ, Edelman R, Grossman RA, Nisalak A, Sullivan MF. Study of Japanese encephalitis in Chiangmai Valley, Thailand. IV. Vector studies. Am J Epidemiol 1974; 100: 49.

Gould EA. Evolution of the Japanese encephalitis serocomplex viruses. Curr Top Microbiol Immunol 2002; 267: 391.

Gould EA, de Lamballerie X, Zanotto PMA, Holmes EC. Evolution, epidemiology and dispersal of flaviviruses revealed by molecular phylogenies. Adv Virus Res 2001; 57: 71.

Gould EA, Moss SR, Turner SL. Evolution and dispersal of flaviviruses. Arch Virol Suppl 2004; 18: 65.

Goverdhan MK, Kulkarni AB, Gupta AK, Tupe CD, Rodrigues JJ. Two-way cross-protection between West Nile and Japanese encephalitis viruses in Bonnet macaques. Acta Virol 1992; 36: 277–283.

Grayston JT, Wang SP, Yen CH. Encephalitis on Taiwan. Am J Trop Med Hyg 1962; 11: 126.

Gresser I, Hardy JL, Hu SMK, Scherer WF. Factors influencing transmission of Japanese B encephalitis virus by a colonized strain of *Culex tritaeniorhynchus* Giles, from infected pigs and chicks to susceptible pigs and birds. Am J Trop Med Hyg 1958; 7: 365.

Grossman RA, Edelman R, Chiewanich P, Voodhikul P, Siriwan C. Study of Japanese encephalitis in Chiangmai Valley, Thailand. II. Human clinical infections. Am J Epidemiol 1973b; 98: 121.

Grossman RA, Edelman R, Gould DJ. Study of Japanese encephalitis in Chiangmai Valley, Thailand. VI. Summary and conclusions. Am J Epidemiol 1974; 100: 69.

Grossman RA, Edelman R, Willhight M, Pantuwatana S, Udomsakdi S. Study of Japanese encephalitis in Chiangmai Valley, Thailand. III. Human seroepidemiology and inapparent infections. Am J Epidemiol 1973c; 98: 133.

Grossman RA, Gould D, Smith T, Johnsen DO, Pantuwatana S. Study of Japanese encephalitis virus in Chiangmai Valley, Thailand. I. Introduction and study design. Am J Epidemiol 1973a; 98: 111.

Hale JH, Colless DH, Lim KA. Investigation of the Malaysian form of *Culex tritaeniorhynchus* as a potential vector of Japanese B encephalitis on Singapore Island. Ann Trop Med Parasitol 1957; 51: 17.

Hale JH, Lee LH. Serological evidence of the incidence of Japanese B encephalitis virus infection in Malaysia. Ann Trop Med Parasitol 1955; 49: 293.

Hale JH, Witherington DH. A serological survey of antibodies to Japanese B encephalitis virus among horses in Malaya. Ann Trop Med Parasitol 1954; 48: 15.

Haley M, Retter AS, Fowler D, Gea-Banacloche J, O'Grady NP. The role for intravenous immunoglobulin in the treatment of West Nile virus encephalitis. Clin Infect Dis 2003; 37: e88.

Halstead SB, Grosz CR. Subclinical Japanese encephalitis. I. Infection of Americans with limited residence in Korea. Am J Hyg 1962; 75: 190.

Halstead SB, Jacobson J. Japanese encephalitis. Adv Virus Res 2003; 61: 103.

Halstead SB, Tsai TF. Japanese encephalitis vaccines. In: Vaccines (Plotkin SA, Orenstein WA, editors). 4th ed. Philadelphia: WB Saunders; 2004; p. 919.

Hammon W, Scharack W, Sather G. Serological survey of arthropod-borne virus infections in the Philippines. Am J Trop Med Hyg 1958a; 7: 323.

Hammon WM, Reeves WC, Sather GE. Japanese B encephalitis virus in the blood of experimentally inoculated birds: epidemiological implication. Am J Hyg 1951; 53: 249.

Hammon WM, Tigertt WD, Sather GE, Berge TO, Meiklejohn G. Epidemiologic studies of concurrent "virgin" epidemics of Japanese B encephalitis and of mumps on Guam, 1947–1948, with subsequent observations including dengue, through 1957. Am J Trop Med Hyg 1958b; 7: 441.

Hanna J, Barnett D, Ewald D. Vaccination against Japanese encephalitis in the Torres Strait. Comm Dis Intell (Aust) 1996a; 19: 447.

Hanna JN, Ritchie SA, Phillips DA, Lee JM, Hills SL, van den Hurk AF, Pyke AT, Johansen CA, Mackenzie JS. Japanese encephalitis in North Queensland, 1998. Med J Aust 1999; 170: 533.

Hanna JN, Ritchie SA, Phillips DA, Shield J, Bailey MC, Mackenzie JS, Poidinger M, McCall BJ, Mills PA. An outbreak of Japanese encephalitis in the Torres Strait, Australia. Med J Aust 1996b; 165: 256.

Hanson JP, Taylor CT, Richards AR, Smith IL, Boutlis CS. Japanese encephalitis acquired near Port Moresby: implications for residents and travelers to Papua New Guinea. Med J Aust 2004; 181: 282.

Hasegawa H, Yoshida M, Kobayashi Y, Fujita S. Antigenic analysis of Japanese encephalitis viruses in Asia by using monoclonal antibodies. Vaccine 1995; 13: 1713.

Hasegawa T, Takehara Y, Takahashi K. Natural and experimental infections of Japanese tree sparrows with Japanese encephalitis virus. Arch Virol 1975; 49: 373.

Heinz FX, Allison SL. Flavivirus structure and membrane fusion. Adv Virus Res 2003; 59: 63.

Heinz FX, Stiasny K, Allison SL. The entry mechanism of flaviviruses. Arch Virol Suppl 2004; 18: 133.

Hennessy S, Liu Z, Tsai TF, Strom BL, Chao-Min W, Hui-Lian L, Tai-Xiang W, Hong-Ji Y, Qi-Mau L, Karabatsos N, Bilker WB, Halstead SB. Effectiveness of live-attenuated Japanese encephalitis vaccine (SA14-14-2): a case–control study. Lancet 1996; 347: 1583.

Hermon YE, Anandarajah M. Isolation of Japanese encephalitis virus from the serum of a child in Ceylon. Ceylon Med J 1974; 19: 93.

Hoke CH, Gingrich JB. Japanese encephalitis. In: Handbook of Zoonoses (Beran GW, editor). 2nd ed. Boca Raton: CRC Press; 1994; p. 59.

Hoke CH, Nisalak A, Sangawhiba N, Jatanasen S, Laorakapongse T, Innis BL, Kotchasenee S, Gingrich JB, Latendresse J, Fukai K, Burke D. Protection against Japanese encephalitis by inactivated vaccines. N Engl J Med 1988; 319: 608.

Hoke CH, Vaughn DW, Nisalak A, Intralawan P, Poolsuppasit S, Jongsawas V, Titsyakorn U, Johnson RT. Effect of high-dose dexamethasone on the outcome of acute encephalitis due to Japanese encephalitis virus. J Infect Dis 1992; 165: 631.

Hombach J, Barrett AD, Cardosa MJ, Deubel V, Guzman M, Kurane I, Roehrig JT, Sabcharoen A, Kieny MP. Review on flavivirus vaccine development: proceedings of a meeting jointly organized by the World Health Organization and the Thai Ministry of Public Health, 26–27 April 2004, Bangkok, Thailand. Vaccine 2005; 23: 2689.

Hotta S, Aoki H, Samoto S, Yasui T, Kawabe M. Virologic-epidemiological studies on Indonesia. II. Measurement of anti-arbovirus antibodies in sera from residents of Lombok, South Sumatra, and West Java, in comparison with results concerning sera from residents of Japanese main islands. Kobe J Med Sci 1970a; 16: 215.

Hotta S, Aoki H, Samoto S, Yasui T, Noerjasin B. Virologic-epidemiological studies on Indonesia. III. HI antibodies against selected arboviruses (Groups A and B) in human and animal sera collected in Surabaja, East Java, in 1968. Kobe J Med Sci 1970b; 16: 235.

Hotta S, Aoki H, Yasui T, Samoto S. Virologic-epidemiological studies on Indonesia. Survey of anti-arboviral antibodies in sera from residents of Lombok, Sumatera and Djawa. Kobe J Med Sci 1967; 13: 221.

Hsu SMK, Grayston JT. Encephalitis on Taiwan. II. Mosquito collection and binomic studies. Am J Trop Med Hyg 1962; 11: 131.

Huang CH. Studies of Japanese encephalitis in China. Adv Virus Res 1982; 27: 71.

Hueston L, Lobo S, Andjaparidze A, Cort Reale E, Slotte A, Kacvinska A, Cartwright M, Tulloch J, Mendes J, Kelly K, Condon R, Lynch C, Brown L. Japanese encephalitis in East Timor. Aust Microbiol 2001; 22(4): A94.

Hullinghorst RL, Burns KF, Choi YT, Whatley LR. Japanese B encephalitis in Korea. The epidemic of 1949. JAMA 1951; 145: 460.

Hurlbut HS. The pig–mosquito cycle of Japanese encephalitis in Taiwan. J Med Entomol 1964; 1: 301.

Hurlbut HS, Thomas JL. Potential vectors of Japanese encephalitis in the Caroline Islands. Am J Trop Med 1949; 29: 215.

ICDDR. Surveillance of encephalitis in Bangladesh: preliminary results. ICDDR B Health Sci Bull 2004; 2(4): 7–11.

Igarashi A. Epidemiology and control of Japanese encephalitis. World Health Stat Q 1992; 45: 229.

Igarashi A. Control of Japanese encephalitis in Japan: immunization of humans and animals, and vector control. Curr Top Microbiol Immunol 2002; 267: 139.

Igarashi A, Tanaka M, Morita A, Takasu T, Ahmed A, Ahmed A, Akram DS, Waqar MA. Detection of West Nile and Japanese encephalitis viral genome sequences in cerebrospinal fluid from acute encephalitis cases in Karachi, Pakistan. Microbiol Immunol 1994; 38: 827.

Ilkal MA, Dhanda V, Rao BU, George S, Mishra AC, Prasanna Y, Gopalkrishna S, Pavri KM. Absence of viraemia in cattle after experimental infection with Japanese encephalitis virus. Trans R Soc Trop Med Hyg 1988; 82: 628–631.

Ilkal MA, Prasanna Y, Jacob PG, Geevarghese G, Banerjee K. Experimental studies on the susceptibility of domestic pigs to West Nile virus followed by Japanese encephalitis virus infection and vice versa. Acta Virol 1994; 38: 157.

Ishii K, Hikiji K, Tsukidate Y, Kono R, Hashimoto N, Takashima I, Sugamata M, Ahmed A, Takasu T. Serological study of acute encephalitis in Karachi, Pakistan, from 1983 to 1985: probable occurrence of JEV infection. In: Virus Diseases in Asia (Thongcharoen P, Kurstak E, editors). Bangkok: Mahidol University; 1988; p. 188.

Islam MN, Kahn AQ, Khan AM. Viral diseases in Bangladesh. In: Viral Diseases in South-East Asia and the Western Pacific (Mackenzie JS, editor). Sydney: Academic Press; 1982; p. 205.

Jacobson J, Sivalenka S. Japanese encephalitis globally and in India. Indian J Public Health 2004; 48: 50.

Johansen C, Ritchie S, Van den Hurk A, Bockarie M, Hanna J, Phillips D, Melrose W, Poidinger M, Scherret J, Hall R, Mackenzie J. The search for Japanese encephalitis virus in the Western province of Papua New Guinea, 1996. In: Arbovirus Research in Australia. Proceedings of the 7th Symposium (Kay BH, Brown MD, Aaskov JG, editors). Brisbane: Queensland Institute of Medical Research and Queensland University of Technology; 1997; p. 131.

Johansen CA, Nisbet DJ, Foley PN, van den Hurk AF, Hall RA, Mackenzie JS, Ritchie SA. Flavivirus isolations from mosquitoes collected from Saibai Island in the northern Torres Strait, Australia, during an incursion of Japanese encephalitis virus. Med Vet Entomol 2004; 18: 281.

Johansen CA, Nisbet DJ, Zborowski P, van den Hurk AF, Ritchie SA, Mackenzie JS. Flavivirus isolations from mosquitoes collected from western Cape York, Australia, 1999–2000. J Am Mosq Control Assoc 2003; 19: 392.

Johansen CA, van den Hurk AF, Pyke AT, Zborowski P, Phillips DA, Mackenzie JS, Ritchie SA. Entomological investigations of an outbreak of Japanese encephalitis virus in the Torres Strait, Australia, in 1998. J Med Entomol 2001; 38: 581.

Johansen CA, van den Hurk AF, Ritchie SA, Zborowski P, Nisbet DJ, Paru R, Bockarie MJ, Macdonald J, Drew AC, Khromykh TI, Mackenzie JS. Isolation of Japanese encephalitis virus from mosquitoes (Diptera: *Culicidae*) collected in the Western Province of Papua New Guinea. Am J Trop Med Hyg 2000; 62: 631.

Johnsen DO, Edelman R, Grossman RA, Muangman J, Pomsdhit J, Gould DJ. Study of Japanese encephalitis in Chiangmai Valley, Thailand. V. Animal infections. Am J Epidemiol 1974; 100: 57.

Jones T. A chimeric live attenuated vaccine against Japanese encephalitis. Exp Rev Vaccines 2004; 3: 143.

Joo HS, Chu RM. Japanese B encephalitis. In: Diseases of Swine (Straw BE, D'Allaire S, Mengeling WL, Taylor DT, editors). 8th ed. Malvern: Blackwell Science Ltd; 1999; p. 173.

Joshi D. Japanese encephalitis in Nepal. JE & HFRS Bull 1986; 1: 5.

Joshi DD. Japanese encephalitis outbreak during the year 1985 and 1986. JE & HFRS Bull 1987; 2: 1.

Joshi DD. Japanese encephalitis in Nepal. Southeast Asian J Trop Med Public Health 1995; 26(Suppl 3): 34.

Kabilan L. Control of Japanese encephalitis in India: a reality. Indian J Pediatr 2004; 71: 707.

Kabilan L, Rajendran R, Arunachalam N, Ramesh S, Srinivasan S, Philip Samuel P, Dash AP. Japanese encephalitis in India: an overview. Indian J Pediatr 2004a; 71: 609.

Kabilan L, Vrati S, Ramesh S, Srinivasan S, Appaiahgari MB, Arunachalam N, Thenmozhi V, Kumaravel SM, Samuel PP, Rajendran R. Japanese encephalitis virus (JEV) is an important cause of encephalitis among children in Cuddalore district, Tamil Nadu, India. J Clin Virol 2004b; 31: 153.

Kalita J, Misra UK. Comparison of CT scan and MRI findings in the diagnosis of Japanese encephalitis. J Neurol Sci 2000; 174: 3.

Kanamitsu M, Taniguchi K, Urasawa S, Ogata T, Wada Y, Wada Y, Saroso JS. Geographic distribution of arbovirus antibodies in indigenous human populations of the Indo-Australian archipelago. Am J Trop Med Hyg 1979; 28: 351.

Kanojia PC, Shetty PS, Geevarghese G. A long-term study on vector abundance & seasonal prevalence in relation to the occurrence of Japanese encephalitis in Gorakhpur district, Uttar Pradesh. Indian J Med Res 2003; 117: 104.

Karabatsos N. (editor). International Catalogue of Arboviruses. 3rd ed. San Antonio, TX: American Society of Tropical Medicine and Hygiene; 1985.

Kaur R, Agarwal CS, Das D. An investigation into the JE epidemic of 2000 in Upper Assam—a prospective study. J Commun Dis 2002; 34: 135.

Kay BH, Boreham PFL, Williams GM. Host preferences and feeding patterns of mosquitoes (Diptera: *Culicidae*) at Kowanyama, Cape York Peninsula, northern Queensland. Bull Entomol Res 1979; 69: 441.

Kedarnath N, Dayaraj C, Gadkari DA, Dandawate CN, Goverdhan MK, Ghosh SN. Monoclonal antibodies against Japanese encephalitis. Indian J Med Res 1986; 84: 125.

Kedarnath N, Prasad SR, Dandawate CN, Koshy AA, George S, Ghosh SN. Isolation of Japanese encephalitis and West Nile viruses from peripheral blood of encephalitis patients. Indian J Med Res 1984; 79: 1.

Keiser J, Maltese MF, Erlanger TE, Bos R, Tanner M, Singer BH, Utzinger J. Effect of irrigated rice agriculture on Japanese encephalitis, including challenges and opportunities for integrated vector management. Acta Trop 2005; 95: 40.

Ketel WB, Ognibene AJ. Japanese B encephalitis in Vietnam. Am J Med Sci 1971; 261: 271.

Khan AM, Khan AQ, Dobrzynski L, Joshi GP, Myat A. A Japanese encephalitis focus in Bangladesh. J Trop Med Hyg 1981; 84: 41.

Khin MM. Viral diseases in Burma. In: Viral Diseases of South-East Asia and the Western Pacific (Mackenzie JS, editor). Sydney: Academic Press; 1982; p. 210.

Kobayashi Y, Hasegawa H, Oyama T, Tamai T, Kusaba T. Antigenic analysis of Japanese encephalitis virus by using monoclonal antibodies. Infect Immun 1984; 44: 117.

Koh YL, Tan BH, Loh JJP, Ooi EE, Su SY, Hsu LY. Japanese encephalitis, Singapore. Emerg Infect Dis 2006; 12: 525.

Konishi E, Shoda M, Kondo T. Analysis of yearly changes in levels of antibodies to Japanese encephalitis virus nonstructural 1 protein in racehorses in central Japan shows high levels of natural virus activity still exist. Vaccine 2006; 24: 516.

Konishi E, Shoda M, Yamamoto S, Arai S, Tanaka-Taya K, Okabe N. Natural infection with Japanese encephalitis virus among inhabitants of Japan: a nationwide survey of antibodies against nonstructural 1 protein. Vaccine, January 19, 2006; 12: 3054.

Konno J, Endo K, Agatsuma H, Ishida N. Cyclic outbreaks of Japanese encephalitis among pigs and humans. Am J Epidemiol 1966; 84: 292.

Ksiazek TG, Trosper JH, Cross JH, Basaca-Sevilla V. Additional isolations of Japanese encephalitis virus from the Philippines. Southeast Asian J Trop Med Public Health 1980; 11: 507.

Kumar R, Misra PK. Japanese encephalitis in India. Indian Pediatr 1988; 25: 354.

Kumar R, Tripathi P, Singh S, Bannerji G. Clinical features in children hospitalized during the 2005 epidemic of Japanese encephalitis in Uttar Pradesh, India. Clin Infect Dis 2006; 73: 123.

Kuno G, Chang GJ, Tsuchiya KR, Karabatsos N, Cropp CB. Phylogeny of the genus Flavivirus. J Virol 1998; 72: 73.

Kuwayama M, Ito M, Takao S, Shimazu Y, Miyazaki K, Kurane I, Takasaki T. Japanese encephalitis in meningitis patients, Japan. Emerg Infect Dis 2005; 11: 471.

Kuzuhara S, Nakamura H, Hayashida K, Obata J, Abe M, Sonoda K, Nishiyama K, Sugawara K, Takeda K, Honda T, Matsui H, Shigaki T, Kino Y, Mizokami H, Tanaka M, Mizuno K, Ueda K. Non-clinical and phase I clinical trials of a Vero cell-derived inactivated Japanese encephalitis vaccine. Vaccine 2003; 21: 4519.

Lacey LA, Lacey CM. The medical importance of rice-land mosquitoes and their control using alternatives to chemical alternatives. J Am Mosq Control Assoc 1990; 2(Suppl): 1.

Lam K, Tsang OTY, Yung RWH, Lau KK. Japanese encephalitis in Hong Kong. Hong Kong Med J 2005a; 11: 182.

Lam KHK, Ellis TM, Williams DT, Lunt RA, Daniels PW, Watkins KL, Riggs CM. Japanese encephalitis in a racing thoroughbred gelding in Hong Kong. Vet Record 2005b; 157: 168.

Lanciotti RS, Roehrig JT, Deubel V, Smith J, Parker M, Steele K, Volpe KE, Crabtree MB, Scherret J, Hall R, Mackenzie J, Cropp CB, Panigrahy B, Malkinson M, Komar N, Savage HM, Stone W, McNamara T, Gubler DJ. Origin of the West Nile virus responsible for an outbreak of encephalitis in the northeastern US. Science 1999; 286: 2333.

Larish LB, Savage HM. Introduction and establishment of *Aedes* (Finlaya) *japonicus japonicus* (Theobald) on the island of Hawaii: implications for arbovirus transmission. J Am Mosq Control Assoc 2005; 21: 318.

Le DH. Clinical aspects of Japanese B encephalitis in North Vietnam. Clin Neurol Neurosurg 1986; 88: 189.

Lee VH, Atmosoedjono S, Rusmiarto S, Aep S, Semendra W. Mosquitoes of Bali Island, Indonesia: common species in the village environment. Southeast Asian J Trop Med Public Health 1983; 14: 298.

Libraty DH, Nisalak A, Endy TP, Suntayakorn S, Vaughn DW, Innis BL. Clinical and immunological risk factors for severe disease in Japanese encephalitis. Trans R Soc Trop Med Hyg 2002; 96: 173.

Lindenbach BD, Rice CM. Molecular biology of flaviviruses. Adv Virus Res 2003; 59: 23.

Liu ZL, Hennessy S, Strom BL, Tsai TF, Wan C-M, Tang S-C, Xiang C-F, Bilker WB, Pan X-P, Tao Y-J, Xu Z-W, Halstead SB. Short-term safety of live-attenuated Japanese encephalitis vaccine (SA14-14-2): results of a 26,239-subject randomized clinical trial. J Infect Dis 1997; 176: 1366.

Loach TR, Narayan KG, Choudhary SP. Sero-epidemiological studies on the 1980 epidemic of human encephalitis in East and West Champaran, Bihar, India. J Commun Dis 1983; 15: 151.

Lounibos LP. Invasions by insect vectors of human disease. Ann Rev Entomol 2002; 47: 233.

Lowry PW, Truong DH, Hinh LD, Ladinsky JL, Karabatsos N, Cropp CB, Martin D, Gubler DJ. Japanese encephalitis among hospitalized pediatric and adult patients with acute encephalitis syndrome in Hanoi, Vietnam 1995. Am J Trop Med Hyg 1998; 58: 324.

Lvov DK, Butenko AM, Gromashevsky VL, Kovtunov AI, Prilipov AG, Kinney R, Arisova VA, Dzharkenov AF, Samokhrasov EI, Savage HM, Shchelkanov MY, Galkina IV, Deryabin PG, Gubler DJ, Kulikova LN, Alkhovsky SK, Moskvina TM, Zlobina LV, Sadykova GK, Shatlov AG, Lvov DN, Usachev VE, Voronina AG. West Nile virus and other zoonotic viruses in Russia: examples of emerging-reemerging situations. Arch Virol Suppl 2004; 18: 85.

Ma SP, Yoshida Y, Makino Y, Tadano M, Ono T, Ogawa M. Short report: a major genotype of Japanese encephalitis virus currently circulating in Japan. Am J Trop Med Hyg 2003; 69: 151.

Macdonald WBG, Tink AR, Ouvrier RA, Menser MA, de Silva LM, Naim H, Hawkes RA. Japanese encephalitis after a two-week holiday in Bali. Med J Aust 1989; 150: 334.

Macdonald WW, Smith CEG, Dawson PS, Ganapathipillai A, Mahadevan S. Arbovirus infections in Sarawak: further observations on mosquitoes. J Med Entomol 1967; 4: 146.

Mackenzie JS The family *Flaviviridae*: a brief overview of the family with particular reference to members of the Asian and Australasian regions. In: Classical Swine Fever and Emerging Viral Diseases in South-East Asia. ACIAR Proceedings No. 94 (Blacksell SD, editor).Canberra: Australian Centre for International Agricultural Research; 2000; p. 48.

Mackenzie JS. Emerging zoonotic encephalitis viruses: lessons learnt from Southeast Asia and Oceania. J Neurovirol 2005; 11: 434.

Mackenzie JS, Barrett ADT, Deubel V. The Japanese encephalitis serological group of flaviviruses: a brief introduction to the group. Curr Top Microbiol Immunol 2002a; 267: 1.

Mackenzie JS, Chua KB, Daniels PW, Eaton BT, Field HE, Hall RA, Halpin K, Johansen CA, Kirkland PD, Lam SK, McMinn P, Nisbet DJ, Paru R, Pyke AT, Ritchie SA, Siba P, Smith DW, Smith GA, van den Hurk AF, Wang LF, Williams DT. Emerging viral diseases of South-East Asia and the Western Pacific: a brief review. Emerg Infect Dis 2001; 7(Suppl 3): 497.

Mackenzie JS, Gubler DJ, Petersen LR. Emerging flaviviruses: the spread and resurgence of Japanese encephalitis, West Nile and Dengue viruses. Nat Med 2004; 10(Suppl 12): S98.

Mackenzie JS, Johansen CA, Ritchie SA, van den Hurk AF, Hall RA. Japanese encephalitis as an emerging virus: the emergence and spread of Japanese encephalitis virus in Australasia. Curr Top Microbiol Immunol 2002b; 267: 49.

Mackenzie JS, Lindsay MD, Coelen RJ, Broom AK, Hall RA, Smith DW. Arboviruses causing human disease in the Australasian zoogeographic region. Arch Virol 1994; 136: 447.

Mackenzie JS, Lindsay MD, Daniels PW. The effect of climate on the incidence of vector-borne viral diseases: the potential value of seasonal forecasting. In: Applications of Seasonal Climate Forecasting in Agriculture and Natural Ecosystems—The Australian Experience (Hammer G, Nicholls N, Mitchell , editors). The Netherlands: Kluwer; 2000; p. 429.

Mackenzie JS, Poidinger M, Phillips D, Johansen CA, Hall RA, Hanna J, Ritchie S, Shield J, Graham R. Emergence of Japanese encephalitis virus in the Australasian region. In: Factors in the Emergence of Arbovirus Diseases (Saluzzo JF, Dodet B, editors). Paris: Elsevier; 1997; p. 191.

Madrid AT, Porterfield JS. The flaviviruses (group B arboviruses): a cross-neutralisation study. J Gen Virol 1974; 23: 91.

Maeda O, Takenokuma K, Karoji Y, Kuroda A, Sasaki O, Karaki T, Ishii T. Epidemiological studies on Japanese encephalitis in Kyoto City area, Japan. IV. Natural infection in sentinel pigs. Jpn J Med Sci Biol 1978; 31: 317–324.

Mani TR, Rao CV, Rajendran R, Devaputra M, Prasanna Y, Hanumaiah, Gajanana A, Reuben R. Surveillance for Japanese encephalitis in villages near Madurai, Tamil Nadu, India. Trans R Soc Trop Med Hyg 1991; 85: 287.

Markoff L. 5′ and 3′ noncoding regions in flavivirus RNA. Adv Virus Res 2003; 59: 177.

Marshall ID. Murray Valley and Kunjin encephalitis. In: The Arboviruses: Epidemiology and Ecology (Monath TP, editor). vol. III. Boca Raton, FL: CRC Press; 1988; p. 151.

Mathur A, Chaturvedi UC, Tandon HO, Agarwal AK, Mathur GP, Nag D, Prasad A, Mittal VP. Japanese encephalitis epidemic in Uttar Pradesh, India, during 1978. Indian J Med Res 1982; 75: 161.

Mathur KK, Bagchi SK, Sehgal CL, Bhardwaj M. Investigation of an outbreak of Japanese encephalitis in Raipur, Madhya Pradesh. J Commun Dis 1981; 13: 257.

May FJ, Lobigs M, Lee E, Gendle DJ, Mackenzie JS, Broom AK, Conlan JV, Hall RA. Biological, antigenic and phylogenetic characterization of the flavivirus Alfuy. J Gen Virol 2006; 87: 329.

McCallum JD. Japanese encephalitis in southeastern Nepal: clinical aspects in the 1986 epidemic. J R Army Med Corps 1991; 137: 8.

Medlock JM, Snow KR, Leach S. Potential transmission of West Nile virus in the British Isles: an ecological review of candidate mosquito bridge vectors. Med Vet Entomol 2005; 19: 221.

Min JG, Xue M. Progress in studies on the overwintering of the mosquito *Culex tritaeniorhynchus*. Southeast Asian J Trop Med Public Health 1996; 27: 810.

Ming CK, Swe T, Thaung U, Lwin TT. Recent outbreaks of Japanese encephalitis in Burma. Southeast Asian J Trop Med Public Health 1977; 8: 113.

Ming JG, Hua J, Riley JR, Reynolds DR, Smith AD, Wang RL, Cheng JY, Cheng XN. Autumn southward 'return' migration of the mosquito *Culex tritaeniorhynchus* in China. Med Vet Entomol 1993; 7: 323.

Mishra AC, Jacob PG, Ramanujam S, Bhat HR, Pavri KM. Mosquito vectors of Japanese encephalitis epidemic (1983) in Mandya district (India). Indian J Med Res 1984; 80: 377.

Mitchell CJ, Chen PS, Boreham PFL. Host-feeding patterns and behaviour of 4 *Culex* species in an endemic area of Japanese encephalitis. Bull World Health Organ 1973; 49: 293.

Mitchell CJ, Savage HM, Smith GC, Flood SP, Castro LT, Roppul M. Japanese encephalitis on Saipan: a survey of suspected mosquito vectors. Am J Trop Med Hyg 1993; 48: 585.

Mohan Rao CVR, Banerjee K, Mandke VB, Dandawate CN, Ilkal MAA, Anand BR, Biswas PN, Ray M. Investigations of the 1978 epidemic of encephalitis in Asansol, West Bengal, and Dhanbad, Bihar. J Assoc Physicians India 1980; 28: 441.

Mohan Rao CVR, Prasad SR, Rodrigues JJ, Sharma NGK, Shaikh BH, Pavri KM. The first laboratory proven outbreak of Japanese encephalitis in Goa. Indian J Med Res 1983; 78: 745.

Monath TP. Japanese encephalitis—a plague of the Orient. N Engl J Med 1988; 319: 641.

Monath TP. Japanese encephalitis vaccines: current vaccines and future prospects. Curr Top Microbiol Immunol 2002; 267: 105.

Monath TP, Guirakhoo F, Nichols R, Yoksan S, Schrader R, Murphy C, Blum P, Woodward S, McCarthy K, Mathis D, Johnson C, Bedford P. Chimeric live, attenuated vaccine against Japanese encephalitis (ChimeriVax-JE): phase 2 clinical trials for safety and immunogenicity, effect of vaccine dose and schedule, and memory response to challenge with inactivated Japanese encephalitis antigen. J Infect Dis 2003; 188: 1213.

Monath TP, McCarthy K, Bedford P, Johnson CT, Nichols R, Yoksan S, Marchesani R, Knauber M, Wells KH, Arroyo J, Guirakhoo F. Clinical proof of principle for ChimeriVax: recombinant live, attenuated vaccines against flavivirus infections. Vaccine 2002; 20: 1004.

Mudur G. Japanese encephalitis outbreak kills 1300 children in India. Brit Med J 2005; 331: 1288.

Mukherjee KK, Chakravarti SK, Mukherjee MK, De PN, Chatterjee S, Chatterjee P, Chakraborty MS. Recurrent outbreaks of Japanese encephalitis in Nagaland (1985–1989)—a seroepidemiological study. J Commun Dis 1991; 23: 11.

Muller MJ, Montgomery BL, Ingram A, Ritchie SA. First records of *Culex gelidus* from Australia. J Am Mosq Control Assoc 2001; 17: 79.

Nam J-H, Chae S-L, Park S-H, Jeong J-S, Joo M-S, Kang C-Y, Cho H-W. High level of sequence variation in the 3' noncoding region of Japanese encephalitis viruses isolated in Korea. Virus Genes 2002; 24: 21.

Nam JH, Chung YJ, Ban SJ, Kim EJ, Park YK, Cho HW. Envelope gene sequence variation among Japanese encephalitis viruses isolated in Korea. Acta Virol 1996; 40: 303.

Nga PT, Parquet MC, Cuong VD, Ma SP, Hasebe F, Inoue S, Makino Y, Takagi M, Nam VS, Morita K. Shift in Japanese encephalitis virus (JEV) genotype circulating in northern Vietnam: implications for frequent introductions of JEV from Southeast Asia to East Asia. J Gen Virol 2004; 85: 1625.

Nguyen HT, Nguyen TY. Japanese encephalitis in Vietnam, 1985–93. Southeast Asian J Trop Med Public Health 1995; 26S: 47.

Nguyen NT JE epidemiology in Vietnam. In: Personal Communication, Presented to the Joint Japanese Encephalitis Meeting of the Global Alliance for Vaccines and Immunization (GAVI) South-East Asia & Western Pacific Regional Working Groups. Setting the Global Agenda on Public Health Solutions and National Needs, June 18–19, 2002, Bangkok.

Nisbet DJ, Lee KJ, van den Hurk AF, Johansen CA, Kuno G, Cheng GJJ, Mackenzie JS, Ritchie SA, Hall RA. Identification of a new Flavivirus in the Kokobera virus complex. J Gen Virol 2005; 86: 121.

Oda K, Igarashi A, Kheong CT, Hong CC, Vijayamalar B, Sinniah M, Hassan SS, Tanaka H. Cross-sectional serosurvey for Japanese encephalitis specific antibody from animal sera in Malaysia 1993. Southeast Asian J Trop Med Public Health 1996; 27: 463.

Ogata M, Nagao Y, Jitsunari F, Kitamura N, Okazaki T. Infection of herons and domestic fowls with Japanese encephalitis virus with specific reference to maternal antibody of hen (epidemiological study on Japanese encephalitis 26). Acta Med Okayama 1970; 24: 175.

Ohrr H, Tandan JB, Sohn YM, Shin SH, Pradhan DP, Halstead SB. Effect of a single dose of SA 14-14-2 vaccine 1 year after immunisation in Nepalese children with Japanese encephalitis: a case–control study. Lancet 2005; 366: 1375.

Okuno T. An epidemiological review of Japanese encephalitis. World Health Stat Q 1978; 31: 120.

Okuno T, Okada T, kondo A, Suzuki M, Kobayashi M, Oya A. Immunotyping of different strains of Japanese encephalitis virus by antibody-absorption, haemagglutination-inhibition and complement-fixation tests. Bull World Health Organ 1968; 38: 547–563.

Okuno T, Tseng PT, Hsu ST, Huang CT, Kuo CC. Japanese encephalitis surveillance in China (Province of Taiwan) during 1968–1971. I. Geographical and season features of case outbreaks. Jpn J Med Sci Biol 1975a; 28: 235.

Okuno T, Tseng PT, Hsu ST, Huang CT, Kuo CC. Japanese encephalitis surveillance in China (Province of Taiwan) during 1968–1971. II Age-specific incidence in connection with Japanese encephalitis vaccination program. Jpn J Med Sci Biol 1975b; 28: 255.

Olson JG, Ksiazek TG, Gubler DJ, See R, Suharyono, Lubis I, Simanjuntak G, Lee V, Nalim S, Juslis J. A survey for arboviral antibodies in sera of humans and animals in Lombok, Republic of Indonesia. Ann Trop Med Parasitol 1983; 77: 131.

Olson JG, Ksiazek TG, Lee VH, Tan R, Shope RE. Isolation of Japanese encephalitis virus from *Anopheles annularis* and *Anopheles vagus* in Lombok, Indonesia. Trans R Soc Trop Med Hyg 1985a; 79: 845.

Olson JG, Ksiazek TG, Tan R, Atmosoedjono S, Lee VH, Converse JD. Correlation of population indicies of female *Culex tritaeniorhynchus* with Japanese encephalitis viral activity in Kapuk, Indonesia. Southeast Asian J Trop Med Public Health 1985b; 16: 337.

Ooi MH Japanese encephalitis in central Sarawak: Sibu Hospital's experience. In: Personal Communication, Presented to the Joint Japanese Encephalitis Meeting of the Global Alliance for Vaccines and Immunization (GAVI) South-East Asia & Western Pacific Regional Working Groups. Setting the Global Agenda on Public Health Solutions and National Needs, June 18–19, 2002, Bangkok.

O'Rourke TF, Hayes CG, San Luis AM, Manaloto CR, Schultz GW, Ranoa CP, Beroy G, Yambao E, Morales V, Bakil L. Epidemiology of Japanese encephalitis in the Philippines. In: Arbovirus Research in Australia. Proceedings of the Fourth Symposium (St George TD, Kay BH, Blok J, editors). Brisane: Queensland Institute for Medical Research; 1986; p. 82.

Ostlund MR, Kan B, Karlsson M, Vene S. Japanese encephalitis in a Swedish tourist after travelling to Java and Bali. Scand J Infect Dis 2004; 36: 312.

Parajuli MB. Status of Japanese encephalitis in Nepal. JE & HFRS Bull 1989; 3: 41.

Paramasivan R, Mishra AC, Mourya DT. West Nile virus: the Indian scenario. Indian J Med Res 2003; 118: 101.

Paterson PY, Ley HL, Wisseman CL, Pond WL, Smadel JE, Diercks FH, Hetherington DG, Sneath PHA, Witherington DH, Lancaster WE. Japanese encephalitis in Malaya. I. Isolation of virus and serologic evidence of human and equine infections. Am J Hyg 1952; 56: 320.

Paul SD, Narasimha Murthy DP, Das M. Isolation of West Nile virus from a human case of febrile illness. Indian J Med Res 1970; 58: 1177.

Paul WS, Moore PS, Karabatsos N, Flood SP, Yamada S, Jackson T, Tsai TF. Outbreak of Japanese encephalitis on the island of Saipan, 1990. J Infect Dis 1993; 167: 1053.

Pavri KM, Singh KRP. Isolation of West Nile virus from *Culex fatigans* mosquitoes from western India. Indian J Med Res 1965; 53: 501.

Peiris JSM, Amerasinghe FP, Amerasinghe PH, Ratnayake CB, Karunaratne SHPP, Tsai TF. Japanese encephalitis in Sri Lanka—the study of an epidemic: vector incrimination, porcine infection and human disease. Trans R Soc Trop Med Hyg 1992; 86: 307.

Peiris JSM, Amerasingje FP, Arunagiri CK, Perera LP, Karunaratne SHPP, Ratnayake CB, Kulatilaka TA, Abeysinghe MRN. Japanese encephalitis in Sri Lanka: comparison of vector and virus ecology in different agro-climatic areas. Trans R Soc Trop Med Hyg 1993; 87: 541.

Petersen LR, Marfin AA. Shifting epidemiology of *Flaviviridae*. J Trav Med 2005; 12(Suppl 1): S3.

Peyton EL, Campbell SR, Candeletti TM, Romanowski M, Crans WJ. *Aedes* (Finlaya) *japonicus japonicus* (Theobald), a new introduction into the United States. J Am Mosq Control Assoc 1999; 15: 238.

Phanthumachinda B. Ecology and biology of Japanese encephalitis vectors. Southeast Asian J Trop Med Public Health 1995; 26(Suppl 3): 11.

Phukan AC, Borah PK, Mahanta J. Japanese encephalitis in Assam, northeast India. Southeast Asian J Trop Med Public Health 2004; 35: 618.

Plesner AM, Arlien-Soborg P, Herning M. Neurological complications to vaccination against Japanese encephalitis. Eur J Neurol 1998; 5: 479.

Plesner AM, Ronne T, Wachmann H. Case–control study of allergic reactions to Japanese encephalitis vaccine. Vaccine 2000; 18: 1830.

Poidinger M, Hall RA, Mackenzie JS. Molecular characterisation of the Japanese encephalitis serocomplex of the flavivirus genus. Virology 1996; 218: 417.

Poland JD, Cropp CB, Craven RB, Monath TP. Evaluation of the potency and safety of inactivated Japanese encephalitis vaccine in US inhabitants. J Infect Dis 1990; 161: 878.

Pond WL, Russ SB, Lancaster WF, Audy JR, Smadel JE. Japanese encephalitis in Malaya. II. Distribution of neutralizing antibodies in man and animals. Am J Hyg 1954; 59: 17.

Pond WL, Smadel JE. Neurotropic viral diseases in the Far East during the Korean war. Med Sci Publ Army Med Serv Graduate Sch 1954; 4: 219.

Potula R, Badrinath S, Srinivasan S. Japanese encephalitis in and around Pondicherry, South India: a clinical appraisal and prognostic indicators for the outcome. J Trop Pediatr 2003; 49: 48.

Prasad SR, George S, Gupta NP. Studies on an outbreak of Japanese encephalitis in Kolar district, Karnataka State, in 1977–1978. Indian J Med Res 1982; 75: 1.

Prasad SR, Kumar V, Marwaha RK, Batra KL, Rath RK, Pal SR. An epidemic of encephalitis in Haryana: serological evidence of Japanese encephalitis in a few patients. Indian Pediatr 1993; 30: 905.

ProMED Posting. Japanese encephalitis—China (Hong Kong) (03), posted on 3 November 2004.

Pyke AT, Williams DT, Nisbet DJ, van den Hurk AF, Taylor CT, Johansen CA, Macdonald J, Hall RA, Simmons RJ, Mason RJV, Lee JM, Ritchie SA, Smith GA, Mackenzie JS. The appearance of a second genotype of Japanese encephalitis virus in the Australasian region. Am J Trop Med Hyg 2001; 65: 747.

Rajendran R, Thenmozhi V, Tewari SC, Balasubramanian A, Ayanar K, Manavalan R, Gajanana A, Kabilan L, Thakare JP, Satyanarayana K. Longitudinal studies in South Indian villages on Japanese encephalitis virus infection in mosquitoes and seroconversion in goats. Trop Med Int Health 2003; 8: 174–181.

Rao BL, Basu A, Wairagkar NS, Gore MM, Arankalle VA, Thakare JP, Jadi RS, Rao KA, Mishra AC. A large outbreak of acute encephalitis with a high fatality rate in children in Andhra Pradesh, India, in 2003, associated with Chandipura virus. Lancet 2004; 364: 869.

Rao CV, Risbud AR, Rodrigues FM, Pinto BD, Joshi GD. The 1981 epidemic of Japanese encephalitis in Tamil Nadu and Pondicherry. Indian J Med Res 1988; 87: 417.

Rao GLNP, Rodrigues FM, Nambiappan M, Nagarajan M, Ghalsasi GR, Rodrigues JJ, Pinto BD, Rao CVRM, Gupta NP. Aetiology of the 1978 outbreak of encephalitis in Tirunelveli and other districts of Tamil Nadu. Indian J Med Res 1982; 76: 36.

Rao GLNP, Rodrigues FM, Nambiappan M, Nagarajan M, Ghalsasi GR, Rodrigues JJ, Pinto BD, Rao CVRM, Gupta NP. Aetiology of the 1978 outbreak of encephalitis in Tirunelveli and other districts of Tamil Nadu. Indian J Med Res 1982; 76: 36.

Rao JS, Misra SP, Patanayak SK, Rao TV, Das Gupta RK, Thapar BR. Japanese encephalitis epidemic in Anantapur district, Andhra Pradesh (October–November, 1999). J Commun Dis 2000; 32: 306.

Rathi AK, Kushwaha KP, Singh YD, Singh J, Sirohi R, Singh RK, Singh UK. JE virus encephalitis: 1988 epidemic at Gorakhpur. Indian Pediatr 1993; 30: 325.

Ratho RK, Sethi S, Prasad SR. Prevalence of Japanese encephalitis and West Nile viral infections in pig population in and around Chandigarh. J Commun Dis 1999; 31: 113.

Reeves WC, Rudnick A. A survey of the mosquitoes of Guam in the two periods in 1948 and 1949 and its epidemiological implications. Am J Trop Med 1951; 31: 633.

Reuben R, Gajanana A. Japanese encephalitis in India. Indian J Pediatr 1997; 64: 243.

Reuben R, Thenmozhi V, Samuel PP, Gajanana A, Mani TR. Mosquito blood feeding patterns as a factor in the epidemiology of Japanese encephalitis in southern India. Am J Trop Med Hyg 1992; 46: 654.

Reynolds DR, Smith AD, Muhhopadhyay S, Chowdhury AK, De BK, Nath PS, Mondal SK, Das BH, Mukhopadhyay S. Atmospheric transport of mosquitoes in northeast India. Med Vet Entomol 1996; 10: 185.

Ritchie SA, Phillips D, Broom A, Mackenzie J, Poidinger M, van den Hurk A. Isolation of Japanese encephalitis virus from *Culex annulirostris* in Australia. Am J Trop Med Hyg 1997; 56: 80.

Ritchie SA, Rochester W. Wind-blown mosquitoes and introduction of Japanese encephalitis into Australia. Emerg Infect Dis 2001; 7: 900.

Rodrigues FM. Epidemiology of arboviral diseases of man in India: known facts and unsolved questions. Bull Nat Instit Virol (Pune) 1988; 6(3 & 4): 3.

Rodrigues FM, Bright Singh P, Dandawate CN, Soman RS, Guttikar SN, Kaul HN. Isolation of Japanese encephalitis and West Nile viruses from mosquitoes collected in Andhra Pradesh. Indian J Parasitol 1980; 4: 149.

Rodrigues JJ, Singh PB, Dave DS, Prasan R, Ayachit V, Shaikh BH, Pavri KM. Isolation of Chandipura virus from the blood in acute encephalopathy syndrome. Indian J Med Res 1983; 77: 303.

Rosen L. The natural history of Japanese encephalitis virus. Ann Rev Microbiol 1986; 40: 395.

Rosen L, Lien JC, Lu LC. A longitudinal study of the prevalence of Japanese encephalitis virus in adult and larval *Culex tritaeniorhynchus* mosquitoes in northern Taiwan. Am J Trop Med Hyg 1989; 40: 557.

Sabin AB, Schlesinger RW, Ginder WR, Matsumoto M. Japanese B encephalitis in an American soldier in Korea. Am J Hyg 1947; 46: 356.

Samuel PP, Hiriyan SJ, Gajanana A. Japanese encephalitis virus infection in mosquitoes and its epidemiological implications. ICMR Bull 2000; 30(4): 37.

Sangkawibha N. Viral diseases in Thailand. In: Viral Diseases in South-East Asia and the Western Pacific (Mackenzie JS, editor). Sydney: Academic Press; 1982; p. 217.

Sangkawibha N, Nakornsri S, Rojanasuphot S. Japanese encephalitis in Thailand. J Dept Med Sci 1982; 24: 1.

Sardelis MR, Turell MJ, Andre RG. Experimental transmission of St Louis encephalitis virus by *Ochlerotatus j. japonicus*. J Am Mosq Control Assoc 2003; 19: 159.

Satake Y, Hasegawa H, Yoshida M, Kobayashi Y. Isolation of anti-Beijing-1 group specific monoclonal antibody and antigenic analysis of Japanese encephalitis viruses in India. Vaccine 1994; 12: 723.

Sazawa H. Japanese encephalitis in domestic animals. Bull Off Int Epiz 1968; 70: 627.

Scherer WF. Ecological studies of Japanese encephalitis virus in Japan. Parts I–IX. Am J Trop Med Hyg 1959; 8: 644.

Scherret JH, Mackenzie JS, Hall RA, Deubel V, Gould EA. Phylogeny and molecular epidemiology of West Nile and Kunjin viruses. Curr Top Microbiol Immunol 2002; 267: 373.

Scherret JH, Poidinger M, Mackenzie JS, Broom AK, Deubel V, Lipkin WI, Briese T, Gould EA, Hall RA. The relationships between West Nile and Kunjin viruses. Emerg Infect Dis 2001; 7: 697.

Scott TW. Vertebrate host ecology. In: The Arboviruses: Epidemiology and Ecology (Monath TP, editor). vol. 1. Boca Raton: CRC Press; 1988; p. 257.

See E, Tan HC, Wang D, Ooi EE, Lee MA. Presence of haemagglutination inhibition and neutralization antibodies to Japanese encephalitis virus in wild pigs on an offshore island in Singapore. Acta Trop 2002; 81: 233.

Sehgal A, Dutta AK. Changing perspectives in Japanese encephalitis in India. Trop Doctor 2003; 33: 131.

Sellers RF. Weather, host and vector—their interplay in the spread of insect-borne animal virus diseases. J Hyg Camb 1980; 85: 65.

Sellers RF. Eastern equine encephalitis in Quebec and Connecticut, 1072: introduction by infected mosquitoes on the wind? Can J Vet Res 1989; 53: 76.

Sellers RF, Maarouf AR. Trajectory analysis of winds and eastern equine encephalitis in USA, 1980–85. Epidemiol Infect 1990; 104: 329.

Sellers RF, Maarouf AR. Weather factors in the prediction of western equine encephalitis epidemics in Manitoba. Epidemiol Infect 1993; 111: 373.

Sharma SN, Panwar BS. An epidemic of Japanese encephalitis in Haryana in the year 1990. J Commun Dis 1991; 23: 168.

Shield J, Hanna J, Phillips D. Reappearance of the Japanese encephalitis virus in the Torres Strait, 1996. Comm Dis Intell (Aust) 1996; 20: 191.

Shlim DR, Solomon T. Japanese encephalitis vaccine for travelers: exploring the limits of risk. Travel Med 2002; 35: 183.

Shortridge KF, Ng MH, Oya A, Kobayashi M, Munro R, Wong F, Lance V. Arbovirus infections in reptiles: immunological evidence for a high incidence of Japanese encephalitis virus in the cobra *Naja naja*. Trans R Soc Trop Med Hyg 1974; 68: 454.

Shortridge KF, Oya A, Kobayashi M, Duggan R. Japanese encephalitis virus in cold blooded animals. Trans R Soc Trop Med Hyg 1977; 71: 261.

Shultz GW, Hayes CG. Ecology of mosquitoes (Diptera: *Culicidae*) at a site endemic with Japanese encephalitis on Luzon, Republic of the Philippines. Southeast Asian J Trop Med Public Health 1993; 24: 157.

Simasathien P, Rohitayodhin S, Nisalak A, Singharaj P, Halstead SB, Russell PK. Recovery of Japanese encephalitis virus from wild caught mosquitoes in Thailand. Southeast Asian J Trop Med Public Health 1972; 3: 52.

Simpson DIH, Bowen ETW, Platt GS, Way H, Smith CEG, Peto S, Kamath S, Lim BL, Lim TW. Japanese encephalitis in Sarawak: virus isolation and serology in a Land Dyak village. Trans R Soc Trop Med Hyg 1970b; 64: 503.

Simpson DIH, Bowen ETW, Way HJ, Platt GS, Hill MN, Kamath S, Wah LT, Bendell PJE, Heathcote OHU. Arbovirus infections in Sarawak, October 1968–February 1970: Japanese encephalitis virus isolations from mosquitoes. Ann Trop Med Parasitol 1974; 68: 393.

Simpson DIH, Smith CEG, Bowen ETW, Platt GS, Way H, McMahon D, Bright WF, Hill MN, Mahadevan S, Macdonald WW. Arbovirus infections in Sarawak: virus isolations from mosquitoes. Ann Trop Med Parasitol 1970a; 64: 137.

Sinniah M. A review of Japanese B virus encephalitis in Malaysia. Southeast Asian J Trop Med Public Health 1989; 20: 581.

Siraprapasiri T, Sawaddiwudhipong W, Rojanasuphot S. Cost–benefit analysis of Japanese encephalitis vaccination program in Thailand. Southeast Asian J Trop Med Public Health 1997; 28: 143.

Smith CEG, Simpson DIH, Bowen ETW, Peto S, McMahon D, Platt GS, Way H, Bright WF, Maidment B. Arbovirus infections in Sarawak: human serological studies. Trans R Soc Trop Med Hyg 1974; 68: 96.

Smithburn KC. Differentiation of the West Nile virus from the viruses of St Louis and Japanese B encephalitis. J Immunol 1942; 44: 25.

Smithburn KC, Kerr JA, Gatne PB. Neutralizing antibodies against certain viruses in the sera of the residents of India. J Immunol 1954; 72: 248.

Sohn YM. Japanese encephalitis immunization in South Korea: past, present and future. Emerg Infect Dis 2000; 6: 17.

Sohn YM, Park MS, Rho HO, Chandler LJ, Shope RE, Tsai TF. Primary and booster immune responses to SA 14-14-2 Japanese encephalitis vaccine in Korean infants. Vaccine 1999; 17: 2259.

Solomon T. Japanese encephalitis. In: Neurobase (Gilman S, Goldstein GW, Waxman SG, editors). San Diego: Medlink Publishing; 2000.

Solomon T. Recent advances in Japanese encephalitis. J Neurovirol 2003; 9: 274.

Solomon T, Dung NM, Kneen R, Gainsborough M, Vaughn DW, Khanh VT. Japanese encephalitis. J Neurol Neurosurg Psychiatry 2000; 68: 405.

Solomon T, Dung NM, Wills B, Kneen R, Gainsborough M, Diet TV, Thuy TT, Loan HT, Khanh VC, Vaughn DW, White NJ, Farrar JJ. Interferon alfa-2a in Japanese encephalitis: a randomised double-blind placebo-controlled trial. Lancet 2003b; 361: 821.

Solomon T, Kneen R, Dung NM, Khanh VC, Thuy TT, Ha DQ, Day NP, Nisalak A, Vaughan DW, Whit NJ. Poliomyelitis-like illness due to Japanese encephalitis virus. Lancet 1998; 351: 1094.

Solomon T, Ni H, Beasley DWC, Ekkelenkamp M, Cardosa MJ, Barrett ADT. Origin and evolution of Japanese encephalitis virus in southeast Asia. J Virol 2003a; 77: 3091.

Solomon T, Winter PM. Neurovirulence and host factors in flavivirus encephalitis—evidence from clinical epidemiology. Arch Virol Suppl 2004; 18: 161.

Soman RS, Rodrigues FM, Guttikar SN, Guru PY. Experimental viraemia and transmission of Japanese encephalitis virus by mosquitoes in ardeid birds. Indian J Med Res 1977; 66: 709.

Spicer PE. Japanese encephalitis in Western Irian Jaya. J Travel Med 1997; 4: 146.

Spicer PE, Phillips D, Pyke A, Johansen C, Melrose W, Hall RA. Antibodies to Japanese encephalitis virus in human sera collected from Irian Jaya. Follow-up of a previously reported case of Japanese encephalitis in that region. Trans R Soc Trop Med Hyg 1999; 93: 511.

Srey VH, Sadones H, Ong S, Mam M, Yim C, Sor S, Grosjean P, Reynes JM. Etiology of encephalitis syndrome among hospitalized children and adults in Takeo, Cambodia, 1999–2000. Am J Trop Med Hyg 2002; 66: 200.

Su HJ, Liang GD. JE epidemics, vaccines and epidemiology in China. In: Personal Communication, Presented to the Joint Japanese Encephalitis Meeting of the Global Alliance for Vaccines and Immunization (GAVI) South-East Asia & Western Pacific Regional Working Groups. Setting the Global Agenda on Public Health Solutions and National Needs, June 18-19, 2002, Bangkok.

Sucharit S, Surathin K, Shrestha SR. Vectors of Japanese encephalitis virus (JEV): species complexes of the vectors. Southeast Asian J Trop Med Public Health 1989; 20: 611.

Sugamata M, Ahmed A, Miura T, Takasu T, Kono R, Ogata T, Kimura-Kuroda J, Yasui K. Seroepidemiological study of infection with West Nile virus in Karachi, Pakistan, in 1983 and 1985. J Med Virol 1988; 26: 243.

Sulkin SE, Allen R. Virus Infections in Bats. Monographs in Virology. vol. 8. Basel: S.Karger; 1974.

Sumarmo, Wuryadi S, Suroso T. Japanese encephalitis in Indonesia. Southeast Asian J Trop Med Public Health 1995; 26(Suppl. 3): 24.

Sunnara Y, Touch S. Japanese encephalitis in the Kingdom of Cambodia. Southeast Asian J Trop Med Public Health 1995; 26(Suppl 3): 22.

Swe T, Thein S, Myint MS. Pilot sero-epidemiological survey on Japanese encephalitis in north-western Burma. Biken J 1979; 22: 125.

Takahashi H, Pool V, Tsai TF, Chen RT, The V.A.E.R.S. Working Group. Adverse events after Japanese encephalitis vaccination: review of the post-marketing surveillance data from Japan and the United States. Vaccine 2000; 18: 2963.

Takashima I, Rosen L. Horizontal and vertical transmission of Japanese encephalitis virus by Aedes japonicus (Diptera: Culicidae). J Med Entomol 1989; 26: 454–458.

Tan LH. Japanese encephalitis in Malaysia. Southeast Asian J Trop Med Public Health 1995; 26(Suppl 3): 31.

Tan R, Nalim S, Suwasono H, Jennings GB. Japanese encephalitis virus isolated from seven species of mosquitoes collected at Semarang Regency, Central Java. Bul Penelit Kesehatan 1993; 21: 1.

Thakare JP, Rao TLG, Padbidri VS. Prevalence of West Nile virus infection in India. Southeast Asian J Trop Med Public Health 2002; 33: 801.

Thakare JP, Shenoy SR, Padbidri VS, Rajput CS, Karmarkar DP, Deo SS. Japanese encephalitis in Sangli District, Maharashtra. Indian J Med Res 1999; 109: 165.

Thein S, Aung H, Sebastian AA. Study of vector, amplifier, and human infection with Japanese encephalitis virus in a Rangoon community. Am J Epidemiol 1988; 128: 1376.

Thiel H-J, Collett MS, Gould EA, Heinz FX, Houghton M, Meyers G, Purcell RH, Rice CM. Family *Flaviviridae*. In: Virus Taxonomy. Classification of Viruses. Eighth Report of the International Committee of the Taxonomy of Viruses (Fauquet CM, Mayo MA, Maniloff J, Desselberger U, Hall LA, editors). San Diego: Elsevier; 2005; p. 981.

Thi-Kim-Thoa N, Ngo-Thi-Vien, Tran-Tuyet-Mai, Thi-Ngoc-Xuan N. Japanese encephalitis vectors: isolation of virus from culicine mosquitoes in the Saigon area. Southeast Asian J Trop Med Public Health 1974; 5: 408.

Thompson JD, Gibson TJ, Plewniak F, Jeanmougin F, Higgins DJ. The CLUSTALX windows interface: flexible strategies for multiple sequence alignments aided by quality analysis tools. Nucleic Acids Res 1997; 25: 4876.

Thongcharoen P. Japanese encephalitis in Thailand. J Med Assoc Thai 1985; 68: 534.

Ting SH, Tan HC, Wong WK, Ng ML, Chan SH, Ooi EE. Seroepidemiology of neutralizing antibodies to Japanese encephalitis virus in Singapore: continued transmission despite the abolishment of pig farming. Acta Trop 2004; 92: 187.

Tiroumourougane SV, Raghava P, Srinivasan S. Japanese viral encephalitis. Postgrad Med J 2002; 78: 205.

Trosper JH, Ksiazek TG, Cross JH. Isolation of Japanese encephalitis virus from the Republic of the Philippines. Trans R Soc Trop Med Hyg 1980; 74: 292.

Tsai TF. Factors in the changing epidemiology of Japanese encephalitis and West Nile fever. In: Factors in the Emergence of Arbovirus Diseases (Saluzzo JF, Dodet B, editors). Paris: Elsevier; 1997; p. 179.

Tsai TF. New initiatives for the control of Japanese encephalitis by vaccination: minutes of a WHO/CVI meeting, Bangkok, Thailand, 13–15 October, 1998. Vaccine 2000; 18(Suppl 2): 1.

Turell MJ, Sardelis MR, O'Guinn ML, Dohm DJ. Potential vectors of West Nile virus in North America. Curr Top Microbiol Immunol 2002; 267: 241.

Twiddy SS, Holmes EC. The extent of homologous recombination in the genus Flavivirus. J Gen Virol 2003; 84: 429.

Uchil PD, Satchidanandam V. Phylogenetic analysis of Japanese encephalitis virus: envelope gene based analysis reveals a fifth genotype, geographic clustering, and multiple introductions of the virus into the Indian subcontinent. Am J Trop Med Hyg 2001; 65: 242.

Umenai T, Krzysko R, Bektimirov TA, Assaad FA. Japanese encephalitis: current worldwide status. Bull World Health Organ 1985; 63: 625.

Vajpayee A, Dey PN, Chakraborty AK, Chakraborty MS. Study of the outbreak of Japanese encephalitis in Lakhimpur district of Assam, 1989. J Indian Med Assoc 1992; 90: 114.

Vajpayee A, Mukherjee MK, Chakraborty AK, Chakraborty MS. Investigation of an outbreak of Japanese encephalitis in Rourkela City (Orissa) during 1989. J Commun Dis 1991; 23: 18.

van den Hurk AF, Johansen CA, Zborowski P, Paru R, Foley PN, Beebe NW, Mackenzie JS, Ritchie SA. Mosquito host feeding patterns and implications for Japanese encephalitis virus transmission in northern Australia and Papua New Guinea. Med Vet Entomol 2003b; 17: 403.

van den Hurk AF, Johansen CA, Zborowski P, Phillips DA, Pyke AT, Mackenzie JS, Ritchie SA. Flaviviruses isolated from mosquitoes collected during the first recorded outbreak of Japanese encephalitis virus on Cape York Peninsula, Australia. Am J Trop Med Hyg 2001b; 64: 125.

van den Hurk AF, Montgomery BL, Northill JA, Smith IL, Zborowski P, Ritchie SA, Mackenzie JS, Smith GA. The first isolation of Japanese encephalitis virus from mosquitoes collected from mainland Australia. Am J Trop Med Hyg 2006; 75: 21.

van den Hurk AF, Nisbet DJ, Hall RA, Kay BH, Mackenzie JS, Ritchie SA. Vector competence of Australian mosquitoes (Diptera: *Culicidae*) for Japanese encephalitis virus. J Med Entomol 2003a; 40: 82.

van den Hurk AF, Nisbet DJ, Johansen CA, Foley PN, Ritchie SA, Mackenzie JS. Japanese encephalitis on Badu Island, Australia: the first isolation of Japanese encephalitis virus from *Culex gelidus* in the Australasian region and the role of mosquito host-feeding patterns in virus transmission cycles. Trans R Soc Trop Med Hyg 2001a; 95: 595.

Van Peenen PFD, Irsiana R, Saroso JS, Joseph SW, Shope RE, Joseph PL. First isolation of Japanese encephalitis virus from Java. Milit Med 1974a; 139: 821.

Van Peenen PFD, Joseph PL, Atmososedjono S, Irsiana R, Saroso JS. Isolation of Japanese encephalitis virus from mosquitoes near Bogor, West Java, Indonesia. J Med Entomol 1975a; 12: 573.

Van Peenen PFD, Joseph PL, Atmosoedjonon S, Irsiana R, Saroso JS. Japanese encephalitis virus from pigs and mosquitoes in Jakarta, Indonesia. Trans R Soc Med Hyg 1975b; 69: 477.

Van Peenen PFD, Joseph SW, Atmosoedjono S, Irsiana R, Saroso JS, Saaroni O. Group B arbovirus antibodies in sentinel pigs near Jakarta, Indonesia. Southeast Asian J Trop Med Public Health 1974b; 5: 1–3.

Vaughn DW, Hoke CH. The epidemiology of Japanese encephalitis: prospects for prevention. Epidemiol Rev 1992; 14: 197.

Venzon EL, Espiritu Campos L, Chan VF, de Castro DS. Arboviruses, meningitis, and encephalitis. Acta Med Philipp 1972; 8: 71.

Vijayarani H, Gajanana A. Low rate of Japanese encephalitis infection in rural children in Thanjavur district (Tamil Nadu), an area with extensive paddy cultivation. Indian J Med Res 2000; 111: 212.

Vitarana T. Viral diseases in Sri Lanka: a national overview. In: Viral Diseases of South-East Asia and the Western Pacific (Mackenzie JS, editor). Sydney: Academic Press; 1982; p. 198.

Vitarana T. Japanese encephalitis in Sri Lanka. Southeast Asian J Trop Med Public Health 1995; 26(Suppl 3): 41.

Vitarana T, Jayasekera N, Wedasinghe N, Senaratne A, Colombage G, Kanapathipillai M, Hettiaratchy L, Ariyaratnam N, Peiris L, Aluthwatte A, Gunasekera HDN. The 1985/86 Japanese encephalitis outbreak in Sri Lanka and the impact of new irrigation schemes. In: Virus Diseases in Asia (Thongcharoen P, Kurstak E, editors). Bangkok: Mahidol University; 1988; p. 193.

Vongxay P. Epidemiology of Japanese encephalitis in Lao PDR. Southeast Asian J Trop Med Public Health 1995; 26(Suppl 3): 28.

Vythilingam I, Oda K, Chew TK, Mahadevan S, Vijayamalaar B, Morita K, Tsuchie H, Igarashi A. Isolation of Japanese encephalitis virus from mosquitoes collected in Sabak Bernam, Selangor, Malaysia in 1992. J Am Mosq Control Assoc 1995; 11: 94.

Vythilingam I, Oda K, Mahadevan S, Abdullah G, Thim CS, Hong CC, Vijayamalar B, Sinniah M, Igarashi A. Abundance, parity, and Japanese encephalitis infection of mosquitoes (Diptera: *Culicidae*) in Sepang district, Malaysia. J Med Entomol 1997; 34: 257.

Vythilingam I, Oda K, Tsuchie H, Mahadevan S, Vijayamalar B. Isolation of Japanese encephalitis virus from *Culex sitiens* mosquitoes in Selangor, Malaysia. J Am Mosq Control Assoc 1994; 10: 228.

Wada Y, Kawai S, Ito S, Oda T, Nishigaki J, Suengaga O, Omori N. Ecology of vector mosquitoes of Japanese encephalitis, especially of *Culex tritaeniorhynchus*. II. Nocturnal activity and host preference based on all-night catches by different methods in 1965 and 1966 near Nagasaki city. Trop Med 1970; 12: 79.

Wang SP, Grayston JT. Encephalitis on Taiwan. IV. Human serology. Am J Trop Med Hyg 1962; 11: 149.

Wang SP, Grayston JT, Chu IH. Encephalitis on Taiwan. V. Animal and bird serology. Am J Trop Med Hyg 1962a; 11: 155.

Wang SP, Grayston JT, Hsu SMK. Encephalitis on Taiwan. III. Virus isolation from mosquitoes. Am J Trop Med Hyg 1962; 11: 141.

Watt G, Jongsakul K. Acute undifferentiated fever caused by infection with Japanese encephalitis virus. Am J Trop Med Hyg 2003; 68: 704.

Webb JKG, Pereira S. Clinical diagnosis of arthropod-borne type virus encephalitis in children of North Arcot District, Madras state, India. Indian J Med Sci 1956; 10: 573.

Weissenbock H, Kolodziejek J, Url A, Lussy H, Rebel-Bauder B, Nowotny N. Emergence of Usutu, an African mosquito-borne flavivirus of the Japanese encephalitis virus group in central Europe. Emerg Infect Dis 2002; 8: 652.

Weng MH, Lien JC, Ji DD. Monitoring Japanese encephalitis virus infection in mosquitoes (Diptera: *Culicidae*) at Guandu Nature Park, Taipei, 2002–2004. J Med Entomol 2005; 42: 1085.

Weng MH, Lien JC, Wang YM, Lin CC, Lin HC, Chin C. Isolation of Japanese encephalitis virus from mosquitoes collected in Northern Taiwan between 1995 and 1996. J Microbiol Immunol Infect 1999; 32: 9.

Westaway EG, Brinton MA, Gaidamovich SY, Horzinek MC, Igarashi A, Kaariainen L, Lvov DK, Porterfield JS, Russell PK, Trent DW. *Flaviviridae*. Intervirology 1985; 24: 183.

Westaway EG, Mackenzie JM, Khromykh AA. Replication and gene function in Kunjin virus. Curr Top Microbiol Immunol 2002; 267: 323.

Whelan P, Hayes G, Carter J, Wilson A, Haigh B. Detection of the exotic mosquito *Culex gelidus* in the Northern Territory. Commun Dis Intell (Aust) 2000; 24(Suppl.): 74.

WHO. The World Health Report 2004—Changing History. Geneva: World Health Organization; 2004.

WHO. Global position advisory committee on vaccine safety, 9–10 June, 2005. Wkly Epidemiol Rec 2005; 80: 242.

Williams DT, Wang L-F, Daniels PD, Mackenzie JS. Molecular characterisation of the first Australian strain of Japanese encephalitis virus, the FU strain. J Gen Virol 2000; 81: 2471.

Wills MR, Sil BK, Cao JX, Yu YX, Barrett AD. Antigenic comparison of the live attenuated Japanese encephalitis vaccine virus SA14-14-2: a comparison with isolates of the virus covering a wide geographic area. Vaccine 1992; 10: 861.

Wittesjo B, Eitrem R, Niklasson B, Vene S, Mangiafico JA. Japanese encephalitis after a 10d holiday in Bali. Lancet 1995; 345: 856.

Wo P. Japanese encephalitis in Singapore children. Singapore Med J 1963; 4: 11.

Work TH, Shah KV. Serological diagnosis of Japanese B type encephalitis in North Arcot district of Madras State, India with epidemiological notes. Indian J Med Sci 1956; 10: 582.

Wu Y-C, Huang W-S, Chien L-J, Lin T-L, Yueh YY, Tseng WL, Chang K-J, Wang G-R. The epidemiology of Japanese encephalitis on Taiwan, 1966–1997. Am J Trop Med Hyg 1999; 61: 78.

Yamada T, Rojanasuphot S, Takagi M, Wungkobkiat S, Hirota T, Yamashita T, Ahandarik S, Pisuthipornkul S, Sawasdikosol S, Sangkawibha N, Tuchinda P, Wacharothal S, Jetanasen S, Hiranniramon S, Laosuthibongse V, Chiowanich P, Roberts CE, Oesawadi P, Bukkavesa S, Gaew-Im M, Shimizu A, Kitaoka M. Studies on an epidemic of Japanese encephalitis in the northern region of Thailand in 1969 and 1970. Biken J 1971; 14: 267.

Yang DK, Kim BH, Kweon CH, Kwon JH, Lim SI, Han HR. Molecular characterization of full-length genome of Japanese encephalitis virus (KV1899) isolated from pigs in Korea. J Vet Sci 2004; 5: 197.

Yoshida M, Igarashi A, Suwendra P, Inada K, Maha MS, Kari K, Suda H, Antonio MT, Arhana BN, Takikawa Y, Maesawa S, Yoshida H, Chiba M. The first report on human cases serologically diagnosed as Japanese encephalitis in Indonesia. Southeast Asian J Trop Med Public Health 1999; 30: 698.

Yu Y. Japanese encephalitis in China. Southeast Asian J Trop Med Public Health. 1995; 26(Suppl. 3): 17.

Yu YX, Ming AG, Pen GY, Ao J, Li HM. Safety of a live-attenuated Japanese encephalitis virus vaccine (SA14-14-2) for children. Am J Trop Med Hyg 1988; 39: 214.

Zimmerman MD, Scott RM, Vaughn DW, Rajbhandari S, Nisalak A, Shrestha MP. Short report: an outbreak of Japanese encephalitis in Kathmandu, Nepal. Am J Trop Med Hyg 1997; 57: 283.

Note in proofs: Since completing this chapter, the Governments of India and Nepal in association with PATH, have initiated historic and immediate, broad-scale campaigns to protect children and adolescents against JEV infection. The programme will immunise 11 million children in India and 2.5 million children in Nepal aged between 1 and 15 as the first part of a phased approach, using the Chinese SA14/14/2 live JE vaccine, produced by the Chengdu Institute of Biological Products in China. Over 9.5 million children have received the vaccine in India. After the earlier successful vaccination programme in Andhra Pradesh, the campaign this year has targeted children in Uttar Pradesh, Assam, West Bengal and Karnataka States. In Nepal, over 1.6 million children have received the vaccine in the districts of Banke, Bardiya, Kailali, Dang, Rupandehi and Kanchanpur. Further information on the campaigns can be obtained from PATH (www.path.org/je).

Emerging Viruses in Human Populations
Edward Tabor (Editor)
© 2007 Elsevier B.V. All rights reserved
DOI 10.1016/S0168-7069(06)16011-5

Dengue and the Dengue Viruses

Ching-Juh Lai[a], Robert Putnak[b]

[a]*Laboratory of Infectious Diseases, National Institute of Allergy and Infectious Diseases, National Institutes of Health, Bethesda, MD 20892, USA*
[b]*Division of Communicable Diseases and Immunology, Department of Virus Diseases, The Walter Reed Army Institute of Research, Silver Spring, MD 20910, USA*

Introduction

The first epidemics of a disease believed to have been dengue occurred in 1779 in Cairo, Egypt and Jakarta, Indonesia. The following year, Benjamin Rush described an epidemic in Philadelphia of a similar disease, which he called break-bone fever (Siler et al., 1926). These epidemics, occurring nearly simultaneously on three continents, were probably part of a pandemic. A global distribution of dengue epidemics was evident by the 19th century, possibly spreading from the east coast of Africa to Asia, to the West Indies, and then to other parts of the Americas. Epidemiologic studies subsequently led to the identification of the etiologic agent and the mosquito vectors. Early attempts to develop inactivated dengue vaccines from infectious human blood and infectious mosquitoes ended in failure (Simmons et al., 1931). It was not until the dengue virus was first isolated in the 1950s (Sabin, 1952) that it became possible to prepare live-attenuated candidate vaccines by serial passage of viral isolates in suckling mouse brain (Sabin and Schlesinger, 1945; Hotta, 1952).

New and more severe forms of dengue, including dengue hemorrhagic fever (DHF) and dengue shock syndrome (DSS), emerged in Southeast Asia in the 1950s, due to intensified transmission of multiple dengue virus serotypes and an increased range of the *Aedes* mosquito vector. The risk of DHF/DSS was shown to increase significantly after a second episode of dengue infection, a phenomenon that was explained by the antibody-dependent enhancement (ADE) hypothesis (Halstead, 1970). A plaque reduction neutralization assay for detecting dengue viruses was developed in the 1960s (Russell et al., 1967).

By the late 1970s, a renewed research effort was undertaken to develop dengue vaccines. The first live-attenuated dengue type 2 virus (DEN2) vaccine candidate was produced in primary fetal rhesus lung (FRhL) cells from plaque-purified dengue virus (Eckels et al., 1976). Dengue virus was attenuated by serial passage in primary dog kidney (PDK) cells (Eckels et al., 1984; Halstead et al., 1984).

In 1980s, sequencing of yellow fever virus (Rice et al., 1985) and the construction of the first infectious cDNA clone of yellow fever virus (Rice et al., 1989) led to greater understanding of the molecular biology of other flaviviruses, including dengue virus. Sequencing of the DEN4 serotype of dengue virus (Zhao et al., 1986; Mackow et al., 1987) and the construction of the first infectious cDNA clone of DEN4 led to the ability to make chimeric dengue viruses (Bray and Lai, 1991a; Lai et al., 1991; Chen et al., 1995). Sequencing and construction of infectious clones of the other dengue virus serotypes soon followed (Hahn et al., 1988; Osatomi and Sumiyoshi, 1990; Fu et al., 1992; Kapoor et al., 1995a; Polo et al., 1997; Puri et al., 2000). This work facilitated research on the pathogenesis of dengue virus and the development of new candidate vaccine strains (Men et al., 1996; Durbin et al., 2001; Guirakhoo et al., 2001).

The virus and the vectors

The dengue viruses belong to the family *flaviviridae*, which consists of some 70 antigenically related viruses (Calisher et al., 1989). Most flaviviruses are arthropod-borne and are sub-divided based on their serological relationships and vector transmissibility (Casals, 1957). Several other flaviviruses are also important human pathogens, including the viruses responsible for yellow fever, tick-borne encephalitis, Japanese encephalitis, and West Nile encephalitis. The existence of shared antigenic determinants between dengue and other flaviviruses complicates serological diagnosis, especially in areas where two or more flaviviruses co-circulate.

Because there are four distinct dengue virus serotypes and because the immune response that develops in an infected host against one serotype results in only brief heterotypic immunity against other serotypes, sequential dengue virus infections with different subtypes can occur. Dengue virus infection in a host who has not been previously infected with dengue virus or other flaviviruses, or previously immunized, is called a "primary infection." Dengue virus infections in a host who has been immunologically sensitized to dengue or other flaviviruses is called a "secondary infection." Individuals residing in areas where multiple dengue virus serotypes are circulating can be infected by two, three, or even four serotypes throughout the course of their lives.

The viral nature of the agent of dengue fever was recognized relatively early; dengue fever was the second human disease after yellow fever to be attributed to a filterable agent (Ashburn and Craig, 1907). An important role of *Aedes aegypti* mosquitoes in dengue transmission was demonstrated (Graham, 1903; Bancroft, 1906) and later confirmed (Cleland et al., 1919; Chandler and Rice, 1923).

The dengue virus was first isolated from human sera during World War II by inoculation of suckling mice (Sabin, 1952).

Two different serotypes were demonstrated by showing that volunteers who recovered from a primary dengue infection were immune, possibly for life, to infection with the same serotype (homotypic immunity), whereas heterotypic immunity to a different serotype was brief, lasting <9 months. Prototype strains of DEN1 (Hawaii strain) and DEN2 (New Guinea B and C strains) were identified and used to produce experimental vaccines attenuated for humans by passage in suckling mice (Sabin and Schlesinger, 1945; Schlesinger and Frankel, 1952). Independently, another DEN1 (Mochizuki strain) was isolated in mouse brain (Kimura and Hotta, 1944) and was also attenuated for humans after serial passage in mice (Hotta, 1952). Two new dengue serotypes, DEN3 (strain H-87) and DEN4 (strain H-241), were isolated (Hammon et al., 1960a,b). Epidemiologic studies of DHF in Thailand provided evidence that all four dengue serotypes were endemic (Halstead et al., 1969) and were responsible for epidemics of dengue fever and DHF.

Dengue virus genome and replication

Virion structure and genome organization

Like other flaviviruses, the dengue virion is an enveloped spherical particle, 50 nm in diameter, with icosahedral symmetry (Lindenbach and Rice, 2003). It contains an inner nucleocapsid core composed of viral RNA (C) capsid protein complexes and an outer shell formed by a lipid bilayer onto which a small membrane (M) protein and a larger envelope (E) protein are inserted. The E protein mediates binding and fusion during viral entry into cells and is the major antigen of dengue virus.

Dengue virus contains a positive-stranded RNA, approximately 10.6 kb in length. The nucleic acid sequence has been determined for each of the four dengue virus serotypes. The genome contains a single open reading frame coding for a long polypeptide that is cleaved during and after translation by cellular and viral proteases, to generate the structural proteins (C, M and its precursor prM, and E) and the non-structural proteins (NS1, NS2A, NS2B, NS3, NS4A, NS4B, and NS5). Cleavage of prM protein to generate M protein by a furin-like cell protease occurs at a late stage in morphogenesis (Stadler et al., 1997), as mature, infectious virions are secreted from the host cell. Non-infectious sub-viral particles containing only E and M or prM proteins, called slow sedimenting hemagglutinin (SHA), are also secreted into the culture fluid of the infected cells (Smith et al., 1970). SHA contains 30 E protein dimers in icosahedral arrangement (Ferlenghi et al., 2001), as do sub-viral particles (similar to SHA) produced by recombinant co-expression of prM and E genes in the absence of dengue infection (Konishi and Mason, 1993; Heinz et al., 1995).

The non-structural proteins are found inside infected cells as part of a complex involved in viral RNA replication. The NS1 protein is also expressed on the surface of infected cells and is secreted extracellularly, often as membrane-associated particles, which are targets for complement-fixing antibodies (Brandt et al., 1970). Mice immunized with NS1 protein or administered anti-NS1 antibodies resist virus challenge, possibly through complement-dependent cytolysis of infected cells, which could play a role in enhancing viral clearance (Schlesinger et al., 1987; Falgout et al., 1990). The NS3 protein exhibits protease, helicase, and NTPase activities (Bazan and Fletterick, 1989; Gorbalenya et al., 1989; Falgout et al., 1991; Wengler and Wengler, 1993). The three-dimensional structure of the NS3 serine protease domain co-crystalized with a protease inhibitor has been determined (Murthy et al., 2000), an important step to understanding substrate recognition and cleavage and the development of inhibitors. The NS3 antigen is a target for cytotoxic T cells, which lyse infected cells and are believed to be involved in viral clearance and the immunopathogenesis of DHF (Kurane et al., 1991a; Livingston et al., 1995). The NS5 protein is the RNA-dependent RNA polymerase (Kapoor et al., 1995b) and also catalyzes methylatrons of the 5'-cap structure (Egloff et al., 2002; Ray et al., 2006). The functions of other small NS proteins are largely unknown, but NS2A is required for the C-terminal proteolytic cleavage of NS1 (Falgout et al., 1989) and NS2B is essential for NS3 protease activity (Falgout et al., 1991).

A 90–100-nucleotide 5'-non-coding region (NCR), which contains secondary structures shared among flaviviruses, might play a regulatory role in translation and packaging of the RNA genome (Brinton and Dispoto, 1988). A conserved, 8-nucleotide cyclization sequence has been identified near the 5'-NCR along with a complimentary sequence in the 3'-NCR of the RNA genomes of dengue and other mosquito-borne flaviviruses (Hahn et al., 1987). Studies using Kunjin virus RNA replicons reveal an essential role for these sequences in viral RNA replication (Khromykh and Westaway, 1997). The dengue virus 3'-NCR contains approximately 500 nucleotides, which exhibit secondary structures and other sequence features common among flaviviruses. A stem-loop structure approximately 90 nucleotides in length is predicted at the 3' end (Rice et al., 1985; Brinton et al., 1986; Zhao et al., 1986; Shi et al., 1996) and conserved sequences (CS), called CS1 and CS2, are located upstream of the 3' stem-loop structure (Hahn et al., 1987). The DEN2 3' stem-loop structure and CS1 element play an essential role in viral replication (Zeng et al., 1998), and DEN4 mutants lacking CS2 have been recovered, but these viruses replicate inefficiently (Men et al., 1996).

Replication

Dengue virus enters the host cell by receptor-mediated endocytosis after its E protein binds to cellular receptors. A conformational change in E protein triggered by low pH induces fusion of the viral membrane and the endosomal membranes (Allison et al., 1995; Stiasny et al., 2002; Modis et al., 2003; Bressanelli et al., 2004).

Replication of viral RNA and assembly of immature virions take place in endoplasmic reticulum. Virion maturation occurs along the exocytotic pathway and mature viruses exit the cell via the *trans*-Golgi network.

The receptors for dengue virus on the cell surface itself have not been fully elucidated, but these appear to include common low-affinity ligands such as heparan sulfate (Chen et al., 1997) and more specific, high-affinity ligands that differ among cell types (Salas-Benito and del Angel, 1997; Bielefeldt-Ohmann et al., 2001). In humans, skin dendritic cells are possibly among the first targets for dengue viruses; attachment is mediated by the cell surface DC-SIGN molecule (Wu et al., 2000; Tassaneetrithep et al., 2003).

Dengue viruses infect a variety of vertebrate and invertebrate cells, both continuous and primary cell lines, including Vero and LLC-MK2 cells (established from monkey kidney), BHK-21 cells (from hamster kidney), FRhL cells (from fetal rhesus lung), PDK cells (from primary dog kidney), and a variety of human cell lines. PDK cells, FRhL cells, and, more recently, Vero cells have been used as substrates for the production of experimental vaccines against dengue virus (Eckels et al., 1984; Halstead et al., 1984; Durbin et al., 2001; Guirakhoo et al., 2001). Several mosquito cell lines have also been used for the isolation and propagation of dengue viruses, including C6/36 cells (from *A. albopictus*) and AP-61 cells (from *A. pseudoscutellaris*) (Varma et al., 1974; Igarashi, 1978), with virus titers as high as 10^8–10^9 pfu/ml in the culture fluid. Cells of the TRA-284 sub-line of mosquito cells (from *T. amboinesis*), grown in serum-free medium, also can be used for virus isolation (Kuno, 1982).

Antigenic and structural models

Epitopes that are flavivirus-specific, dengue complex-specific, and type-specific have been identified on the E protein using mouse monoclonal antibodies against dengue virus and other flaviviruses. These epitopes are generally consistent with the serotype classification determined using polyclonal antisera (Heinz, 1986). Mouse monoclonal antibodies have been used to map and spatially locate three major non-overlapping antigenic domains (Henchal et al., 1982; Guirakhoo et al., 1989; Roehrig, 2003), which correlate well with the three physical domains of the three-dimensional structure of the E protein identified by X-ray crystallographic analysis at 2 Å resolution, first for the flavivirus tick-borne encephalitis virus (Rey et al., 1995) and later for DEN2 and DEN3 (Modis et al., 2003, 2005). These studies reveal that the E monomeric subunit protein consists of three structurally distinct domains. The central domain I consists of an 8-stranded central beta-barrel structure and a flavivirus-conserved glycosylation site. Domain II is an elongated structure containing at its distal end the fusion peptide sequence, which is conserved among flaviviruses. Domain III, which is folded like an immunoglobulin, is located on the lateral side of the subunit and is believed to be involved in binding to cellular receptors. The surface structure of the DEN2 virion has been determined at a resolution of 24 Å by cryo-electron microscopy and is consistent with the known structure of E protein (Kuhn et al., 2002); it appears as a smooth surface comprised of 90 E protein dimers tightly arranged in a herring-bone-like pattern with icosahedral symmetry. The flat, homodimeric E protein lies parallel to the viral membrane. The location of M protein also fits an electron dense space on the surface. It is suggested that the E dimers are poised for rotational rearrangement at low pH to form a fusogenic trimer, which mediates fusion of the virus membrane with the host cell endosomal membrane.

Mosquito vectors and virus transmission cycles

A. aegypti is the principal vector for dengue virus and a high incidence of epidemic dengue activity always occurs where this mosquito is prevalent. However, a number of mosquito species belonging to the genus *Aedes* (subgenus *Stegomyia*), such as *A. albopictus* and *A. polynesiensis*, also have been shown to transmit dengue virus (Rodhain and Rosen, 1997; Gubler, 1998). *A. aegypti* is a highly anthropophilic mosquito, which can rapidly populate natural or man-made habitats, the latter being generally water containers in close proximity to human dwellings (Platt et al., 1997; Scott et al., 2000). The incubation period for the virus in mosquitoes has been described (Simmons et al., 1931).

The female *A. aegypti* can feed upon multiple people in succession, thus infecting several people. The infected individuals often become viremic; further transmission to uninfected *Aedes* mosquitoes feeding on these individuals initiates an *A. aegypti*-human-*A. aegypti* transmission cycle, called the "urban cycle." This maintains dengue virus in the human population with the occasional emergence of epidemics in large cities of the tropics.

DEN2 has been isolated from forest *Aedes* species, *A. furcifer*, *A. taylori*, and *A. luteocephalus* in Africa during epidemic and non-epidemic periods (Traore-Lamizana et al., 1994). While sylvatic mosquitoes may play a role in maintaining dengue viruses in a primitive enzootic transmission cycle, this cycle is not considered important for the global resurgence of dengue fever/DHF. An African sylvatic DEN2 isolate was shown to be distinct from dengue viruses isolated from epidemics in other areas (Rico-Hesse, 1990). The endemic/epidemic lineages of dengue viruses probably evolved independently from their sylvatic progenitors (Wang et al., 2000; Shurtleff et al., 2001). A study comparing the replication efficiency of epidemic and sylvatic DEN2 isolates suggests that epidemic dengue viruses emerged upon adaptation to *A. aegypti* and *A. albopictus* mosquitoes that were living near human dwellings (Moncayo et al., 2004).

A. aegypti probably originated in Africa and probably spread to South and Central America as a result of international trade in the 18th century. It was mostly eradicated in the 1950s but has since re-infested those countries, usually within 20 years of the end of the eradication programs in the 1960s. *A. aegypti* was probably introduced into tropical Asia in the 19th century. Today, it has spread to most large tropical cosmopolitan cities (Fig. 1A). *A. albopictus*, originally indigenous to Southeast Asia, has become established in areas of the Pacific, North and

South Americas, Australia, Africa, and Europe. Although this species is considered to be an inefficient dengue vector (because it is less anthropophilic and not as well adapted to urban domestic environments), it was responsible for a dengue fever outbreak (DEN1) in Hawaii in 2001–2002 affecting 1644 persons (Effler et al., 2005). Such native dengue infection had last been reported in Hawaii in 1944. In Puerto Rico, *A. mediovittatus* might also be a vector of dengue virus (Gubler et al., 1985).

There may also be an enzootic cycle of dengue virus transmission involving non-human primates in the rain forests of Asia and Africa (Rodhain, 1991; de Silva et al., 1999). This enzootic transmission cycle may represent a retrograde infection from dengue epidemic(s) in humans (Rodhain and Rosen, 1997; Gubler, 1998). Studies in monkeys with DEN2 show that the infection rate and transmission efficiency by *A. aegypti* are temperature dependent (Watts et al., 1987), with the most efficient transmission occurring at or above 30°C. The results reveal that the incubation period for the virus in mosquitoes is approximately 12 days when the mosquito vectors are kept at 30°C, but only 7 days at 32°C and 35°C, which provides a possible explanation for the seasonal variation in incidence and the cyclic pattern of DHF epidemics.

Epidemic patterns of dengue

Dengue is an expanding public health problem worldwide with nearly 100 million new cases each year (Monath, 1994). This pandemic status is expected to continue unless vigorous and extensive applications of vector control methods are implemented or until an effective vaccine is developed (Thomas et al., 2003).

Dengue in Asia

It is believed that ecological destruction due to World War II, as well as unplanned urban population growth in Southeast Asian cities and the Pacific Islands, led to resurgence of *A. aegypti* mosquitoes. Increased dengue transmission favored co-circulation of multiple serotypes (hyper-endemicity). The first recorded DHF epidemic occurred in 1953–1954 in Manila (Quintos et al., 1954), then in 1956 and again in 1958 in Bangkok (Halstead and Yamarat, 1965). The disease quickly spread to other major cities in the next 20 years. In 1980s and 1990s, major dengue virus epidemics occurred in other countries, including Sri Lanka (Lucas et al., 2000), India (Kabra et al., 1999), Pakistan (Paul et al., 1998), China (southern coastal cities Hainan and Hong Kong) (Qiu et al., 1991), Taiwan (King et al., 2000; Liu et al., 2003), and the south and central Pacific islands (Hales et al., 1996). In the last decade, there has been a significant increase in the number of dengue cases in Asia, and DHF has become the leading cause of hospitalization and death among young children there. In Singapore, with a population of about 4.2 million, there were 13,984 cases of dengue fever and 19 deaths in 2005.

Dengue in the Americas

A. aegypti re-infested most of Central and South America and the Caribbean after eradication programs were discontinued in the 1960s and dengue subsequently emerged in Jamaica, Puerto Rico, and Venezuela (Morens et al., 1986). The first major epidemic caused by DEN1 occurred in Cuba in 1977. The 1981 dengue epidemic in Cuba was caused by a new strain of DEN2, later found to be the same as the Southeast Asian DEN2 genotype. More than 10,000 cases of DHF occurred during this epidemic, and in most instances (95%) these were a result of secondary dengue infections (Kouri et al., 1989). Other major DHF epidemics occurred in Cuba in 1997, also caused by secondary infections with DEN2 (Guzman et al., 1999), and in Venezuela in 1989–1990, with 3108 DHF cases and 73 deaths. Venezuela has suffered epidemics of dengue and DHF every year since then (Isturiz et al., 2000). Brazil has experienced dengue outbreaks involving multiple serotypes since 1986 (Siqueira et al., 2005). Brazil reported a record of 780,644 cases of dengue caused by DEN3, including 2607 cases of DHF in 2002 (Fig. 1B), representing more than 70% of dengue fever cases reported in the Americas. Hyper-endemicity has now been documented in nearly all countries in the Americas, increasing the risk that dengue virus infections will be clinically severe (Wilson and Chen, 2002).

Clinical features

The incubation period and clinical features of dengue virus infection in humans have been described (Siler et al., 1926; Simmons et al., 1931; Sabin 1952). Dengue infection in adults may be inapparent or may lead to a range of illnesses from undifferentiated fever, clinically indistinguishable from many other viral or bacterial infections, to mild dengue fever, to severe DHF/DSS with hypovolemic shock. Primary dengue virus infections in infants and young children are usually present as an undifferentiated febrile illness, whereas secondary dengue infections are more often clinically severe.

Dengue fever

Classical dengue fever, usually a disease of older children and adults, can occur during primary or secondary dengue virus infections. The incubation period varies from 3 to 14 or more days (average 5–7 days). Typically, the disease begins with a sudden onset of fever with temperature rising to 103–106°F (39–41°C) accompanied by a variety of signs and symptoms, including severe headache, retro-orbital pain, photophobia, conjunctival hyperemia, bradycardia, and a transient macular rash. Flushing commonly appears on the face, neck, and chest. Initial symptoms are followed by althralgia, myalgia, anorexia, bone pain, abdominal discomfort, vomiting, and general weakness. Severe muscle and bone pain are characteristic of dengue fever in adults but are rare in children (George and Lum, 1997). Fever may continue for 2–7 days or may be biphasic with a return to near normal for 12–24 h and then rising again. Coincident with defervescence or shortly thereafter a second rash may appear, maculopapular or morbilliform and non-irritating. Although less common, mild hemorrhagic manifestations, such as petechiae, purpura, hematuria, gingival bleeding, epistaxis, menorrhagia, and gastrointestinal breading may occur in dengue fever patients. Severe gastrointestinal bleeding associated with DEN1 infection has been reported in patients with peptic ulcers (Wang et al., 1990; Tsai et al., 1991). Myocarditis (Promphan et al., 2004), ocular abnormalities, and neurologic manifestations including Guillain–Barré syndrome (Santos et al., 2004), and encephalopathy have also been reported in dengue fever patients (Chotmongkol and Sawanyawisuth, 2004). Dengue fever is rarely fatal, but convalescence may be prolonged and associated with fatigue and depression, especially in adults.

Clinical laboratory tests reveal a reduced leukocyte count with an absolute granulocytopenia. Mild elevations in serum liver enzyme levels may also occur.

Dengue hemorrhagic fever

DHF and DSS are increasingly common in dengue endemic areas. In children under age 15, DHF is now the major cause of hospitalization in Southeast Asia and DHF may also occur in adults in certain regions (Gonzalez et al., 2005; Dietz et al., 1990; Liu et al., 2003). DHF usually follows secondary dengue infections, but may also occur during primary infections, especially in infants (Halstead et al., 1969). Regardless of age, the clinical manifestations of DHF are similar and begin with sudden rise of temperature and generalized constitutional symptoms that are indistinguishable from classical dengue fever. Clinical deterioration is usually coincident with the time of defervescence, when temperature falls to normal or below, and when plasma leakage and hemorrhage become manifest. Typically, tachycardia and hypotension characterize the onset of plasma leakage, which may lead to prolonged capillary refill time, narrow pulse pressure and shock. Ascites and pleural effusions occur.

Hemorrhagic features are characterized by petechiae, purpuric lesions, ecchymoses, bleeding at venipuncture sites, and a positive tourniquet test indicating increased capillary fragility. Epistaxis, gingival bleeding, hematuria, and GI bleeding may also occur, accompanied by increased vascular permeability. Blood tests show thrombocytopenia (platelet counts $<100,000/mm^3$) and evidence of hematoconcentration (hematocrit increased by $\geqslant 20\%$ due to plasma leakage). (Later, in the event of severe hemorrhage, the hematocrit will drop.) Acute abdominal pain and persistent vomiting with a progressive decrease in platelet count and rise in hematocrit are warning signs for the development of DSS. The duration of shock is short, with patients either dying in the first 24 h or recovering rapidly. The fatality rate of DSS is 10–50%, depending on the level of supportive care in the hospital.

Hepatomegaly is observed more frequently in DHF than in dengue fever (Mohan et al., 2000) and the degree of enlargement varies from country to country, possibly reflecting variations in measurement technique, virus virulence, or population susceptibility (George and Lum, 1997). Elevations in serum aminotransferase levels also are observed more frequently in DHF than in dengue fever. Encephalopathy occurs rarely in dengue virus infection, as a consequence of either intracranial hemorrhage, cerebral edema, hyponatremia, cerebral anoxia, fulminant hepatic failure, or microcapillary hemorrhage. The WHO has issued guidelines for classification of DHF into four grades (Grade I–IV) of increasing severity, applicable to childhood DHF in Asia as well as adult DHF in the Americas. Grade III is characterized by cold, clammy skin, weak pulse, narrowing of the pulse pressure (<20 mm Hg) and hypotension, and may progress to profound shock (Grade IV).

Laboratory diagnosis

Laboratory diagnosis of dengue infection is based on the detection of dengue virus or dengue virus-specific antibodies. Assays for antibodies can provide reliable diagnosis of current or recent infection from properly timed serum samples. Appropriately standardized assays can differentiate between primary and secondary dengue infections, which are important because secondary dengue infection has a greater risk of developing DHF. Molecular methods such as RT-PCR allow for rapid detection and serotype specificity. The method of choice is indicated by the objectives of the clinician and the available specimens.

Serologic tests

A variety of tests are available to detect anti-dengue antibodies. These include hemagglutination inhibition (HI), complement fixation (CF), IgM capture (MAC), and indirect IgG ELISA assays, and the virus neutralization test (NT).

The HI test is widely used for diagnosis of recent infection and for seroepidemiological studies (Clarke and Casals, 1958). By day 5 of febrile illness during primary dengue virus infection, HI antibodies are generally detectable at a titer greater than the cut-off titer of 1 : 10. In convalescent sera, HI titers may reach 1 : 640 or greater. Paired sera collected at the time of hospital admission (acute phase) and discharge (convalescent phase) that exhibit a fourfold or greater rise in titer in the same assay run are diagnostic for dengue virus infection. Primary dengue virus infection is characterized by a slow rise in HI antibody titers to about 1 : 1280 within at least 7 days. In secondary dengue virus infection, there is a rapid anamnestic antibody response with HI titers increasing to 1 : 2560 or greater within a few days of infection. An HI titer greater than 1 : 1280 in an acute or early convalescent-phase serum sample is presumptively diagnostic for secondary dengue infection. HI titers generally fall to below 1 : 640 after 1–2 months but remain detectable for many years. HI antibodies are broadly flavivirus cross-reactive so that virus-specific diagnosis is usually not possible, although mono-specific responses may be detected using other assays during primary infection.

The CF assay detects dengue complement-fixing antibodies with a positive cut-off titer of 1:2. Like HI, antibodies measured by CF are flavivirus cross-reactive and the assay is difficult to standardize; therefore, CF is no longer widely used.

The MAC-ELISA assay measures dengue-specific IgM antibodies and is the most widely used diagnostic test for primary dengue infection. Anti-dengue IgM antibodies are generally detectible by day 5 of illness, reach a peak by 2 weeks, and wane after 2–3 months. In contrast, in secondary dengue virus infection, IgM antibody only rises transiently and to a low peak titer. Detection of anti-dengue IgM indicates a recent infection, though not necessarily a current infection (Vorndam and Kuno, 1997). MAC-ELISA is also useful for population-based surveillance. Efforts have been made to standardize the MAC-ELISA test by using mammalian cell-derived virus-like particles containing prM-E (Holmes et al., 2005) or synthetic peptides (Videa et al., 2005). The specificity of the MAC-ELISA test for IgM antibodies in a single serum sample is similar to that of the HI test using paired sera.

NT is the only test for anti-dengue antibodies that is serotype-specific. A variety of newer formats of NT are being developed to increase assay speed (Vorndam and Beltran, 2002; Martin et al., 2006).

Virus isolation and identification

Dengue viremia usually begins around 24 h before onset of fever and ends as fever subsides. In a prospective study of children with DHF as a result of secondary infection, titers of dengue virus in serum ranged from $10^{1.8}$ to 10^8 pfu/ml, with titers in DEN4 infections being about 100-fold lower than those of the other three serotypes (Gubler et al., 1981). In dengue fever patients with primary infection, virus titers in serum are generally $<10^6$ pfu/ml.

Laboratory isolation of dengue viruses is usually performed by inoculation of C6/36 cells or Vero cells, which are incubated for up to 14 days, and infection is detected either by plaque assay of culture supernatants or by immunofluorescence assay of infected cells to detect viral-associated antigen. Virus serotype can be determined using type-specific mouse monoclonal antibodies.

Dengue viruses can also be isolated by intra-thoracic inoculation of live mosquitoes (most commonly *Tox. amboinensis*) (Rosen and Gubler, 1974). It is important that virus isolation be conducted in reference laboratories skilled in virus typing and characterization.

Virus detection by PCR and other molecular methods

PCR permits rapid and accurate differential diagnosis of dengue infection crucial for effective treatment, disease surveillance, and control. The method for nested RT-PCR is about 10 times more sensitive than most real-time RT-PCR assays, but the real-time RT-PCR assay is about 4 times faster (Lanciotti, 2003; Shu and Huang, 2004). Methods are available to detect viremia as 0.02 pfu of virus per reaction (0.4 pfu/ml). (Johnson et al., 2005), but lack standardization and validation (Teles et al., 2005). A highly sensitive immuno-capture ELISA has been described that can specifically detect the NS1 protein even when the virus genome cannot be detected by RT-PCR (Alcon et al., 2002).

Pathogenesis and pathology

Studies of DHF/DSS tissue specimens have shown no obvious pathognomonic lesions at the organ level (Bhamaraparati, 1997). Diffuse petechial hemorrhages of most organs and serous effusions into pericardial, pleural, and peritoneal cavities are common, consistent with the clinical features. Microscopically, swelling of endothelial cells, gap formation in the vascular wall, and perivascular edema with little or no infiltration are observed, consistent with loss of integrity of the tight junctions (Sahaphong et al., 1980). Proliferation of plasma cells or lymphocytes is observed in spleen, lymph node, and lung tissues. Microscopic examination of the enlarged liver reveals mild-to-moderate zonal necrosis and Councilman bodies. Dengue antigens are shown to be present in Kupfler cells and hepatocytes. Direct identification of cells where dengue virus replication takes place in humans has been difficult. The presence of viral RNA within cells that stain positive for viral antigen in spleen and blood-clot samples suggests the presence of active viral replication in these tissues (Jessie et al., 2004). Two main hypotheses have emerged to explain the pathogenesis of DHF/DSS. The first hypothesis is that it is caused by dengue virus strains that possess increased virulence. The second hypothesis, which arose from the observation that most cases of DHF occur after a secondary dengue infection, proposes a key role for ADE of infection in the disease process. These hypotheses are not mutually exclusive, and most likely both are valid.

Viral virulence factors

Dengue viruses undergo genetic and structural changes that may affect their virulence, as a result of replication and selection pressure in both mosquito and human hosts. An increase in viral virulence has been proposed to explain severe dengue associated with primary infection that occurs late in dengue epidemics (Rosen, 1977). For instance, a large outbreak of severe dengue in Greece in 1927–1928 was thought to be due to primary DEN1 infection, with no evidence of previous dengue infections in the population for at least 13 years previously (Rosen, 1986).

Increased viral replication, resulting in high levels of viremia and virus sequence diversity may play a role in dengue virulence (Wang et al., 2002, 2003). A prospective study in young children with secondary DEN2 virus infection in Thailand revealed a correlation between disease severity and high virus titers in serum (Vaughn et al., 2000). Specific virulence determinants have not been found, although a unique 3′ RNA secondary structure appears to be present in isolates from DSS patients (Mangada and Igarashi, 1998). In the Americas, DEN2 and other serotypes caused mainly mild cases of dengue fever prior to 1981; introduction of a new strain of DEN2 in Cuba in 1981 resulted in an epidemic with DHF, followed by other major DHF epidemics in other countries in the region. Molecular analysis of virus isolates from these DHF outbreaks has identified strains with increased pathogenecity (Rico-Hesse et al., 1997). Phylogenetic studies suggest that two distinct DEN2 genotypes from Southeast Asia were introduced and replaced the native American genotype in at least four countries.

Sequence analysis of viruses isolated from dengue fever and DHF patients in Thailand and the Americas has identified distinct structures that correlate with increased pathogenesis (Leitmeyer et al., 1999). The American genotype structures appear to be associated with lower ability to replicate than the Southeast Asian genotype structures (Cologna and Rico-Hesse, 2003). In contrast, infection with an American genotype of DEN2 in Iquitos, Peru, in 1999 was not associated with much disease in a population of that was immune to DEN1 (Kochel et al., 2002). The American DEN2 virus from the Iquitos outbreak was neutralized *in vitro* by serum from the patients who were immune to DEN1, whereas the Southeast Asia DEN2 virus was poorly neutralized by anti-DEN1 sera. This suggests that neutralizing epitopes shared by the DEN1 virus and the American DEN2 virus conferred some degree of cross-protection, in contrast to the non-neutralizing, cross-reactive epitopes, which might have led to enhanced infection with a DEN2 strain.

The secondary dengue hypothesis and the concept of antibody-dependent enhancement

According to the secondary dengue hypothesis, individuals experiencing a secondary infection with a serotype different from their primary infection have a significantly greater risk for developing severe disease (Halstead, 1970). Data to support this hypothesis are derived in part from maternal–infant studies in Thailand.

Extensive studies of DHF/DSS in the 1960s in Thailand demonstrated a bimodal age-dependent incidence pattern of dengue virus infections in children, with one disease peak at 7–8 months for infants 3–11 months of age, mainly associated with primary dengue infections, and another peak at 6–7 years, mainly associated with secondary dengue infections (Halstead et al., 1969). Since most of the infants with DHF were born to mothers who had antibodies from earlier dengue infections, it appeared that low levels of maternally transferred antibodies might be sensitizing them, similar to the way a primary infection would, making them more likely to develop DHF and DSS (Kliks et al., 1988). These observations, together with the finding that multiple dengue virus serotypes were co-circulating in the endemic region, form the basis for the hypothesis.

Additional support for this hypothesis comes from a study mentioned earlier, in which nearly 95% of the DHF cases were associated with secondary infections (Guzman et al., 1987). Prior to this epidemic, there was a primary DEN1 epidemic without DHF in 1977 in the same population affecting 4.5 million people. DHF did not occur in individuals too young to have lived through the earlier DEN1 epidemic and therefore are unlikely to have been sensitized by an earlier heterologous infection. Studies of other dengue epidemics generally support the increased occurrence of DHF in secondary dengue infections (Sangkawibha et al., 1984; Qiu et al., 1991; Nogueira et al., 1993; Liu et al., 2003; Guzman, 2005). A prior dengue infection has been calculated to increase the risk for subsequent development of DHF by at least 6.5 times (Burke et al., 1988).

A good animal model for DHF is still not available to confirm the secondary infection hypothesis. Non-human primates exhibit viremia without overt disease after dengue virus infection, but only 1 of 118 monkeys infected sequentially with a different serotype developed DHF-like disease or exhibited laboratory abnormalities similar to those seen in humans with DHF (Halstead et al., 1973).

Peripheral mononuclear lymphocytes from humans and monkeys appear to be important targets for dengue infection. Viral replication in these cells can be enhanced by non-neutralizing or sub-neutralizing, serotype cross-reactive antibodies (Halstead et al., 1976; Marchette et al., 1976), presumably by the formation of virus-IgG complexes, which are internalized by monocytes via Fcγ receptors on the cell surface. These observations provide evidence for the occurrence of ADE in dengue virus infection (Halstead, 1989). It was also hypothesized that the formation of circulating immune complexes could lead to complement activation (Bokisch et al., 1973). Depression of serum C3 and C5 and elevation of complement activation products C3a and C5a and circulating immune complexes were detected in DHF patients at the onset of shock (Ruangjirachuporn et al., 1979; Malasit, 1987).

Dengue-specific CD4+ and CD8+ T-lymphocytes have been detected following infection in humans (Bukowski et al., 1989; Livingston et al., 1994). These are both dengue serotype-specific and cross-reactive and lyse autologous dengue-infected cells in an HLA class-restricted manner (Kurane et al., 1991a). It has been hypothesized that excessive T-lymphocyte activation plays a major role in DHF (Kurane et al., 1991b), as the levels of soluble interleukin-2 (IL2) receptor, soluble CD4, soluble CD8, and interferon gamma are higher in DHF patients than in dengue fever patients.

A model linking ADE and T-cell activation has been proposed to explain the mechanisms of DHF (Kurane and Ennis, 1992; Rothman, 1997). According to this model, secondary infection with a heterologous dengue serotype produces excessive T-cell activation, leading to high levels of cytokines and chemical mediators. Memory CD4+ and CD8+ T-cells proliferate in the presence of dengue antigens and produce interferon gamma, and the cytokines TNFα, interleukin-2 (IL2), and IL6 (Chen and Wang, 2002). Interferon gamma up-regulates expression of FcγR and HLA class I and II molecules on monocytes and macrophages, making these cells more permissive for viral replication and susceptible to lysis by effector T cells. Lysis of dengue virus-infected monocytes or macrophages may also produce vasoactive cytokines TNFα, IL1, IL6, and chemical mediators such a platelet-activating factor and histamine, resulting in disturbances in vascular permeability. In DHF patients, elevated levels of TNFα, IL-1, and IL-6 can be demonstrated on the day of onset of shock (Hober et al., 1993).

Treatment

There are no effective anti-viral drugs for dengue and treatment is mainly supportive. Individuals who have traveled or lived in areas endemic for dengue virus, who have febrile illnesses should seek health care, but since dengue fever is generally acute and self-limited, most cases require no hospitalization. WHO guidelines for the management of DHF and DSS are available; their adoption in 1979 by regional hospitals in Thailand reduced the case mortality rate from 13.9% to <1% (Nimmannitya, 1997; Kalayanarooj, 1999).

Control and prevention

Vector control programs aimed at reducing the mosquito population in the affected and surrounding areas are the only available control measures. There are no licensed dengue vaccines, but experimental vaccines are under development. It is clear that a dengue vaccine must be able to induce balanced immunity to all four virus serotypes to minimize dengue infection in a region.

Vector control

A. aegypti and *A. albopictus* now have a wide geographical distribution, and various vector control measures, such as chemical and biological targeting of adult mosquitoes and larvae, have been developed. Space applications of 4% malathion or 1% fenitrothion are widely used, and ultra-low-volume spraying with bifenetrin has been shown to be effective (Lee et al., 1997). Conventional chemical fogging in a natural environment is ineffective (Chua et al., 2005). Owing to the development of vector resistance to the chemicals, regular monitoring is essential (Huong and Ngoc, 1999; Katyal et al., 2001).

   Biological control methods have been described using a variety of organisms such as larvivorous fish and endotoxin-producing *Bacillus thuringiensis* serotype H-14, which target the larvae of *A. aegypti* and *A. albopictus* (Lee et al., 1996). The use of *Mesocyclops copods* (a crustacean) for mosquito eradication in Vietnam resulted in the reduction of *A. aegypti* by approximately 90% in the first year, 93–99% by the second year, and almost complete elimination from two of three communes by the third year, compared to regions without intervention (Kay and Vu, 2005). Owing to these measures, the incidence of dengue was reduced from 14.4–112.8 cases per 100,000 people to no reported cases at the district level (Vu et al., 2005). The elimination of dengue outbreaks in Cuba from 1981 to 1990 is likely due to successful government-led campaigns to control *A. aegypti* (Gessa and Gonzalez, 1986).

   However, programs consisting solely of insecticide spraying have been generally unsuccessful in controlling mosquitoes in Southeast and South Asia. Long-term vector control appears to be feasible by relatively simple measures such as the elimination or regular cleaning of water containers and other habitats to decrease larval burden. Public education and community participation are considered essential (Gubler, 1989).

Immunization strategies

Experimental inactivated virus, recombinant subunit, and DNA vaccines

A partially purified, formalin-inactivated DEN2 vaccine (DEN2 PIV) with alum adjuvant elicits virus-neutralizing antibodies and partially protects rhesus monkeys against challenge virus of the same serotype and strain (Putnak, 1994). The DEN2 PIV and a *Drosophila*-expressed antigen consisting of the N-terminal 80% of the E antigen formulated with adjuvants, consisting of a mixture of alum and saponin with or without monophosphoryl lipid A, elicit higher-titered virus-neutralizing antibodies and protect monkeys against viremia, although sterile immunity was not observed (Putnak et al., 2005).

Recombinant prM, E, or NS1 proteins, alone or in combination, are also immunogenic and confer protection against dengue virus challenge in animal models (Zhang et al., 1988; Falgout et al., 1990; Bray and Lai, 1991a; Putnak, 1994). Expression of a truncated E gene to produce a C-terminal truncated protein approximately 80% of the full length E protein increases its immunogenicity and protective efficacy (Men et al., 1991). A recombinant vaccinia virus expressing 80% E has also been shown to protect monkeys against homologous DEN2 virus challenge (Men et al., 2000). DNA vaccines expressing the prM and E genes induce moderate levels of neutralizing antibody and at least partial protection against dengue virus challenge. A DNA vaccine expressing the prM-E gene region of DEN3 is immunogenic and protective for *Aotus* spp. monkeys (Kochel et al., 2000; Blair et al., 2006). Antibody responses and protection are improved by the co-expression of the cytokine GM-CSF (Raviprakash et al., 2001).

Live-attenuated virus vaccines

The first candidate live-attenuated dengue virus vaccines prepared by serial passage of wild-type isolates in suckling mouse brain were immunogenic and attenuated for humans. One such vaccine, MD-1, tested in 1100 volunteers, appeared to give some protection against a concurrent DEN3 epidemic (Wisseman et al., 1963; Wisseman et al., unpublished results). The first candidate live-attenuated vaccine made from cloned DEN2 (DEN2 PR 159/S1) was produced in FRhL cells using a virus selected for a small plaque, temperature-sensitive phenotype; it reduced the viremia of infection in rhesus monkeys (Eckels, et al., 1976; Scott et al., 1980) but encountered other problems later that resulted in its abandonment (Bancroft et al., 1984). It has not been possible to produce a DEN1 live-attenuated vaccine by *in vitro* chemical mutagenesis or a DEN3 vaccine by plaque cloning (McKee et al., 1987).

Candidate monovalent live vaccines produced by serial passage in PDK cells showed acceptable levels of reactogenicity and immunogenicity in Phase I clinical trials, and were subsequently combined to produce tetravalent formulations (Sun et al., 2003). This vaccine resulted in seroconversion to each serotype at rates ranging from approximately 40–80%, with up to 70% of recipients exhibiting seroconversion against three or four serotypes, depending upon the formulation (Edelman et al., 2003). Further clinical development of this dengue vaccine is ongoing. Table 1 summarizes the current status of tetravalent vaccine candidates.

Additional candidate live-attenuated vaccines (Vaughn et al., 1996; Bhamarapravati and Sutee, 2000) demonstrated that the monovalent vaccines were safe and immunogenic. Tetravalent formulations have also been tested in clinical trials (Kanesa-Thasan et al., 2001; Sabchareon et al., 2004). The tetravalent vaccines in some cases produced an unbalanced immune response with antibody primarily against DEN3 and a high frequency of DEN3 viremia, and an unacceptable level of reactogenicity (Kitchener et al., 2006).

It appears that putative *in vitro* markers of dengue virus attenuation, e.g., small plaque morphology or temperature sensitivity, and *in vivo* markers, e.g., reduced viremia in non-human primates, are poor predictors of attenuation for humans (Innis et al., 1988). Furthermore, the reactogenicity and immunogenicity of tetravalent vaccine formulations cannot always be predicted from clinical evaluation of the individual monovalent vaccine components.

Genetic engineering has been used as an alternative to conventional cell passage. These have been used to create intertypic chimeras from DEN4 deletion mutants, in which the antigen-encoding genes C-prM-E or prM-E of DEN4 are replaced by the corresponding genes from DEN1, DEN2, or DEN3 (Bray and Lai, 1991b; Chen et al., 1995). Protective immunity was produced by immunization with these chimeras in non-human primates (Bray et al., 1996). A 30-nucleotide deletion mutation within the conserved 3'-NCR that leads to attenuation of wild-type DEN4 for both non-human primates and humans has been identified (Men et al., 1996; Durbin et al., 2001; Durbin et al., 2005). This attenuating mutation was used to produce vaccine candidates for DEN1, DEN2, and DEN3 in the DEN4 backbone (Blaney et al., 2005). Intertypic dengue chimeras have also been constructed using the DEN2 PDK53 vaccine as the backbone (Huang et al., 2003). Mutations within the DEN2 5'-NCR, NS1 and NS3, selected for by passage in PDK cells, have been identified that led to reduced viral replication in cell culture and in mice (Butrapet et al., 2000) and might be suitable for future experimental vaccines. Chimeric vaccine candidates were also constructed using the attenuated 17D yellow fever vaccine as a backbone to express the PrM-E genes of all dengue virus serotypes for use in pre-clinical studies (Guirakhoo et al., 2001; Guirakhoo et al., 2004) and clinical trials (Guirakhoo et al., 2005). Genetically engineered dengue vaccines may, by virtue of their targeted mutations, produce an acceptable safety profile and may elicit a balanced immune response (Lai and Monath, 2003).

Passive immunization

Passive immunization with humanized monoclonal antibodies offers an alternative to vaccines for short-term prevention of dengue fever. Fab antibody fragments that efficiently neutralize one or more dengue viruses have been obtained from chimpanzees infected with all four dengue virus serotypes. A humanized IgG was produced that neutralizes DEN4 strains at a titer of 0.03–0.05 μg/ml by plaque reduction neutralization test (PRNT) (Men et al., 2004) and another, IgG 1A5, that cross-neutralizes DEN1 and DEN2 at PRNT titers of 0.48 and 0.98 μg/ml, respectively (Goncalvez et al., 2004). Interestingly, IgG 1A5 also neutralizes DEN3, DEN4, and West Nile virus at PRNT titers ranging from 3.2 to 4.3 μg/ml. The major classes of Fc receptor have been identified and their interacting sequences in the Fc region of IgG mapped (Chappel et al., 1993) so that it should be possible to alter the FcγR binding sequences such that these antibodies would not enhance virus replication *in vitro*, thus reducing the risk for inducing ADE when the antibodies are used clinically.

Conclusions

Studies over the past three-quarters of a century have led to the accumulation of knowledge invaluable to our understanding of the dengue viruses and the diseases they cause. However, the goals of a safe, effective vaccine and vector eradication have been elusive. One might ask why the control of dengue has been so difficult to achieve. First, there are lack of good animal models for dengue disease and for evaluation of vaccine safety and efficacy. Second, it has been difficult to develop vaccines capable of inducing balanced immunity to all four serotypes, and a tetravalent vaccine will be necessary in order to minimize the risk for severe disease resulting from secondary dengue virus infections. Third, the dengue viruses and mosquito vectors are becoming increasingly widespread and the incidence of DHF is rising. A better understanding of vector–virus–human host interactions and the development of new rapid diagnostic assays should help in devising more effective measures for monitoring and controlling outbreaks. Data from vaccine trials are promising, and new developments in this area are expected. Genetically engineered vaccine candidates, such as chimeric dengue viruses, offer hope for more predictable attenuation of virulence and balanced immunogenicity.

References

Alcon S, Talarmin A, Debruyne M, Falconar A, Deubel V, Flamand M. Enzyme-linked immunosorbent assay specific to Dengue virus type 1 nonstructural protein NS1 reveals circulation of the antigen in the blood during the acute phase of disease in patients experiencing primary or secondary infections. J Clin Microbiol 2002; 40: 376.

Allison SL, Schalich J, Stiasny K, Mandl CW, Kunz C, Heinz FX. Oligomeric rearrangement of tick-borne encephalitis virus envelope proteins induced by an acidic pH. J Virol 1995; 69: 695.

Ashburn PM, Craig CF. Experimental investigations regarding the etiology of dengue fever. J Infect Dis 1907; 4: 776.

Bancroft TL. On the aetiology of dengue fever. Aust Med Gaz 1906; 25: 17.

Bancroft WH, Scott RM, Eckels KH, Hoke Jr. CH, Simms TE, Jesrani KD, Summers PL, Dubois DR, Tsoulos D, Russell PK. Dengue virus type 2 vaccine: reactogenicity and immunogenicity in soldiers. J Infect Dis 1984; 149: 1005–1010.

Bazan JF, Fletterick RJ. Detection of a trypsin-like serine protease domain in flaviviruses and pestiviruses. Virology 1989; 171: 637.

Bhamaraparati N. Pathology of dengue infections. In: Dengue and Dengue Hemorrhagic Fever (Gubler DJ, Kuno G, editors). London: CAB International; 1997; p. 115.

Bhamarapravati N, Sutee Y. Live attenuated tetravalent dengue vaccine. Vaccine 2000; 18(Suppl 2): 44.

Bielefeldt-Ohmann H, Meyer M, Fitzpatrick DR, Mackenzie JS. Dengue virus binding to human leukocyte cell lines: receptor usage differs between cell types and virus strains. Virus Res 2001; 73: 81.

Blair PJ, Kochel TJ, Raviprakash K, Guevara C, Salazar M, Wu SJ, Olson JG, Porter KR. Evaluation of immunity and protective efficacy of a dengue-3 premembrane and envelope DNA vaccine in *Aotus nancymae* monkeys. Vaccine 2006; 24: 1427.

Blaney Jr. JE, Matro JM, Murphy BR, Whitehead SS. Recombinant, live-attenuated tetravalent dengue virus vaccine formulations induce a balanced, broad, and protective neutralizing antibody response against each of the four serotypes in rhesus monkeys. J Virol 2005; 79: 5516.

Bokisch VA, Top Jr. FH, Russell PK, Dixon FJ, Muller-Eberhard HJ. The potential pathogenic role of complement in dengue hemorrhagic shock syndrome. N Engl J Med 1973; 289: 996.

Brandt WE, Chiewslip D, Harris DL, Russell PK. Partial purification and characterization of a dengue virus soluble complement-fixing antigen. J Immunol 1970; 105: 1565.

Bray M, Lai CJ. Dengue virus premembrane and membrane proteins elicit a protective immune response. Virology 1991a; 185: 505.

Bray M, Lai CJ. Construction of intertypic chimeric dengue viruses by substitution of structural protein genes. Proc Natl Acad Sci USA 1991b; 88: 10342.

Bray M, Men R, Lai CJ. Monkeys immunized with intertypic chimeric dengue viruses are protected against wild-type virus challenge. J Virol 1996; 70: 4162.

Bressanelli S, Stiasny K, Allison SL, Stura EA, Duquerroy S, Lescar J, Heinz FX, Rey FA. Structure of a flavivirus envelope glycoprotein in its low-pH-induced membrane fusion conformation. EMBO J 2004; 23: 728.

Brinton MA, Dispoto JH. Sequence and secondary structure analysis of the 5′-terminal region of flavivirus genome RNA. Virology 1988; 162: 290.

Brinton MA, Fernandez AV, Dispoto JH. The 3′-nucleotides of flavivirus genomic RNA form a conserved secondary structure. Virology 1986; 153: 113.

Bukowski JF, Kurane I, Lai CJ, Bray M, Falgout B, Ennis FA. Dengue virus-specific cross-reactive CD8+ human cytotoxic T lymphocytes. J Virol 1989; 63: 5086.

Burke DS, Nisalak A, Johnson DE, Scott RM. A prospective study of dengue infections in Bangkok. Am J Trop Med Hyg 1988; 38: 172.

Butrapet S, Huang CY, Pierro DJ, Bhamarapravati N, Gubler DJ, Kinney RM. Attenuation markers of a candidate dengue type 2 vaccine virus, strain 16681 (PDK-53), are defined by mutations in the 5' noncoding region and nonstructural proteins 1 and 3. J Virol 2000; 74: 3011.

Calisher CH, Karabatsos N, Darlymple JM, Shope RE, Porterfield JS, Westaway EG, Brandt WE. Antigenic relationships between flaviviruses as determined by cross-neutralization tests with polyclonal sera. J Gen Virol 1989; 70: 37.

Casals J. The arthropod-borne group of animal viruses. Trans N Y Acad Sci 1957; 19: 219.

Chandler AC, Rice L. Observations on the etiology of dengue fever. Am J Trop Med 1923; 3: 233.

Chappel MS, Isenman DE, Oomen R, Xu YY, Klein MH. Identification of a secondary Fc gamma RI binding site within a genetically engineered human IgG antibody. J Biol Chem 1993; 268: 25124.

Chen Y, Maguire T, Hileman RE, Fromm JR, Esko JD, Linhardt RJ, Marks RM. Dengue virus infectivity depends on envelope protein binding to target cell heparan sulfate. Nat Med 1997; 3: 866.

Chen YC, Wang SY. Activation of terminally differentiated human monocytes/macrophages by dengue virus: productive infection, hierarchical production of innate cytokines and chemokines, and the synergistic effect of lipopolysaccharide. J Virol 2002; 76: 9877.

Chen W, Kawano H, Men R, Clark D, Lai CJ. Construction of intertypic chimeric dengue viruses exhibiting type 3 antigenicity and neurovirulence for mice. J Virol 1995; 69: 5186.

Chotmongkol V, Sawanyawisuth K. Case report: dengue hemorrhagic fever with encephalopathy in an adult. Southeast Asian J Trop Med Public Health 2004; 35: 160.

Chua KB, Chua IL, Chua IE, Chua KH. Effect of chemical fogging on immature *Aedes* mosquitoes in natural field conditions. Singapore Med J 2005; 46: 639.

Clarke DH, Casals J. Techniques for hemagglutination and hemagglutination inhibition with arthropod-borne viruses. Am J Trop Med Hyg 1958; 7: 561.

Cleland JB, Bradley B, McDonald W. Further experiments in the etiology of dengue fever. J Hyg 1919; 18: 217.

Cologna R, Rico-Hesse R. American genotype structures decrease dengue virus output from human monocytes and dendritic cells. J Virol 2003; 77: 3929.

Dietz VJ, Gubler DJ, Rigau-Perez JG, Pinheiro F, Schatzmayr HG, Bailey R, Gunn RA. Epidemic dengue 1 in Brazil, 1986: evaluation of a clinically based dengue surveillance system. Am J Epidemiol 1990; 131: 693.

Durbin AP, Karron RA, Sun W, Vaughn DW, Reynolds MJ, Perreault JR, Thumar B, Men R, Lai CJ, Elkins WR, Chanock RM, Murphy BR, Whitehead SS. Attenuation and immunogenicity in humans of a live dengue virus type-4 vaccine candidate with a 30 nucleotide deletion in its 3'-untranslated region. Am J Trop Med Hyg 2001; 65: 405.

Durbin AP, Whitehead SS, McArthur J, Perreault JR, Blaney Jr. JE, Thumar B, Murphy BR, Karron RA. rDEN4 delta30, a live attenuated dengue virus type 4 vaccine candidate, is safe, immunogenic, and highly infectious in healthy adult volunteers. J Infect Dis 2005; 191: 710.

de Silva AM, Dittus WP, Amerasinghe PH, Amerasinghe FP. Serologic evidence for an epizootic dengue virus infecting toque macaques (*Macaca sinica*) at Polonnaruwa, Sri Lanka. Am J Trop Med Hyg 1999; 60: 300.

Eckels KH, Brandt WE, Harrison VR, McCown JM, Russell PK. Isolation of a temperature-sensitive dengue-2 virus under conditions suitable for vaccine development. Infect Immun 1976; 14: 1221.

Eckels KH, Scott RM, Bancroft WH, Brown J, Dubois DR, Summers PL, Russell PK, Halstead SB. Selection of attenuated dengue 4 viruses by serial passage in primary kidney cells. V. Human response to immunization with a candidate vaccine prepared in fetal rhesus lung cells. Am J Trop Med Hyg 1994; 33: 684.

Edelman R, Wasserman SS, Bodison SA, Putnak RJ, Eckels KH, Tang D, Kanesa-Thasan N, Vaughn DW, Innis BL, Sun W. Phase I trial of 16 formulations of a tetravalent live-attenuated dengue vaccine. Am J Trop Med Hyg 2003; 69(6 Suppl): 48.

Effler PV, Pang L, Kitsutani P, Vorndam V, Nakata M, Ayers T, Elm J, Tom T, Reiter P, Rigau-Perez JG, Hayes JM, Mills K, Napier M, Clark GG, Gubler DJ. Dengue fever, Hawaii, 2001–2002. Emerg Infect Dis 2005; 11: 742.

Egloff MP, Benarroch O, Selisko B, Romette JL, Canard B. An RNA Cap (nucleoside-2′-0-)-methyltransferase in the flavivirus RNA polymerase NS5: Crystal structure and functional characterization. EMBO J. 2002; 21: 2757.

Falgout B, Bray M, Schlesinger JJ, Lai CJ. Immunization of mice with recombinant vaccinia virus expressing authentic dengue virus nonstructural protein NS1 protects against lethal dengue virus encephalitis. J Virol 1990; 64: 4356.

Falgout B, Chanock R, Lai CJ. Proper processing of dengue virus nonstructural glycoprotein NS1 requires the N-terminal hydrophobic signal sequence and the downstream nonstructural protein NS2a. J Virol 1989; 63: 1852.

Falgout B, Pethel M, Zhang YM, Lai CJ. Both nonstructural proteins NS2B and NS3 are required for the proteolytic processing of dengue virus nonstructural proteins. J Virol 1991; 65: 2467.

Ferlenghi I, Clarke M, Ruttan T, Allison SL, Schalich J, Heinz FX, Harrison SC, Rey FA, Fuller SD. Molecular organization of a recombinant subviral particle from tick-borne encephalitis virus. Mol Cell 2001; 7: 593.

Fu J, Tan B-H, Yap E-U, Chan Y-C, Tan Y-H. Full-length cDNA sequence of dengue type 1 virus (Singapore strain S275/90). Virology 1992; 188: 953.

George R, Lum LCS. Clinical spectrum of dengue infection. In: Dengue and Dengue Hemorrhagic Fever (Gubler DJ, Kuno G, editors). London: CAB International; 1997; p. 89.

Gessa JAA, Gonzalez RF. Application of governmental management principles in the program for eradication of *Aedes (Stegomyia) aegypti* (linneaus 1762) in the Republic of Cuba. Bull Pan Am Health Organ 1986; 186.

Goncalvez AP, Men R, Wernly C, Purcell RH, Lai CJ. Chimpanzee Fab fragments and a derived humanized immunoglobulin G1 antibody that efficiently cross-neutralize dengue type 1 and type 2 viruses. J Virol 2004; 78: 12910.

Gonzalez D, Castro OE, Kouri G, Perez J, Martinez E, Vazquez S, Rosario D, Cancio R, Guzman MG. Classical dengue hemorrhagic fever resulting from two dengue infections spaced 20 years or more apart: Havana, dengue 3 epidemic, 2001–2002. Int J Infect Dis 2005; 9: 280.

Gorbalenya AE, Donchenko AP, Koonin EV, Blinov VM. N-terminal domains of putative helicases of flavi- and pestiviruses may be serine proteases. Nucleic Acids Res 1989; 17: 3889.

Graham H. The dengue: a study of its pathology and mode of propagation. J Trop Med 1903; 6: 209.

Gubler DJ. *Aedes aegypti* and *Aedes aegypti*-borne disease control in the 1990s: top down or bottom up. Am J Trop Med Hyg 1989; 40: 571.

Gubler DJ. Dengue and dengue hemorrhagic fever. Clin Microbiol Rev 1998; 11: 480.

Gubler DJ, Novak RJ, Vergne E, Colon NA, Velez M, Fowler J. *Aedes* (*Gymnometopa*) *mediovittatus* (Diptera: *Culicidae*), a potential maintenance vector of dengue viruses in Puerto Rico. J Med Entomol 1985; 22: 469.

Gubler DJ, Suharyono W, Tan R, Abidin M, Sie A. Viremia in patients with naturally acquired dengue infection. Bull World Health Organ 1981; 59: 623.

Guirakhoo F, Arroyo J, Pugachev KV, Miller C, Zhang ZX, Weltzin R, Georgakopoulos K, Catalan J, Ocran S, Soike K, Ratterree M, Monath TP. Construction, safety, and immunogenicity in nonhuman primates of a chimeric yellow fever-dengue virus tetravalent vaccine. J Virol 2001; 75: 7290.

Guirakhoo F, Lang J, Monath TP. Chimeric yellow fever-dengue tetravalent vaccine. Pediatric Dengue Vaccine Initiative. Meeting abstract, 2005; p. 9.

Guirakhoo F, Pugachev K, Zhang Z, Myers G, Levenbook I, Draper K, Lang J, Ocran S, Mitchell F, Parsons M, Brown N, Brandler S, Fournier C, Barrere B, Rizvi F, Travassos A, Nichols R, Trent D, Monath T. Safety and efficacy of chimeric yellow fever-dengue virus tetravalent vaccine formulations in nonhuman primates. J Virol 2004; 78: 4761.

Guzman MG. Global voices of science. Deciphering dengue: the Cuban experience. Science 2005; 309: 1495.

Guzman MG, Alvarez M, Rodriguez R, Rosario D, Vazquez S, Vald SL, Cabrera MV, Kouri G. Fatal dengue hemorrhagic fever in Cuba, 1997. Int J Infect Dis 1999; 3: 130.

Guzman MG, Kouri G, Martinez E, Bravo J, Riveron R, Soler M, Vazquez S, Morier L. Clinical and serologic study of Cuban children with dengue hemorrhagic fever/dengue shock syndrome (DHF/DSS). Bull Pan Am Health Organ 1987; 21: 270.

Hahn CS, Hahn YS, Rice CM, Lee E, Dalgarno L, Strauss EG, Strauss JH. Conserved elements in the 3′ untranslated region of flavivirus RNAs and potential cyclization sequences. J Mol Biol 1987; 198: 33.

Hahn YS, Galler R, Hunkapiller T, Dalrymple JM, Strauss JH, Strauss EG. Nucleotide sequence of dengue 2 RNA and comparison of the encoded proteins with those of other flaviviruses. Virology 1988; 162: 167.

Hales S, Weinstein P, Woodward A. Dengue fever epidemics in the South Pacific: driven by El Nino Southern Oscillation? Lancet 1996; 348(9042): 1664.

Halstead SB. Observations related to pathogenesis of dengue hemorrhagic fever. VI. Hypotheses and discussion. Yale J Biol Med 1970; 42: 350.

Halstead SB. Antibody, macrophages, dengue virus infection, shock, and hemorrhage: a pathogenetic cascade. Rev Infect Dis 1989; 11(Suppl 4): 830.

Halstead SB, Eckels KH, Putvatana R, Larsen LK, Marchette NJ. Selection of attenuated dengue 4 viruses by serial passage in primary kidney cells. IV. Characterization of a vaccine candidate in fetal rhesus lung cells. Am J Trop Med Hyg 1984; 33: 679.

Halstead SB, Marchette NJ, Sung Chow JS, Lolekha S. Dengue virus replication enhancement in peripheral blood leukocytes from immune human beings. Proc Soc Exp Biol Med 1976; 151: 136.

Halstead SB, Scanlon JE, Umpaivit P, Udomsakdi S. Dengue and chikungunya virus infection in man in Thailand, 1962–1964. IV. Epidemiologic studies in the Bangkok metropolitan area. Am J Trop Med Hyg 1969; 18: 997.

Halstead SB, Shotwell H, Casals J. Studies on the pathogenesis of dengue infection in monkeys. II. Clinical laboratory responses to heterologous infection. J Infect Dis 1973; 128: 15.

Halstead SB, Yamarat C. Recent epidemics of hemorrhagic fever in Thailand: observations related to pathogenesis of a 'new' dengue disease. Am J Public Health 1965; 5: 386.

Hammon W, Rudnick A, Sather GE. Viruses associated with hemorrhagic fever of the Philippines and Thailand. Science 1960a; 131: 1102.

Hammon WM, Rudnick A, Sather G, Rogers KD, Morse LJ. New hemorrhagic fevers of children in the Philippines and Thailand. Trans Assoc Am Physicians 1960b; 73: 140.

Heinz FX. Epitope mapping of flavivirus glycoproteins. Adv Virus Res 1986; 31: 103.

Heinz FX, Allison SL, Stiasny K, Schalich J, Holzmann H, Mandl CW, Kunz C. Recombinant and virion-derived soluble and particulate immunogens for vaccination against tick-borne encephalitis. Vaccine 1995; 13: 1636.

Henchal EA, Gentry MK, McCown JM, Brandt WE. Dengue virus-specific and flavivirus group determinants identified with monoclonal antibodies by indirect immunofluorescence. Am J Trop Med Hyg 1982; 31: 830.

Hober D, Poli L, Roblin B, Gestas P, Chungue E, Granic G, Imbert P, Pecarere JL, Vergez-Pascal R, Wattre P, Maniez-Montreuil. Serum levels of tumor necrosis factor-alpha (TNF-alpha), interleukin-6 (IL-6), and interleukin-1 beta (IL-1 beta) in dengue-infected patients. Am J Trop Med Hyg 1993; 48: 324.

Holmes DA, Purdy DE, Chao DY, Noga AJ, Chang GJ. Comparative analysis of immunoglobulin M (IgM) capture enzyme-linked immunosorbent assay using virus-like particles or virus-infected mouse. J Clin Microbiol 2005; 43: 3227.

Hotta S. Experimental studies on dengue. I. Isolation, identification, and modification of the virus. J Infect Dis 1952; 90: 1.

Huang CY, Butrapet S, Tsuchiya KR, Bhamarapravati N, Gubler DJ, Kinney RM. Dengue 2 PDK-53 virus as a chimeric carrier for tetravalent dengue vaccine development. J Virol 2003; 77: 11436.

Huong VD, Ngoc NTB. Susceptibility of *Aedes aegypti* to insecticides in south Vietnam. WHO Dengue Bull 1999; 23: 85.

Igarashi A. Isolation of a Singh's *Aedes albopictus* cell clone sensitive to dengue and chikungunya viruses. J Gen Virol 1978; 40: 531.

Innis BL, Eckels KH, Kraiselburd E, Dubois DR, Meadors GF, Gubler DJ, Burke DS, Bancroft WH. Virulence of a live dengue virus vaccine candidate: a possible new marker of dengue virus attenuation. J Infect Dis 1988; 158: 876.

Isturiz RE, Gubler DJ, Brea del Castillo J. Dengue and dengue hemorrhagic fever in Latin America and the Caribbean. Infect Dis Clin North Am 2000; 14: 121.

Jessie K, Fong MY, Devi S, Lam SK, Wong KT. Localization of dengue virus in naturally infected human tissues, by immunohistochemistry and *in situ* hybridization. J Infect Dis 2004; 189: 1411.

Johnson BW, Russell BJ, Lanciotti RS. Serotype-specific detection of dengue viruses in a fourplex real-time reverse transcriptase PCR assay. J Clin Microbiol 2005; 43: 4977.

Kabra SK, Jain Y, Pandey RM, Madhulika, Singhal T, Tripathi P, Broor S, Seth P, Seth V. Dengue haemorrhagic fever in children in the 1996 Delhi epidemic. Trans R Soc Trop Med Hyg 1999; 93: 294.

Kalayanarooj S. Standardized clinical management: evidence of reduction of dengue haemorrhagic fever case-fatality rate in Thailand. WHO Dengue Bull 1999; 23.

Kanesa-thasan N, Sun W, Kim-Ahn G, Van Albert S, Putnak JR, King A, Raengsakulsrach B, Christ-Schmidt H, Gilson K, Zahradnik JM, Vaughn DW, Innis BL, Saluzzo JF, Hoke Jr. CH. Safety and immunogenicity of attenuated dengue virus vaccines (Aventis Pasteur) in human volunteers. Vaccine 2001; 19: 3179.

Kapoor M, Zhang L, Mohan PM, Padmanabhan R. Synthesis and characterization of an infectious dengue virus type-2 RNA genome (New Guinea C strain). Gene 1995a; 162: 175.

Kapoor M, Zhang L, Ramachandra M, Kusukawa J, Ebner KE, Padmanabhan R. Association between NS3 and NS5 proteins of dengue virus type 2 in the putative RNA replicase is linked to differential phosphorylation of NS5. J Biol Chem 1995b; 270: 19100.

Katyal R, Tewari P, Rahman SJ, Pajni HR, Kumar K, Gill KS. Susceptibility status of immature and adult stages of *Aedes aegypti* against conventional insecticides in Delhi, India. WHO Dengue Bull 2001; 25: 84.

Kay B, Vu SN. New strategy against *Aedes aegypti* in Vietnam. Lancet 2005; 365: 613.

Khromykh AA, Westaway EG. Subgenomic replicons of the flavivirus Kunjin: construction and applications. J Virol 1997; 71: 1497.

Kimura R, Hotta S. On the inoculation of dengue virus into mice. Nippon Igaku 1944; 3379: 629.

King CC, Wu YC, Chao DY, Lin TH, Chow L, Wang HT, Ku CC, Kao CL, Chien LJ, Chang HJ, Huang JH, Twu SJ, Huang KP, Lam SK, Gubler DJ. Major epidemics of dengue in Taiwan in 1981–2000: related to intensive virus activities in Asia. WHO Dengue Bull 2000; 24: 1.

Kitchener S, Nissen M, Nasveld P, Forrat R, Yoksan S, Lang J, Saluzzo JF. Immunogenicity and safety of two live-attenuated tetravalent dengue vaccine formulations in healthy Australian adults. Vaccine 2006; 24: 1238.

Kliks SC, Nimmanitya S, Nisalak A, Burke DS. Evidence that maternal dengue antibodies are important in the development of dengue hemorrhagic fever in infants. Am J Trop Med Hyg 1988; 38: 411.

Kochel TJ, Raviprakash K, Hayes CG, Watts DM, Russell KL, Gozalo AS, Phillips IA, Ewing DF, Murphy GS, Porter KR. A dengue virus serotype-1 DNA vaccine induces virus neutralizing antibodies and provides protection from viral challenge in *Aotus* monkeys. Vaccine 2000; 18: 3166.

Kochel TJ, Watts DM, Halstead SB, Hayes CG, Espinoza A, Felices V, Caceda R, Bautista CT, Montoya Y, Douglas S, Russell KL. Effect of dengue-1 antibodies on American dengue-2 viral infection and dengue haemorrhagic fever. Lancet 2002; 360: 310.

Konishi E, Mason PW. Proper maturation of the Japanese encephalitis virus envelope glycoprotein requires cosynthesis with the premembrane protein. J Virol 1993; 67: 1672.

Kouri GP, Guzman MG, Bravo J, Triana C. Dengue haemorrhagic fever/dengue shock syndrome: lessons from the Cuban epidemic, 1981. Bull World Health Organ 1989; 67: 375.

Kuhn RJ, Zhang W, Rossmann MG, Pletnev SV, Corver J, Lenches E, Jones CT, Mukhopadhyay S, Chipman PR, Strauss EG, Baker TS, Strauss JH. Structure of dengue virus: implications for flavivirus organization, maturation, and fusion. Cell 2002; 108: 717.

Kuno G. Dengue virus replication in a polyploid mosquito cell culture grown in serum-free medium. J Clin Microbiol 1982; 16: 851.

Kurane I, Brinton MA, Samson AL, Ennis FA. Dengue virus-specific, human CD4 + CD8-cytotoxic T-cell clones: multiple patterns of virus cross-reactivity recognized by NS3-specific T-cell clones. J Virol 1991a; 65: 1823.

Kurane I, Ennis FA. Immunity and immunopathology in dengue virus infections. Semin Immunol 1992; 4: 121.

Kurane I, Innis BL, Nimmannitya S, Nisalak A, Meager A, Janus J, Ennis FA. Activation of T lymphocytes in dengue virus infections. High levels of soluble interleukin 2 receptor, soluble CD4, soluble CD8, interleukin 2, and interferon-gamma in sera of children with dengue. J Clin Invest 1991b; 88: 1473.

Lai CJ, Monath TP. Chimeric flaviviruses: novel vaccines against dengue fever, tick-borne encephalitis, and Japanese encephalitis. Adv Virus Res 2003; 61: 469.

Lai CJ, Zhao BT, Hori H, Bray M. Infectious RNA transcribed from stably cloned full-length cDNA of dengue type 4 virus. Proc Natl Acad Sci USA 1991; 88: 5139.

Lanciotti RS. Molecular amplification assays for the detection of flaviviruses. Adv Virus Res 2003; 61: 67.

Lee HL, Gregorio Jr. R, Khadri MS, Seleena P. Ultra-low volume application of *Bacillus thuringiensis* spp. israelensis for the control of mosquitoes. J Am Mosq Control Assoc 1996; 12: 651.

Lee HL, Khadri MS, Chiang YF. Preliminary field evaluation of the combined adulticidal, larvicidal, and wall residual activity of ULV-applied bifenthrin against mosquitoes. J Vector Ecol 1997; 22: 146.

Leitmeyer KC, Vaughn DW, Watts DM, Salas R, Villalobos I, de Chacon X, Ramos C, Rico-Hesse R. Dengue virus structural differences that correlate with pathogenesis. J Virol 1999; 73: 4738.

Lindenbach RD, Rice CM. Molecular biology of flaviviruses. Adv Virus Res 2003; 59: 23.

Liu JW, Khor BS, Lee CH, Lee IK, Chen RF, Yang KD. Dengue hemorrhagic fever in Taiwan. WHO Dengue Bull 2003; 27: 19.

Livingston PG, Kurane I, Dai LC, Okamoto Y, Lai CJ, Men R, Karaki S, Takiguchi M, Ennis FA. Dengue virus-specific, HLA-B35-restricted, human CD8 + cytotoxic T lymphocyte (CTL) clones. Recognition of NS3 amino acids 500 to 508 by CTL clones of two different serotype specificities. J Immunol 1995; 154: 1287.

Livingston PG, Kurane I, Lai CJ, Bray M, Ennis FA. Recognition of envelope protein by dengue virus serotype-specific human CD4 + CD8- cytotoxic T-cell clones. J Virol 1994; 68: 3283.

Lucas GN, Amerasinghe A, Sriranganathan S. Dengue haemorrhagic fever in Sri Lanka. Indian J Pediatr 2000; 67: 503.

Mackow E, Makino Y, Zhao BT, Zhang YM, Markoff L, Buckler-White A, Guiler M, Chanock R, Lai CJ. The nucleotide sequence of dengue type 4 virus: analysis of genes coding for nonstructural proteins. Virology 1987; 159: 217.

Malasit P. Complement and dengue haemorrhagic fever/shock syndrome. Southeast Asian J Trop Med Public Health 1987; 18: 316.

Mangada M, Igarashi A. Molecular and *in vitro* analysis of eight dengue type 2 viruses isolated from patients exhibiting different disease severity. Virology 1998; 244: 458.

Marchette NJ, Halstead SB, Chow JS. Replication of dengue viruses in cultures of peripheral blood leukocytes from dengue-immune rhesus monkeys. J Infect Dis 1976; 133: 274.

Martin NC, Pardo J, Simmons M, Tjaden JA, Widjaja S, Marovich MA, Sun W, Porter KR, Burgess TH. An immunocytometric assay based on dengue infection via DC-SIGN permits rapid measurement of anti-dengue neutralizing antibodies. J Virol Methods 2006; 134: 74.

McKee Jr. KT, Bancroft WH, Eckels KH, Redfield RR, Summers PL, Russell PK. Lack of attenuation of a candidate dengue 1 vaccine (45AZ5) in human volunteers. Am J Trop Med Hyg 1987; 36: 435.

Men R, Bray M, Clark D, Chanock RM, Lai CJ. Dengue type 4 virus mutants containing deletions in the 3' noncoding region of the RNA genome: analysis of growth restriction in cell culture and altered viremia pattern and immunogenicity in rhesus monkeys. J Virol 1996; 70: 3930.

Men R, Bray M, Lai CJ. Carboxy-terminally truncated dengue virus envelope glycoproteins expressed on the cell surface and secreted extracellularly exhibit increased immunogenicity in mice. J Virol 1991; 65: 1400.

Men R, Wyatt L, Tokimatsu I, Arakaki S, Shameem G, Elkins R, Chanock R, Moss B, Lai CJ. Immunization of rhesus monkeys with a recombinant of modified vaccinia virus Ankara expressing a truncated envelope glycoprotein of dengue type 2 virus induced resistance to dengue type 2 virus challenge. Vaccine 2000; 18: 3113.

Men R, Yamashiro T, Goncalvez AP, Wernly C, Schofield DJ, Emerson SU, Purcell RH, Lai CJ. Identification of chimpanzee Fab fragments by repertoire cloning and production of a full-length humanized immunoglobulin G1 antibody that is highly efficient for neutralization of dengue type 4 virus. J Virol 2004; 78: 4665.

Modis Y, Ogata S, Clements D, Harrison SC. A ligand-binding pocket in the dengue virus envelope glycoprotein. Proc Natl Acad Sci USA 2003; 100: 6986.

Modis Y, Ogata S, Clements D, Harrison SC. Variable surface epitopes in the crystal structure of dengue virus type 3 envelope glycoprotein. J Virol 2005; 79: 1223.

Mohan B, Patwari AK, Anand VK. Hepatic dysfunction in childhood dengue infection. J Trop Pediatr 2000; 46: 40.

Monath TP. Dengue: the risk to developed and developing countries. Proc Natl Acad Sci USA 1994; 91: 2395.

Moncayo AC, Fernandez Z, Ortiz D, Diallo M, Sall A, Hartman S, Davis CT, Coffey L, Mathiot CC, Tesh RB, Weaver SC. Dengue emergence and adaptation to peridomestic mosquitoes. Emerg Infect Dis 2004; 10: 1790.

Morens DM, Rigau-Perez JG, Lopez-Correa RH, Moore CG, Ruiz-Tiben EE, Sather GE, Chiriboga J, Eliason DA, Casta-Velez A, Woodall JP. Dengue in Puerto Rico, 1977: public health response to characterize and control an epidemic of multiple serotypes. Am J Trop Med Hyg 1986; 35: 197.

Murthy HM, Judge K, DeLucas L, Padmanabhan R. Crystal structure of dengue virus NS3 protease in complex with a Bowman–Birk inhibitor: implications for flaviviral polyprotein processing and drug design. J Mol Biol 2000; 301: 759.

Nimmannitya S. Dengue haemorrhagic fever: diagnosis and management. In: Dengue and Dengue Haemorrhagic Fever (Gubler DJ, Kuno G, editors). London: CAB International; 1997; p. 133.

Nogueira RM, Miagostovich MP, Lampe E, Souza RW, Zagne SM, Schatzmayr HG. Dengue epidemic in the stage of Rio de Janeiro, Brazil, 1990–1: co-circulation of dengue 1 and dengue 2 serotypes. Epidemiol Infect 1993; 111: 163.

Osatomi K, Sumiyoshi H. Complete nucleotide sequence of dengue type 3 virus genome RNA. Virology 1990; 176: 643.

Paul RE, Patel AY, Mirza S, Fisher-Hoch SP, Luby SP. Expansion of epidemic dengue viral infections to Pakistan. Int J Infect Dis 1998; 2: 197.

Platt KB, Linthicum KJ, Myint KSA, Innis BL, Lerdthusnee K, Vaughn DW. Impact of dengue virus infection on feeding behavior of *Aedes aegypti*. Am J Trop Med Hyg 1997; 57: 119.

Polo S, Ketner G, Levis R, Falgout B. Infectious RNA transcripts from full-length dengue virus type 2 cDNA clones made in yeast. J Virol 1997; 71: 5366.

Promphan W, Sopontammarak S, Pruekprasert P, Kajornwattanakul W, Kongpattanayothin A. Dengue myocarditis. Southeast Asian J Trop Med Public Health 2004; 35: 611.

Puri B, Polo S, Hayes CG, Falgout B. Construction of a full length infectious clone for dengue-1 virus Western Pacific, 74 strain. Virus Genes 2000; 20: 57.

Putnak R. Progress in the development of recombinant vaccines against and other arthropod-borne flaviviruses. In: Modern Vaccinology (Kurstak E, editor). New York: Plenum Medical; 1994; p. 231.

Putnak R, Coller BA, Voss G, Vaughn DW, Clements D, Peters I, Bignami G, Houng HS, Chen RC, Barvir DA, Seriwatana J, Cayphas S, Garcon N, Gheysen D, Kanesa-Thasan N, McDonell M, Humphreys T, Eckels KH, Prieels JP, Innis BL. An evaluation of dengue type-2 inactivated, recombinant subunit, and live-attenuated vaccine candidates in the rhesus macaque model. Vaccine 2005; 23: 4442.

Qiu FX, Chen QQ, Ho QY, Chen WZ, Zhao ZG, Zhao BW. The first epidemic of dengue hemorrhagic fever in the People's Republic of China. Am J Trop Med Hyg 1991; 44: 364.

Quintos FM, Lim LE, Juliano L, Reyes A, Lacson P. Hemorrhagic fever observed among children in the Philippines. Philipp J Pediatr 1954; 3: 1.

Raviprakash K, Marques E, Ewing D, Lu Y, Phillips I, Porter KR, Kochel TJ, August TJ, Hayes CG, Murphy GS. Synergistic neutralizing antibody response to a dengue virus type 2 DNA vaccine by incorporation of lysosome-associated membrane protein sequences and use of plasmid expressing GM-CSF. Virology 2001; 290: 74.

Ray D, Shah A, Tilgner M, Guo Y, Zhao Y, Dong H, Deas TS, Zhou Y, Li H, Shi PY. West Nile virus 5'-Cap structure is formed by sequential guanine N-7 and ribose 2'-0 methylations by nonstructural protein 5. J Virol 2006; 8362.

Rey FA, Heinz FX, Mandl C, Kunz C, Harrison SC. The envelope glycoprotein from tick-borne encephalitis virus at 2 Å resolution. Nature 1995; 375: 291.

Rice CM, Grakoui A, Galler R, Chambers TJ. Transcription of infectious yellow fever RNA from full-length cDNA templates produced by *in vitro* ligation. Nat New Biol 1989; 1: 285.

Rice CM, Lenches EM, Eddy SR, Shin SJ, Sheets RL, Strauss JH. Nucleotide sequence of yellow fever virus: implications for flavivirus gene expression and evolution. Science 1985; 229: 726.

Rico-Hesse R. Molecular evolution and distribution of dengue viruses type 1 and 2 in nature. Virology 1990; 174: 479.

Rico-Hesse R, Harrison LM, Sala RA, Tovar D, Nisalak A, Ramos C, Boshell J, de Mesa MT, Noguiera RM, da Rosa AT. Origins of dengue viruses associated with increased pathogenicity in the Americas. Virology 1997; 230: 244.

Rodhain F. The role of monkeys in the biology of dengue and yellow fever. Comp Immunol Microbiol Inf Dis 1991; 14: 9.

Rodhain F, Rosen L. Mosquito vectors and dengue virus–vector relationships. In: Dengue and Dengue Hemorrhagic Fever (Gubler DJ, Kuno G, editors). London: CAB International; 1997; p. 46.

Roehrig JT. Antigenic structure of flavivirus proteins. Adv Virus Res 2003; 59: 141.

Rosen L. The Emperor's New Clothes revisited, or reflections on the pathogenesis of dengue hemorrhagic fever. Am J Trop Med Hyg 1977; 26: 337.

Rosen L. Dengue in Greece in 1927 and 1928 and the pathogenesis of dengue hemorrhagic fever: new data and a different conclusion. Am J Trop Med Hyg 1986; 35: 642.

Rosen L, Gubler D. The use of mosquitoes to detect and propagate dengue viruses. Am J Trop Med Hyg 1974; 23: 1153.

Rothman A. Viral pathogenesis of dengue infection. In: Dengue and Dengue Hemorrhagic Fever (Gubler DJ, Kuno G, editors). London: CAB International; 1997; p. 245.

Ruangjirachuporn W, Boonpucknavig S, Nimmanitya S. Circulating immune complexes in serum from patients with dengue haemorrhagic fever. Clin Exp Immunol 1979; 36: 46.

Russell PK, Nisalak A, Sukhavachana P, Vivona S. A plaque reduction test for dengue virus neutralizing antibodies. J Immunol 1967; 99: 285.

Sabchareon A, Lang J, Chanthavanich P, Yoksan S, Forrat R, Attanath P, Sirivichayakul C, Pengsaa K, Pojjaroen-Anant C, Chambonneau L, Saluzzo JF, Bhamarapravati N. Safety and immunogenicity of a three dose regimen of two tetravalent live-attenuated dengue vaccines in five- to twelve-year-old Thai children. Pediatr Infect Dis J 2004; 23: 99.

Sabin AB. Research on dengue during World War II. Am J Trop Med Hyg 1952; 1: 30.

Sabin AB, Schlesinger RW. Production of immunity to dengue with virus modified by propagation in mice. Science 1945; 101: 640.

Sahaphong S, Riengrojpitak S, Bhamarapravati N, Chirachariyavej T. Electron microscopic study of the vascular endothelial cell in dengue hemorrhagic fever. Southeast Asian J Trop Med Public Health 1980; 11: 194.

Salas-Benito JS, del Angel RM. Identification of two surface proteins from C6/36 cells that bind dengue type 4 virus. J Virol 1997; 71: 7246.

Sangkawibha N, Rojanasuphot S, Ahandrik S, Viriyapongse S, Jatanasen S, Salitul V, Phanthumachinda B, Halstead SB. Risk factors in dengue shock syndrome: a prospective epidemiologic study in Rayong, Thailand. I. The 1980 outbreak. Am J Epidemiol 1984; 120: 653.

Santos NQ, Azoubel AC, Lopes AA, Costa G, Bacellar A. Guillain–Barré syndrome in the course of dengue: case report. Arq Neuropsiquiatr 2004; 62: 144.

Schlesinger JJ, Brandriss MW, Walsh EE. Protection of mice against dengue 2 virus encephalitis by immunization with the dengue 2 virus non-structural glycoprotein NS1. J Gen Virol 1987; 68: 853.

Schlesinger RW, Frankel JW. Adaptation of the "New Guinea B" strain of dengue virus to suckling and to adult Swiss mice: a study in viral variation. J Am Trop Med Hyg 1952; 1: 66.

Scott RM, Nisalak A, Eckels KH, Tingpalapong M, Harrison VR, Gould DJ, Chapple FE, Russell PK. Dengue-2 vaccine: viremia and immune responses in rhesus monkeys. Infect Immun 1980; 27: 181.

Scott TW, Amerasinghe PH, Morrison AC, Lorenz LH, Clark GG, Strickman D, Kittayapong P, Edman JD. Longitudinal studies of Aedes aegypti (Diptera: Culicidae) in Thailand and Puerto Rico: blood feeding frequency. J Med Entomol 2000; 37: 89.

Shi PY, Brinton MA, Veal JM, Zhong YY, Wilson WD. Evidence for the existence of a pseudoknot structure at the 3′ terminus of the flavivirus genomic RNA. Biochemistry 1996; 35: 4222.

Shu PY, Huang JH. Current advances in dengue diagnosis. Clin Diagn Lab Immunol 2004; 11: 642.

Shurtleff AC, Beasley DW, Chen JJ, Ni H, Suderman MT, Wang H, Xu R, Wang E, Weaver SC, Watts DM, Russell KL, Barrett AD. Genetic variation in the 3′ non-coding region of dengue viruses. Virology 2001; 281: 75.

Siler JF, Hall MW, Hitchens AP. Dengue: its history, epidemiology, mechanism of transmission, etiology, clinical manifestations, immunity, and prevention. Philipp J Sci 1926; 29: 1.

Simmons JS, St. John JH, Reynolds FHK. Experimental studies of dengue. Philipp J Sci 1931; 44: 1.

Siqueira Jr. JB, Martelli CM, Coelho GE, Simplicio AC, Hatch DL. Dengue and dengue hemorrhagic fever, Brazil, 1981–2002. Emerg Infect Dis 2005; 1: 48.

Smith TJ, Brandt WE, Swanson JL, McCown JM, Buescher EL. Physical and biological properties of dengue-2 virus and associated antigens. J Virol 1970; 5: 524.

Stadler K, Allison SL, Schalich J, Heinz FX. Proteolytic activation of tick-borne encephalitis virus by furin. J Virol 1997; 71: 8475.

Stiasny K, Allison SL, Schalich J, Heinz FX. Membrane interactions of the tick-borne encephalitis virus fusion protein E at low pH. J Virol 2002; 76: 3784.

Sun W, Edelman R, Kanesa-Thasan N, Eckels KH, Putnak JR, King AD, Houng HS, Tang D, Scherer JM, Hoke Jr. CH, Innis BL. Vaccination of human volunteers with monovalent and tetravalent live-attenuated dengue vaccine candidates. Am J Trop Med Hyg 2003; 69(Suppl): 24.

Tassaneetrithep B, Burgess TH, Granelli-Piperno A, Trumpfheller C, Finke J, Sun W, Eller MA, Pattanapanyasat K, Sarasombath S, Birx DL, Steinman RM, Schlesinger S, Marovich MA. DC-SIGN (CD209) mediates dengue virus infection of human dendritic cells. J Exp Med 2003; 197: 823.

Teles FRR, Prazeres DMF, Lima-Filho JL. Trends in dengue diagnosis. Rev Med Virol 2005; 15: 287.

Thomas SJ, Strickman D, Vaughn DW. Dengue epidemiology: virus epidemiology, ecology, and emergence. Adv Virus Res 2003; 61: 235.

Traore-Lamizana M, Zeller H, Monlun E, Mondo M, Hervy JP, Adam F, Digoutte JP. Dengue 2 outbreak in southeastern Senegal during 1990: virus isolations from mosquitoes (Diptera: *Culicidae*). J Med Entomol 1994; 31: 623.

Tsai CJ, Kuo CH, Chen PC, Chang Cheng CS. Upper gastrointestinal bleeding in dengue fever. Am J Gastroenterol 1991; 86: 33.

Varma MG, Pudney M, Leake CJ. Cell lines from larvae of *Aedes* (Stegomyia) malayensis Colless and *Aedes* (S) *pseudoscutellaris* (Theobald) and their infection with some arboviruses. Trans R Soc Trop Med Hyg 1974; 68: 374.

Vaughn DW, Green S, Kalayanarooj S, Innis BL, Nimmannitya S, Suntayakorn S, Endy TP, Raengsakulrach B, Rothman AL, Ennis FA, Nisalak A. Dengue viremia titer, antibody response pattern, and virus serotype correlate with disease severity. J Infect Dis 2000; 181: 2.

Vaughn DW, Hoke Jr. CH, Yoksan S, LaChance R, Innis BL, Rice RM, Bhamarapravati N. Testing of a dengue 2 live-attenuated vaccine (strain 16681 PDK 53) in ten American volunteers. Vaccine 1996; 14: 329.

Videa E, Coloma MJ, Dos Santos FB, Balmaseda A, Harris E. Immunoglobulin M enzyme-linked immunosorbent assay using recombinant polypeptides for diagnosis of dengue. Clin Diagn Lab Immunol 2005; 12: 882.

Vorndam V, Beltran M. Enzyme-linked immunosorbent assay-format microneutralization test for dengue viruses. Am J Trop Med Hyg 2002; 66: 208.

Vorndam V, Kuno G. Laboratory diagnosis of dengue virus infections. In: Dengue and Dengue Hemorrhagic Fever (Gubler DJ, Kuno G, editors). London: CAB International; 1997; p. 313.

Vu SN, Nguyen TY, Tran VP, Truong UN, Le QM, Le VL, Le TN, Bektas A, Briscombe A, Aaskov JG, Ryan PA, Kay BH. Elimination of dengue by community programs using Mesocyclops (Copepoda) against *Aedes aegypti* in central Vietnam. Am J Trop Med Hyg 2005; 72: 67.

Wang E, Ni H, Xu R, Barrett AD, Watowich SJ, Gubler DJ, Weaver SC. Evolutionary relationships of endemic/epidemic and sylvatic dengue viruses. J Virol 2000; 74: 3227.

Wang WK, Chao DY, Kao CL, Wu HC, Liu YC, Li CM, Lin SC, Ho ST, Huang JH, King CC. High levels of plasma dengue viral load during defervescence in patients with dengue hemorrhagic fever: implications for pathogenesis. Virology 2003; 305: 330.

Wang WK, Lin SR, Lee CM, King CC, Chang SC. Dengue type 3 virus in plasma is a population of closely related genomes: quasispecies. J Virol 2002; 76: 4662.

Wang JY, Tseng CC, Lee CS, Cheng KP. Clinical and gastro-endoscopic feature of patients with dengue virus infection. J Gastroenteriol Hepatol 1990; 5: 701.

Watts DM, Burke DS, Harrison BA, Whitmire RE, Nisalak A. Effect of temperature on the vector efficiency of *Aedes aegypti* for dengue 2 virus. Am J Trop Med Hyg 1987; 36: 143.

Wengler G, Wengler G. The NS3 nonstructural protein of flaviviruses contains an RNA triphosphatase activity. Virology 1993; 197: 265.

Wilson ME, Chen LH. Dengue in the Americas. WHO Dengue Bull 2002; 26: 44.

Wisseman Jr. CL, Sweet BH, Rosenzweig EC, Eylar OR. Attenuated living type 1 dengue vaccines. Am J Trop Med Hyg 1963; 12: 620.

Wu SJ, Grouard-Vogel G, Sun W, Mascola JR, Brachtel E, Putvatana R, Louder MK, Filgueira L, Marovich MA, Wong HK, Blauvelt A, Murphy GS, Robb ML, Innes BL, Birx DL, Hayes CG, Frankel SS. Human skin Langerhans cells are targets of dengue virus infection. Nat Med 2000; 6: 816.

Zeng L, Falgout B, Markoff L. Identification of specific nucleotide sequences within the conserved 3'-SL in the dengue type 2 virus genome required for replication. J Virol 1998; 72: 7510.

Zhang YM, Hayes EP, McCarty TC, Dubois DR, Summers PL, Eckels KH, Chanock RM, Lai CJ. Immunization of mice with dengue structural proteins and nonstructural protein NS1 expressed by baculovirus recombinant induces resistance to dengue virus encephalitis. J Virol 1988; 62: 3027.

Zhao B, Mackow E, Buckler-White A, Markoff L, Chanock RM, Lai CJ, Makino Y. Cloning full-length dengue type 4 viral DNA sequences: analysis of genes coding for structural proteins. Virology 1986; 155: 77.

Emerging Viruses in Human Populations
Edward Tabor (Editor)
DOI 10.1016/S0168-7069(06)16012-7

Crimean–Congo Hemorrhagic Fever Virus

Pierre Nabeth

Institut Pasteur de Dakar, 36 avenue Pasteur, BP 220, Dakar, Senegal

Historical review

Crimean–Congo hemorrhagic fever (CCHF) may have been reported as early as 1110 AD. In the *Thesaurus of the Shah of Khwarazm*, compiled by Dzhurzhoni, a disease in Tajikistan similar to CCHF and transmitted by an arthropod was described. Symptoms were presence of blood in the urine, rectum, gums, vomitus, sputum, and abdominal cavity. The arthropod associated with the disease was said to be tough, small, resembling a louse or tick, and normally a parasite of a black bird. Over the course of the following centuries, the disease was reported in what is now Uzbekistan, and it was called either *khungribta* (blood taking), *khunymuny* (nose bleeding), or *harak halak* (black death) (Hoogstraal, 1979).

The first modern description of CCHF was the report of an outbreak in the West Crimea region of the USSR (Chumakov, 1945, 1947) during World War II. At that time, agricultural activities were disrupted, pastures were overgrown, and hares with ticks proliferated. During the summer of 1944, about 200 cases of fever with hemorrhage (called "acute infectious capillarotoxicosis") occurred among farmers and soldiers assisting with the harvest.

When new cases appeared in 1945–1946, Chumakov was able to describe the viral nature of the agent after reproducing the disease in psychiatric patients inoculated with infected blood for pyrogenic therapy. He was also able to identify the nymphal *Hyalomma marginatum marginatum* tick as the disease vector, after inducing a mild clinical course of CCHF in healthy human volunteers by inoculation of tick suspensions (Chumakov, 1974). In 1956, a virus was isolated from the blood of a patient in the Belgian Congo and became the prototype strain of Congo virus (Simpson et al., 1967; Williams et al., 1967). In 1967, the Drozdov strain of the Crimean hemorrhagic fever virus was isolated from a patient in Astrakhan region and became the prototype strain for much later experimental work (Butenko et al., 1968; Chumakov et al., 1968). In 1969, Casals showed that the viruses detected in the Crimea and in the Congo were antigenically similar (Casals, 1969), and the name "Crimean–Congo hemorrhagic fever virus" gradually came into use.

Cases of CCHF have been reported throughout the Eastern Hemisphere (Table 1). More than 2000 cases have been reported in the Ukraine, Russia, and central Asia (Hoogstraal, 1979). In Africa, the disease has continued to occur in recent years; for instance, an outbreak occurred in Mauritania with 38 recorded cases through August 2003 (Nabeth et al., 2004a). In the Middle East, the presence of the virus has been recognized since 1950 (Semyatkovskaya and Sudtdykova, 1950), but large-scale human epidemics have only been reported recently.

In 2006, two countries have experienced a sudden increase of CCHF cases: in the Southern Federal District of Russia, a total of 192 CCHF cases have been reported until August, representing an increase of 43% in comparison to the same period of 2005 (ProMED (2006b)) while in Turkey, 242 cases were reported during the 7 first months of the year (ProMED (2006a)).

Virus description

CCHFV is a member of the *Nairovirus* genus of the *Bunyaviridae* family. Like the 33 other members of the *Nairovirus* genus, CCHFV is transmitted by ixodid ticks (hard ticks) or argasid ticks (soft ticks) (Elliott et al., 2000). CCHFV, along with the Hazara virus and the Khasan virus that have been isolated from ixodid ticks in Pakistan (Begum et al., 1970a) and the USSR (Lvov et al., 1978), respectively, constitute the CCHF serogroup. The only other viruses in the *Nairovirus* genus that are infectious for humans, the Dugbe virus (discovered in Nigeria in 1964 [Causey, 1970]) and the Nairobi sheep virus (discovered in Kenya in 1910 [Montgomery, 1917]), belong to a different serogroup (Fig. 1).

CCHFV is a single-stranded RNA virus, with a genome that consists of three negative-stranded segments designated S (small), M (medium), and L (large), which encode the nucleocapsid (N) protein, two envelope glycoproteins (G1 and G2), and the polymerase, respectively. The molecular weights of the nucleocapsid protein, the G1 and G2 glycoproteins, and the polymerase proteins, respectively, are 48–54 kD, 72–84 kD, 30–40 kD, and 180–200 kD (Schmaljohn and Hooper, 2001).

CCHFV is a spherical virus with a diameter of about 100 nm, with a lipid bilayer envelope approximately 5–7 nm thick, with glycoprotein spikes (Martin et al., 1985). Since CCHFV is enveloped, it can be inactivated by lipid solvents and detergents (Kolman, 1970). It can be inactivated at 56°C and by low pH. The disappearance of the virus from infected tissues after death may be due to the action of a decrease in tissue pH (Swanepoel, 1995). The infectivity of the virus is maintained in serum for several days at ambient temperature and for > 3 weeks at 4°C (Hoogstraal, 1979).

Table 1

Geographical distribution of human cases of CCHF occurring during the last 25 years in Europe, Asia, and Africa

Country	CCHFV presence first detected	Period	Number of cases	References
Europe				
Albania	1981	1981–2001	More than 60 cases	Eltari et al. (1988), Papa et al. (2002a)
Bulgaria	1951	1975–2003	403 cases	Donchev et al. (1967), Papa et al. (2004)
Greece	1978	1980–1981	4 cases	Papadopoulos and Koptopoulos (1978), Antoniadis and Casals (1982)
Russia	1944	1999–2004	More than 300 cases	Hoogstraal (1979), Onishchenko (2001), Onishchenko et al. (2001), ProMED (2003b, 2004a, 2005c,d), Yashina et al. (2003a,b),
		1999–2006	More than 500 cases	
Serbia and Montenegro	1954–1967	1990–2004	More than 130 cases	Gligic et al. (1977), ProMED (2000d, 2004d), WHO (2001a), Drosten et al. (2002b), USACHPPM (2002), ProMED-mail (2006b)
Asia				
Afghanistan	1950	1998–2002	More than 100 cases	Semyatkovskaya and Sudtdykova (1950), WHO (1998), Ahmad (2000), WHO (2001b), ProMED (2002b), FAS (2002)
China	1965	1965–2002	More than 340 cases	Han et al. (2002), Papa et al. (2002c), Tang et al. (2003)
Iran	1970	1999–2004	More than 250 cases	Chumakov et al. (1970), Chinikar et al. (2004, 2005), ProMED (2005a)
Iraq	1979	1979–2000	More than 12 cases	Al-Tikriti et al. (1981), ProMED (2000e)
Kazakhstan	1948	1999–2004	More than 50 cases	Rybalko et al. (1963), ProMED (1999, 2001, 2004e), Kazakov et al. (2001), Yashina et al. (2003a)

Table 1 (continued)

Country	CCHFV presence first detected	Period	Number of cases	References
Kuwait	1979	1979–1982	17 cases	Al-Nakib et al. (1984)
Oman	1995	1995–1999	7 cases	Schwarz et al. (1995), Scrimgeour et al. (1999), Williams et al. (2000)
Pakistan	1970	1979–2004	More than 150 cases	Begum et al. (1970b), Darwish et al. (1983), Altaf et al. (1998), Bosan et al. (2000), NICD (2003), ProMED (2003a, 2004b,c,f, 2005b), Sheikh et al. (2005)
Saudi Arabia	1990	1989–1990	40 cases	el-Azazy and Scrimgeour (1997)
Tajikistan	1943	2000	At least 1 case	Pak (1975), ProMED (2000c)
Turkey	1974	2002–2003	134 cases	Casals (1977), Ergonul et al. (2004), Bakir et al. (2005), ProMED-mail (2006a)
		2002–2006	376 cases	
United Arab Emirates	1979	1979–2000	More than 150 cases	Suleiman et al. (1980), Khan et al. (1997), ProMED (2000a,b)
Africa				
Burkina Faso	1983	1983	1 case	Saluzzo et al. (1984)
D.R. Congo	1956	1981–2002	1 case	Simpson et al. (1967), NICD (2003)
Kenya	1965	2000	1 case	Woodall et al. (1965), Dunster et al. (2002)
Mauritania	1983	1983–2003	More than 40 cases	Saluzzo et al. (1985a), Gonzalez et al. (1990), Nabeth et al. (2004a)
Namibia	1984	1984–2005	15 cases	ProMED (2002a), NICD (2003, 2005b)
Senegal	1969	2003–2004	2 cases	Chunikhin et al. (1969), Nabeth et al. (2004b), Jaureguiberry et al. (2005)
South Africa	1981	1981–2004	160 cases	Gear et al. (1982), NICD (2003, 2005a), ProMED-mail (2005e)
Tanzania	1974–1975	1981–2002	1 case	Hoogstraal (1979), NICD (2003)

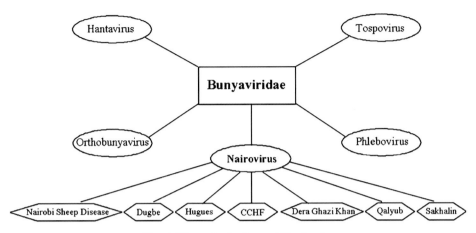

Fig. 1 Viruses in the *Bunyaviridae* family.

Molecular biology and phylogenetic relationships

The sequences of 19 complete S segments from CCHFV have been deposited in Genbank (Hewson et al., 2004). The first CCHFV sequence to be published was an analysis of the S segment of a Chinese sheep strain of the virus (Marriott and Nuttall, 1992). The genetic characterization of the CCHFV M segment from two other Chinese strains of CCHFV isolated from a patient and from *Hyalomma* ticks (Papa et al., 2002c) was important because the M gene appears to be critical for immunity and pathogenicity; it also may be useful for future vaccine development. Characterization of the CCHFV genome was completed with determination of the L segment sequence (Honig et al., 2004; Kinsella et al., 2004).

Little is known about the molecular heterogeneity of CCHFV strains in different parts of the world, but it seems that genetic differences between strains are sometimes considerable (Marriott and Nuttall, 1992; Schwarz et al., 1996; Rodriguez et al., 1997). It has been stated that nucleotide variability between strains can reach up to 20% (Marriott and Nuttall, 1992; Burt and Swanepoel, 2005). Although comparison of CCHFV strains based on the analysis of the M segment has been proposed (Yashina et al., 2003b; Chinikar et al., 2004), most phylogenetic trees are based on the analysis of a 220–260 bp fragment of the S segment (Schwarz et al., 1996; Rodriguez et al., 1997; Papa et al., 2002b, 2004).

There is no clear correlation between genetic variants and epidemiological features such as year of isolation, host species, or geographic origin of the strain (Marriott and Nuttall, 1992; Rodriguez et al., 1997; Burt and Swanepoel, 2005). The greatest genetic variability was seen between isolates from different tick species rather than from geographically distinct areas, suggesting that a long-term association with a particular tick species plays a role in genetic variation (Yashina et al., 2003a).

The potential roles of migratory birds and the movements of infected livestock and ticks in the geographic spread of the virus have been hypothesized and studied (Hoogstraal, 1979; Khan et al., 1997; Rodriguez et al., 1997).

CCHFV has been reported to consist of from three to eight major genetic lineages. The phylogenetic relationships among 70 geographically distinct CCHFV isolates are shown in Fig. 2. Burt and Swanepoel (2005) have reported three sub-types of CCHFV, including subtype A, consisting of two clades circulating in Asia and Madagascar; subtype B circulating in southern and western Africa; and sub-type C consisting of a unique isolate from Greece. Other authors (Drosten et al., 2002b; Chinikar et al., 2004; Hewson et al., 2004) have reported seven major genetic groups, and one has reported eight (Papa et al., 2004), with the Nigerian strain IbAr10200 and the central African strain ArB604 making up the additional genetic group.

Disease cycle

Reservoir

Although CCHFV has never been definitively isolated from large mammals in the wild, antibodies to CCHFV have been found in foxes in Central Europe and in baboons and gazelles in Africa (Chumakov, 1974; Zarubinski et al., 1975). Exper-imental infection of African nonhuman primates leads to infection with no more than moderate clinical signs (Butenko et al., 1970; Fagbami et al., 1975). Natural infection of large domestic mammals does occur, such as in camels, horses, and donkeys; in fact, cattle in Central Europe (Pak et al., 1975) and goats and sheep in western Africa (Gonzalez et al., 1998) are the primary reservoirs for CCHFV in-fection in those areas. Symptoms have been rarely observed in animals: dullness, lassitude, and decreased appetite have been reported in inoculated calves (Causey et al., 1970) and fever has been reported in a cow (Woodall et al., 1965).

However, CCHFV or antibodies to it have been found in numerous smaller wild mammalian species, including hedgehogs (Causey et al., 1970), bats (Tkachenko et al., 1969), hares (Chumakov, 1974), mice and rats (Saluzzo et al., 1985b), squirrels and eland antelopes (Swanepoel et al., 1983), gerbils (Darwish et al., 1983), and genets (Hoogstraal, 1979). These animals rarely have large numbers of ticks, but the large populations of these animals may indirectly create a strong density of ticks.

Antibodies to CCHFV have been detected in many species of wild birds (hornbills, guinea fowl, and blackbirds) (Hoogstraal, 1979) and in one domestic bird (ostriches) (Shepherd et al., 1987). Their role in virus transmission has been demonstrated experimentally (Swanepoel et al., 1998).

The role of birds was underestimated until recent years, and it was only after the detection of antibodies in certain wild species (hornbills, guinea fowl, and

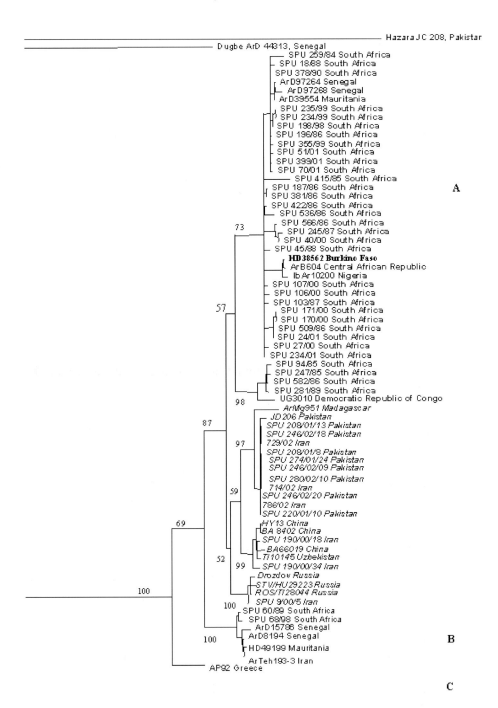

blackbirds) (Hoogstraal, 1979) and domestically-bred species (ostriches) (Shepherd et al., 1987) that their role in virus transmission could be demonstrated experimentally (Swanepoel et al., 1998).

The CCHFV multiplies during viremia in animals with short lives (small rodents, birds, and animals meant for slaughter). It is present during short viraemic phases in the first days of infection, which would normally limit its impact in terms of propagation and geographic distribution. But, it is present during the entire lifecycle of the tick vector, and can be passed to future generations through transovarial transmission (Gonzalez et al., 1992).

CCHFV is present in a short viremic phase in the first days of infection in many animals. It multiplies during this viremic period, allowing the tick vector to acquire the virus by feeding on the animal.

Vector

CCHFV has been detected in at least 30 tick species throughout the world (Camicas et al., 1990). The virus has been isolated from two tick species in the family Argasidae ("Soft" ticks) and from 28 species of Ixodidae ("hard" ticks) distributed among 7 genera of the family *Ixodidae*. Most are either two or three host ticks. It is present in the tick during the entire life cycle of the tick, and it can be passed to future generations through transovarial transmission (Gonzalez et al., 1992). Despite virus isolation from ticks, this alone does not incriminate a given tick species as a vector; further studies are needed, particularly to confirm transovarial transmission by some of these tick species (Burgdorfer and Varma, 1967).

The principal vectors of CCHFV are in the genus *Hyalomma* (Hoogstraal, 1979). The only exception shown so far is *Ixodes ricinus* as the principal vector in the forests of Moldavia. Within enzootic foci, *Hyalomma* ticks are found only in lowlands, foothills, low mountain belts with arid to semi-arid climates, and areas with long dry seasons including deserts, steppes, and tropical savannahs and grasslands (Watts et al., 1989a).

Hyalomma marginatum rufipes, one of the principal vectors in Senegal, has a life cycle that is ditropic (two hosts) and biphasic (two stages for the first host). The fasting larva parasitizes a bird or hare, gorges itself, and then molts (transforms to produce a nymph) on its host. The nymph gorges itself in turn, and then falls to the

Fig. 2 Phylogenetic relationship among 70 geographically distinct CCHFV isolates was determined for a 450-nucleotide region of the S segment of the viral genome using a weighted maximum parsimony method, with Phylogenetic Analysis Using Parsimony (PAUP). Two nairoviruses, Dugbe and Hazara, were included as outgroups. Numbers at each branch indicate the percent bootstrap support for that node generated from 100 replicates (heuristic search). Tree topology indicates the existence of three groups of genetically related isolates, A, B, and C, with two clades within group A: an African clade (shown in bold type) and a predominantly Asian clade, which includes isolates from Pakistan, China, Russia, Iran, and Madagascar (shown in italics). Reproduced from Burt and Swanepoel (2005), with permission.

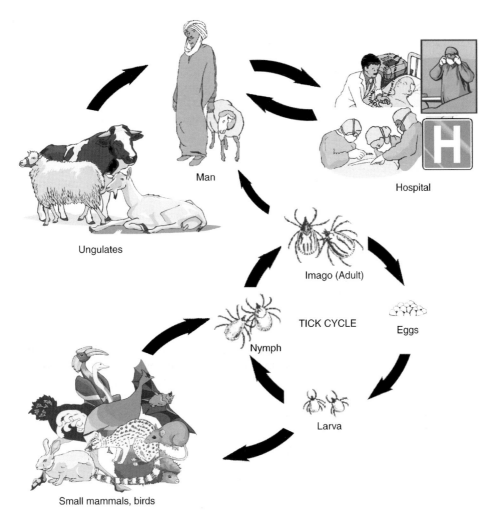

Fig. 3 Example of CCHF virus circulation: transmission by the *Hyalomma marginatum rufipes* tick. (For colour version: see Colour Section on page 356).

ground, where it transforms into an imago, taking shelter in a crevice or other physically protected location before actively seeking a new host, generally an ungulate (Fig. 3). Certain imagos attach themselves readily to humans (Camicas et al., 1990).

CCHF in humans: modes of transmission and risk factors

The greatest risk of transmission of CCHF to humans occurs in areas where ticks of the genus *Hyalomma* are the predominant species (Watts et al., 1989a). During an epidemic in Rostov, Russia, it was found that the risk of human infection was directly proportional to the rate of attachment of *Hyalomma marginatum marginatum* on humans (Goldfarb et al., 1980).

The risk of seropositivity for CCHFV among humans increases with age, sleeping outdoors, history of tick bites, handling young or sick animals, and having contact with confirmed cases of CCHFV infection (Chapman et al., 1991; Fisher-Hoch et al., 1992). Human males and females appear to be equally susceptible to CCHFV infection, although a preponderance of males sometimes occurs due to differences in occupational activities associated with increased exposure to the virus (Burney et al., 1980; Suleiman et al., 1980; Swanepoel et al., 1983, 1985).

CCHFV is transmitted to humans through one of the following modes: (1) the bite of a tick (Chapman et al., 1991); (2) contact with the tissues or blood of a recently slaughtered infected animal in the viremic phase of infection (butchers are particularly at risk) (Williams et al., 2000); and (3) contact with the blood of viremic-phase patients, most frequently in a hospital setting (Papa et al., 2002b; Athar et al., 2003; Nabeth et al., 2004a). Human epidemics of CCHF rarely affect more than a few individuals.

Secondary cases are rare and tertiary cases are very rarely reported (Papa et al., 2002b). It has been suggested that subpopulations of less-virulent strains of the virus, with an altered transmission capacity, are selected during transmission from animal or tick to man (Gonzalez et al., 1995).

Human-to-human transmission of CCHFV is rare, except in the presence of hemorrhage, unsafe injections, unprotected venipuncture, or other types of hospital exposures. It is believed that infected blood plays an important role; in Pakistan in 1976, 10 hospital staff members who had contact with a patient with CCHF became ill (Burney et al., 1980), and all those infected had been heavily exposed to blood from the infected patient (Burney, et al., 1980). In Mauritania in 2003, a patient with CCHF infected five hospital staff members and 10 patients and visitors in the hospital emergency ward (Nabeth et al., 2004a); the absence of basic protection measures for blood exposure were felt to be the primary factor in transmission. It has been suggested that CCHFV infections resulting from human-to-human transmission may be more severe than disease contracted by tick bites (Hoogstraal, 1979). However, this may reflect the fact that all deaths related to human-to-human transmission in hospitals get reported while deaths caused by the disease in other locations may be under-reported.

Pathophysiology

The physiopathology of CCHF is not well understood (Joubert et al., 1985; Swanepoel et al., 1987, 1989; Swanepoel, 1995; Burt et al., 1997). As with other hemorrhagic fever viruses, lesions of CCHFV infection are not severe enough to account for terminal shock and death of the patient. However, in fatal cases, a fulminant shock-like syndrome occurs, suggesting that inflammatory mediators may play an important role in the pathogenesis (Geisbert and Jahrling, 2004).

The virus mainly infects endothelial cells and monocytes, which in turn contribute to the viremic phase of the disease. Hepatocytes are also infected. It appears that virus exploits the host cell's endocytic machinery to enter the cell.

After inoculation by tick bite or other mechanism, CCHFV is thought to replicate at the inoculation site and spread to lymphoid tissues, the liver, and the adrenals. Endothelial damage, evidenced in the skin by a rash, contributes to stimulating platelet aggregation and activation of the intrinsic coagulation cascade. Organ lesions cause the release of procoagulants and disruption of the capacity to regenerate the consumed clotting factors. Vascular disruption during the first days of infection appears to be due to mechanisms similar to those of disseminated intravascular coagulopathy.

The formation of circulating immune complexes with complement activation probably contributes to the alteration of the capillary bed particularly in renal, pulmonary, central nervous system (congestion, hemorrhages, and localized cerebral necrosis), and adrenal tissues. Liver lesions vary from disseminated necrotic foci to massive necrosis involving 75% of hepatocytes, with hemorrhages of varying degree and little or no inflammatory response.

Clinical findings

CCHFV causes clinical manifestations in humans but these are inconsistent, with a 5:1 ratio of asymptomatic to symptomatic cases (Goldfarb et al., 1980). The incubation period is variable depending on the mode of transmission: from 1 to 3 days with a maximum of 9 days when infection is caused by the bite of a tick, and from 5 to 6 days with a maximum of 13 days when the infection is caused by contact with infected tissues or blood (Hoogstraal, 1979; Swanepoel et al., 1987, 1989). The disease progresses rapidly. The first symptoms include fever, chills, stiffness, myalgia and arthralgia, vertigo, severe headache, ocular pain, photophobia, dizziness, nausea, vomiting, general abdominal pain, and diarrhea. The fever then becomes intermittent and is accompanied by mood swings. Between the second and fourth day, intense asthenia and drowsiness appear. Conjunctival injection and/or chemosis can be observed. Hepatomegaly can be present, with abdominal pain becoming localized in the right upper quadrant of the abdomen. Tachycardia, hypotension, lymphadenopathy, and enanthema (and petechiae in the throat, tonsils, and the oral mucous membranes) can also be observed. Between the third and sixth day, petechial subcutaneous hemorrhages or ecchymoses appear on the trunk and limbs. Between the fourth and fifth day, epistaxis, hematemesis, hematuria, melena, vaginal bleeding, or bleeding from other orifices occur. Internal hemorrhages can also occur, notably retroperitoneal or intracranial. In the most severe, life-threatening forms, hepatorenal failure and/or pulmonary failure can occur. During the second week, icterus can appear. Recovery, if it occurs, usually begins after 9 or 10 days. The recovery period can be long, accompanied by asthenia, confusion, alopecia, and localized neuralgia (Swanepoel, 1995).

In the absence of specific treatment, from 30% to 50% of cases are fatal (Hoogstraal, 1979; Swanepoel, 1995; Nichol, 2001; Nabeth et al., 2004a). Death usually occurs between the fifth and the fourteenth days (Swanepoel et al., 1987, 1989).

Laboratory findings

In the initial days of the disease, either a leukocytosis or a leukopenia occurs (Joubert et al., 1985; Swanepoel et al., 1987, 1989). Next, a rapid increase in liver enzymes (AST, ALT, gamma-GT, LDH, or alkaline phosphatase) or muscle enzymes (creatine kinase) is observed (Ergonul et al., 2004).

Disruption of the coagulation mechanisms is reflected in thrombocytopenia, elevated prothrombin time, kaolin cephalin clotting time, thrombin time, an increase in fibrin degradation products, and a decrease in fibrinogen and hemoglobin levels (Swanepoel, 1995; Karti et al., 2004).

Diagnosis

CCHFV infected samples are processed in biosafety level 4 (BSL4) laboratories. The infection can be diagnosed by: (1) virus isolation; (2) the detection of genome fragments by reverse transcription polymerase chain reaction (RT-PCR); (3) the detection of the viral antigen; (4) seroconversion; (5) the detection of specific IgM antibodies; or (6) a fourfold increase in antibody titer between two successive blood draws. These methods can be performed on peripheral blood, cardiac blood, or on a postmortem liver sample (Swanepoel et al., 1987, 1989).

Viral isolation

It has been shown that CCHFV can be isolated from the blood of patients for 8 days and occasionally for up to 12 days after the onset of disease (Butenko, 1971). Isolation is performed in cell culture (Vero, PS, LLC-MK2, CER, BHK21, or SW13 cells) (Watts et al., 1989a; Swanepoel, 1995) or by intracerebral inoculation of newborn mice. Cell culture is a faster method than inoculation of newborn mice (1–6 days versus 5–10 days), but it is less sensitive (Shepherd et al., 1986). Longer incubation times for growing the virus in cell lines have been reported by other authors, e.g. maximum virus yields (10^7–10^8 PFU/ml) after 4–7 days of incubation (Nichol 2001). Isolation must be followed by a virus identification by immunofluorescence, complement fixation, and/or neutralization assays.

Molecular diagnosis

The diagnosis can also be made during the first week after onset of the disease by RT-PCR of the S segment. RT-PCR can be nested (Schwarz et al., 1996) or one-step (Drosten et al., 2002a). More recently, a one-step real time RT-PCR assay using primers for the nucleoprotein gene was developed (Drosten et al., 2002a). This method has higher sensitivity and specificity than conventional PCR, and it is more rapid (results are obtained in minutes instead of hours).

Serological diagnosis

Serologic tests such as indirect immunofluorescence assay (IFA) and ELISA can be used to make the diagnosis. However, IgM and IgG antibodies are not detectable by IFA before the third day of illness (Burt et al., 1994). On the fourth and fifth days, antibodies are detectable in 10% of patients, in 65% of patients at day 6, 83% of patients at day 7, 94% of patients at day 8, and all patients by day 9. The IgM titer is maximal at the end of the second or third week; IgM generally disappears before the fifth month; IgG starts to decrease in the fourth month and stays detectable for at least 5 years.

IgM and IgG ELISA capture assays also have been developed (Garcia et al., 2005; Saijo et al., 2005) for detecting IgM antibodies to CCHFV. In ELISA, IgM and IgG are detectable as early as the third day of illness (Burt et al., 1994). ELISA is the most widely used method for rapid diagnosis and epidemiological surveillance at present, although genetic techniques may be more widely used in future field interventions. In fatal cases, it is rare to detect antibodies (Burt et al., 1994); viral isolation or RT-PCR are needed for diagnosis (Swanepoel et al., 1989; Ergonul et al., 2004; Karti et al., 2004; Nabeth et al., 2004a)

Prognostic factors

Several aspects of the clinical and laboratory test status of patients infected with CCHFV can provide an indication of the patient's prognosis. Deterioration in the clinical status occurs earlier and is more marked for patients who die. Leukocytosis, severe thrombocytopenia, and low fibrinogen have been reported to be associated with fatal outcome (Swanepoel et al., 1989). The ratio of AST level to ALT levels has been reported to be higher for patients with severe disease during the first days of infection (Ergonul et al., 2004), and the LDH and CPK levels are higher in patients with severe disease (Ergonul et al., 2004). The incubation period is shorter among fatal cases, probably because the viremic load is higher (Nabeth et al., 2004a).

Treatment and prevention

Treatment

Treatment includes administration of specific intravenous immunoglobulins and/ or ribavirin. In an uncontrolled study, seven patients with severe CCHFV infection received a specific immunoglobulin prepared from the plasma of donors who had been given one dose of a CCHFV vaccine to boost pre-existing antibodies; all recovered quickly (Vassilenko et al., 1990). More targeted human monoclonal antibodies to CCHFV may be available for therapy in the future (Jahrling, 1997).

Ribavirin inhibits CCHFV replication in cell culture and in mice (Berezina et al., 1983). In Vero cells, ribavirin appears to be even more effective against CCHF than its known efficacy against Rift Valley Fever (RVF), inhibiting CCHFV replication at doses nine times less than those needed to inhibit RVFV (Watts et al., 1989b). In newborn mice, ribavirin decreases the case–fatality ratio of CCHF, increases survival time, reduces viral replication in the liver, and decreases the viral load in the circulation. It also seems to select for hepatotropic subpopulations: there is no cerebral or cardiac infection in treated newborn mice (Tignor and Hanham, 1993).

No clinical trials have been conducted of ribavirin for the treatment of human CCHFV infections. In an uncontrolled study in Iran, of 69 patients with CCHFV infection who were treated with ribavirin, only 11.6% died (Mardani et al., 2003). None of the seven patients who were treated with Ribavirin before the fourth day of illness in South Africa died, while three of the five patients treated after the fifth day died (Swanepoel et al., 1990). However, in Karachi, Pakistan, five of nine died despite ribavirin therapy (Smego et al., 2004).

Intravenous ribavirin is recommended for treatment of CCHFV infection, while an oral dosage form is recommended for postexposure prophylaxis (CDC, 1995). However, ribavirin taken orally has been shown to attain blood levels comparable to *in vitro* sensitivity levels (Watts et al., 1989b). The 10-day treatment course can be administered (Mardani et al., 2003) as an initial dose: 30 mg/kg; day 1–4: 15 mg/kg every 6 h; day 5–10: 7.5 mg/kg every 8 h. Side effects of ribavirin are anemia, hyperbilirubinemia (due to a mild hemolysis), and reversible block of erythropoiesis (Jahrling, 1997). Despite its impact on the treatment costs (Bakir et al., 2005), and the absence of clear proof about its efficiency, ribavirin should be used to treat CCHF. The case fatality ratio of the disease is high and all means of increasing the chances of survival should be employed.

New experimental treatments for CCHFV have been investigated. Pullikotil et al. (2004) have proposed the use of inhibitors that affect the processing and the stability of the CCHFV glycoprotein. Several other investigators (Peters et al., 1986; Tamura et al., 1987; Temonen et al., 1995; Andersson et al., 2004) have shown that human MxA inhibits the replication of other Bunyaviridae only Andersson et al. have shown that it has an action on CCHFV.

Patients infected with CCHFV infection need close medical supervision; most severe cases require admission to an intensive care unit. Actions must be taken to reduce the risk of contamination of other patients and medical staff. Sedatives should be used in some cases with psychiatric symptoms. Aspirin and steroids should be avoided. Patients who are not sick enough to require continuous use of intravenous catheters should not be given these, since their use results in increased exposure to infectious blood for hospital staff. Lost red blood cells, platelets, coagulation factors, and proteins must be replaced, however. Heparin can be used for prophylaxis and treatment of DIC, particularly if appropriate laboratory support is available (Jahrling, 1997).

Prevention

In endemic zones, prevention should include systematic disinfection of affected households, animals, stables, and holding pens to kill ticks; treatment of herds with tick disinfection before export; education of meat industry personnel and veterinarians for careful handling of blood and flesh of slaughtered animals; and education of potentially affected populations about when to notify health personnel of suspected CCHF symptoms. Patients should be treated in a private isolation room, with negative pressure and tight surveillance of all entrances and exits (CDC, 1995). If possible, an intermediary transition room between the safe zone and the contaminated zone should be provided.

Experimental vaccines have been reported (Tkachenko et al., 1971, 1972), but the effectiveness has not been demonstrated. Vassilenko (1973) vaccinated 583 volunteers with an experimental CCHFV vaccine in Bulgaria, producing antibodies to CCHFV in up to 96% of recipients.

Ribavirin has been proposed for the prevention of CCHF, but its effectiveness for this purpose has not yet been tested in controlled trials (van de Wal et al., 1985).

The risk of CCHFV as an agent of bioterrorism

At the present time, CCHFV has not been listed as a likely agent of bioterrorism, because it does not meet the criteria for such an agent (Borio et al., 2002). CCHFV, as it exists in nature, is not extremely contagious, seems to lose virulence after transmission to man and is not easily transmitted from person to person, does not have documented airborne transmission, is difficult to obtain in elevated titers in culture, and has a low case–fatality ratio compared to many other infectious agents. Even in the absence of effective treatment, it could be contained by the implementation of simple hygiene measures. Nevertheless, it is conceivable that biological engineering could produce a variant in the future that would make it necessary to list CCHFV as such an agent.

Emerging CCHF

During recent years, several countries have reported human CCHF cases for the first time, even though the presence of the virus in animals had been known for years. In Senegal, the virus had been isolated in 1969 (Chunikhin et al., 1969), but no human case was reported until 2003 (Nabeth et al., 2004b). In 2004, two other sporadic cases, unrelated to each other, occurred in Senegal (Jaureguiberry et al., 2005; also personal communication). A case was detected in 1983 in Mauritania (Saluzzo et al., 1985a), but no further cases were detected there until 2003 (Nabeth et al., 2004a). In Kenya, CCHFV was detected in a cow in 1965 (Woodall et al., 1965), but the first human case was not detected until 2000 (Dunster et al., 2002). In Turkey, antibodies to the virus were found in 1974 (Casals, 1977), but the first human case was reported in outbreaks in 2002–2003 outbreaks (134 cases) (Bakir et al., 2005). In Iran, the virus had been isolated from ticks in 1970 (Chumakov et al., 1970), but the first human cases were detected in 1999, and more than 250 human cases have now been reported (Chinikar et al., 2005).

Human cases have also been reported in countries where the virus had not been previously found. Forty cases have been reported in Saudi Arabia since 1989 and seven cases in Oman since 1995 (Schwarz et al., 1995; el-Azazy and Scrimgeour, 1997; Scrimgeour et al., 1999; Williams et al., 2000).

It is very likely that the increasing access to health facilities and the reinforcement of epidemiological surveillance systems have contributed to a better detection of cases. There are now health posts even in remote African areas, supervision and training of health staff are well organized, diagnostic procedures are defined, and, most of the time, reference laboratories are available.

According to officials in Iran, the first human CCHF cases there followed the increase of importation of cattle, sheep, and goats from neighboring countries that resulted from the fall-back sale of animals there because they could not be sold in Europe due to the BSE crisis there, and because of the indirect effects of droughts in Afghanistan and Pakistan where several CCHF outbreaks occurred, resulting in the sale of animals to Iran (personal communications).

The appearance of new high-risk regions for CCHF are more likely to be caused by demographic and social changes in endemic regions rather than by bioterrorism. Because the tick vector of CCHFV is found in many geographical regions of the world, increases in international travel and livestock exportation may contribute to an increase in the risks of disease transmission in new regions.

References

Ahmad K. Outbreak of Crimean–Congo haemorrhagic fever in Pakistan. Lancet 2000; 356: 1254.

Al-Nakib W, Lloyd G, El-Mekki A, Platt G, Beeson A, Southee T. Preliminary report on arbovirus-antibody prevalence among patients in Kuwait: evidence of Congo/Crimean virus infection. Trans R Soc Trop Med Hyg 1984; 78: 474–476.

Altaf A, Luby S, Ahmed AJ, Zaidi N, Khan AJ, Mirza S, McCormick J, Fisher-Hoch S. Outbreak of Crimean–Congo haemorrhagic fever in Quetta, Pakistan: contact tracing and risk assessment. Trop Med Int Health 1998; 3: 878–882.

Al-Tikriti SK, Al-Ani F, Jurji FJ, Tantawi H, Al-Moslih M, Al-Janabi N, Mahmud MI, Al-Bana A, Habib H, Al-Munthri H, Al-Janabi S, K AL-J, Yonan M, Hassan F, Simpson DI. Congo/Crimean haemorrhagic fever in Iraq. Bull World Health Organ 1981; 59: 85–90.

Andersson I, Bladh L, Mousavi-Jazi M, Magnusson KE, Lundkvist A, Haller O, Mirazimi A. Human MxA protein inhibits the replication of Crimean–Congo hemorrhagic fever virus. J Virol 2004; 78: 4323–4329.

Antoniadis A, Casals J. Serological evidence of human infection with Congo-Crimean hemorrhagic fever virus in Greece. Am J Trop Med Hyg 1982; 31: 1066–1067.

Athar MN, Baqai HZ, Ahmad M, Khalid MA, Bashir N, Ahmad AM, Balouch AH, Bashir K. Short report: Crimean–Congo hemorrhagic fever outbreak in Rawalpindi, Pakistan, February 2002. Am J Trop Med Hyg 2003; 69: 284–287.

Bakir M, Ugurlu M, Dokuzoguz B, Bodur H, Tasyaran MA, Vahaboglu H. Crimean–Congo haemorrhagic fever outbreak in Middle Anatolia: a multicentre study of clinical features and outcome measures. J Med Microbiol 2005; 54: 385–389.

Begum F, Wisseman Jr. CL, Casals J. Tick-borne viruses of West Pakistan. II. Hazara virus, a new agent isolated from *Ixodes redikorzevi* ticks from the Kaghan Valley, W. Pakistan. Am J Epidemiol 1970a; 92: 192–194.

Begum F, Wisseman CL, Casals J. Tick-borne viruses of West Pakistan. IV. Viruses similar to or identical with, Crimean hemorrhagic fever (Congo-Semunya), Wad Medani and Pak Argas 461 isolated from ticks of the Changa Manga Forest, Lahore District, and of Hunza, Gilgit Agency, W. Pakistan. Am J Epidemiol 1970b; 92: 197–202.

Berezina LK, Leont'eva NA, Kondrashina NG, L'vov DK, Gagelov GA. Effect of ribavirin on bunyavirus reproduction in cell culture and in an experiment on white mice. Voprosy Virusologii 1983; 28: 627–629.

Borio L, Inglesby T, Peters CJ, Schmaljohn AL, Hughes JM, Jahrling PB, Ksiazek T, Johnson KM, Meyerhoff A, O'Toole T, Ascher MS, Bartlett J, Breman JG, Eitzen Jr. EM, Hamburg M, Hauer J, Henderson DA, Johnson RT, Kwik G, Layton M, Lillibridge S, Nabel GJ, Osterholm MT, Perl TM, Russell P, Tonat K. Hemorrhagic fever viruses as biological weapons: medical and public health management. JAMA 2002; 287: 2391–2405.

Bosan AH, Kakar F, Dil AS, Asghar HA, Zaidi S. Crimean–Congo hemorrhagic fever (CCHF) in Pakistan. Dis Surveillance 2000; 2: 4–5.

Burgdorfer W, Varma MG. Trans-stadial and transovarial development of disease agents in arthropods. Annu Rev Entomol 1967; 12: 347–376.

Burney MI, Ghafoor A, Saleen M, Webb PA, Casals J. Nosocomial outbreak of viral hemorrhagic fever caused by Crimean hemorrhagic fever-Congo virus in Pakistan, January 1976. Am J Trop Med Hyg 1980; 29: 941–947.

Burt FJ, Leman PA, Abbott JC, Swanepoel R. Serodiagnosis of Crimean–Congo haemorrhagic fever. Epidemiol Infect 1994; 113: 551–562.

Burt FJ, Swanepoel R. Molecular epidemiology of African and Asian Crimean–Congo haemorrhagic fever isolates. Epidemiol Infect 2005; 133: 659–666.

Burt FJ, Swanepoel R, Shieh WJ, Smith JF, Leman PA, Greer PW, Coffield LM, Rollin PE, Ksiazek TG, Peters CJ, Zaki SR. Immunohistochemical and *in situ* localization of Crimean–Congo hemorrhagic fever (CCHF) virus in human tissues and implications for CCHF pathogenesis. Arch Pathol Lab Med 1997; 121: 839–846.

Butenko AM. Data from studying etiology, laboratory diagnosis, and immunology of Crimean hemorrhagic fever; questions of ecology of the viral agent. (Atvorev Diss Soisk Uchen Step Dokt Biol Nauk), Inst Polio Virus Entsefalitov Akad Med Nauk SSSR 1971. (In English, NAMRU3-T1152).

Butenko AM, Chumakov MP, Bashkirtsev VN, Zavodova TI, Tkachenko EA, Rubin SG, Stolbov DN. Isolation and investigation of Astrakhan strain ("Drozdov") of Crimean hemorrhagic fever virus and data on serodiagnosis of this infection. Mater 15 Nauchn Sess Inst Polio Virus Entsefalitov (Moscow, October 1968) 1968; 3: 88–90 (In English, NAMRU3-T866).

Butenko AM, Chumakov MP, Smirnova SE, Vassilenko SM, Zavodova TI, Tkachenko EA, Zarubina LV, Bashkirtsev VN, Zgurskaia GN, Vyshnivetskaya LK. Isolation of Crimean hemorrhagic fever virus from blood of patients and corpse material (from 1968–1969 investigation data) in Rostov, Astrakhan Oblast, and Bulgaria. Mater 3 Oblast Nauchn Prakt Konf (Rostov-on-Don, May 1970) 1970; 6–25. (In English, NAMRU3-T522).

Camicas JL, Wilson ML, Cornet JP, Digoutte JP, Calvo MA, Adam F, Gonzalez JP. Ecology of ticks as potential vectors of Crimean–Congo hemorrhagic fever virus in Senegal: epidemiological implications. Arch Virol 1990; (Suppl 1): 303–322.

Casals J. Antigenic similarity between the virus causing Crimean hemorrhagic fever and Congo virus. Exp Biol Med 1969; 131: 233–236.

Casals J. Crimean–Congo hemorrhagic fever: in Ebola virus haemorrhagic fever. In: Proceedings of an International Colloquium on Ebola Virus Infection and other haemorrhagic fevers held in Antwerp, Belgium, 6–8 December, 1977 (Pattyn SR, editor). Amsterdam, The Netherlands, Elsevier/North-Holland; 1977; pp. 201–210.

Causey OR. Dugbe (DUG) strain AR 1792. Supplement to the catalogue of arthropod-borne viruses. Am J Trop Med Hyg 1970; 19: 1123–1124.

Causey OR, Kemp GE, Madbouly MH, David-West TS. Congo virus from domestic livestock, African hedgehog, and arthropods in Nigeria. Am J Trcp Med Hyg 1970; 19(5): 846–850.

Centers for Disease Control and Prevention (CDC). Update: management of patients with suspected viral hemorrhagic fever: United States. MMWR 1995; 44: 475–479.

Chapman LE, Wilson ML, Hall DB, LeGuenno B, Dykstra EA, Ba K, Fisher-Hoch SP. Risk factors for Crimean–Congo hemorrhagic fever in rural northern Senegal. J Infect Dis 1991; 164: 686–692.

Chinikar S, Mazaheri V, Mirahmadi R, Nabeth P, Saron MF, Salehi P, Hosseini N, Bouloy M, Mirazimi A, Lundkvist A, Nilsson M, Mehrabi-Tavana A. A serological survey in suspected human patients of Crimean–Congo hemorrhagic fever in Iran by determination of IgM-specific ELISA method during 2000–2004. Arch Iran Med 2005; 8: 52–55.

Chinikar S, Persson SM, Johansson M, Bladh L, Goya M, Houshmand B, Mirazimi A, Plyusnin A, Lundkvist A, Nilsson M. Genetic analysis of Crimean–Congo hemorrhagic fever virus in Iran. J Med Virol 2004; 73: 404–411.

Chumakov MP. A new tick-borne virus disease—Crimean hemorrhagic fever. In: Crimean hemorrhagic fever (acute infectious capillary toxicosis) (Sokolov AA, Chumakov MP, Kolachev AA, editors). Simferopol: Izd. Otd. Primorskoi Armii; 1945; pp. 13–43.

Chumakov MP. A new virus disease—Crimean hemorrhagic fever (in Russian). Nov Med 1947; 4: 9–11 (In English, NAMRU3-T900).

Chumakov MP. On 30 years of investigation of Crimean hemorrhagic fever (in Russian). Tr Inst Polio Virusn Entsefalitov Akad Med Nauk SSSR 1974; 22: 5–18 (In English, NAMRU3-T950).

Chumakov MP, Belyaeva AP, Voroshilova MK, Butenko AM, Shalunova NV, Semashko IV, Mart'ianova LI, Smirnova SE, Bashkirtsev VN, Zavodova TI, Rubin SG, Tkachenko EA, Karmysheva VI, Reingol'd VN, Popov GV, Kirov DN, Stolbov DN, Perelatov VD. Progress in studying the etiology, immunology, and laboratory diagnosis of Crimean hemorrhagic fever in the USSR and Bulgaria. Mater 15 Nauchn Sess Inst Polio Virus Entsefalitov (Moscow, October 1968) 1968; 3: 100–103 (In English, NAMRU3-T613).

Chumakov MP, Ismailova ST, Rubin SG, Smirnova SE, Zgurskaia GN, Khankishiev A Sh, Berezin VV, Solovei EA. Detection of Crimean hemorrhagic fever foci in Azerbaijan SSR from results from serological investigations of domestic animals (in Russian). Tr Inst Polio Virusn Entsefalitov Akad Med Nauk SSSR 1970; 18: 120–122. (In English, NAMRU3-T941).

Chunikhin SP, Chumakov MP, Butenko AM, Smirnova SE, Taufflieb R, Camicas JL, Robin Y, Cornet JP, Shabon Zh. Results from investigating human and domestic and wild animal blood sera in the Senegal Republic (western Africa) for antibodies to Crimean hemorrhagic fever virus. Mater 16 Nauchn Sess Inst Polio Virus Entsefalitov (Moscow, October 1969) 1969; 2: 158–160 (In English, NAMRU3-T810).

Darwish MA, Hoogstraal H, Roberts TJ, Ghazi R, Amer T. A sero-epidemiological survey for *Bunyaviridae* and certain other arboviruses in Pakistan. Trans R Soc Trop Med Hyg 1983; 77: 446–450.

Donchev D, Kebedzhiev G, Rusakiev M. Hemorrhagic fever in Bulgaria. Bulg Akad Nauk Mikrobiol Inst 1. Kongr Mikrobiol (1965) 1967; 777–784. (In English, NAMRU3-T465).

Drosten C, Gottig S, Schilling S, Asper M, Panning M, Schmitz H, Gunther S. Rapid detection and quantification of RNA of Ebola and Marburg viruses, Lassa virus, Crimean–Congo hemorrhagic fever virus, Rift Valley fever virus, dengue virus, and yellow fever virus by real-time reverse transcription-PCR. J Clin Microbiol 2002a; 40: 2323–2330.

Drosten C, Minnak D, Emmerich P, Schmitz H, Reinicke T. Crimean–Congo hemorrhagic fever in Kosovo. J Clin Microbiol 2002b; 40: 1122–1123.

Dunster L, Dunster M, Ofula V, Beti D, Kazooba-Voskamp F, Burt F, Swanepoel R, DeCock KM. First documentation of human Crimean–Congo hemorrhagic fever, Kenya. Emerg Infect Dis 2002; 8: 1005–1006.

el-Azazy OM, Scrimgeour EM. Crimean–Congo haemorrhagic fever virus infection in the western province of Saudi Arabia. Trans R Soc Trop Med Hyg 1997; 91: 275–278.

Elliott RM, Bouloy M, Calisher CH, Goldbach R, Moyer JT, Nichol ST, Pettersson R, Plyusnin A, Schmaljohn CS. Bunyaviridae. In: Virus Taxonomy. VII Report of the International Committee on Taxonomy of Viruses (van Regenmortel MHV, Fauquet CM, Bishop DHL, Carsten EB, Estes MK, Lemon SM, Maniloff J, Mayo MA, McGeoch DJ, Pringle CR, Wickner RB, editors). San Diego, CA: Academic Press; 2000; pp. 599–621.

Eltari E, Cani M, Cani K, Gina A. Crimean–Congo hemorrhagic fever in Albania. Abstracts of 1st International Symposium on Hantaviruses and Crimean–Congo Hemorrhagic Fever Virus, Halkidiki, Greece; 1988; p. 34.

Ergonul O, Celikbas A, Dokuzoguz B, Eren S, Baykam N, Esener H. Characteristics of patients with Crimean–Congo hemorrhagic fever in a recent outbreak in Turkey and impact of oral ribavirin therapy. Clin Infect Dis 2004; 39: 284–287.

Fagbami AH, Tomori O, Fabiyi A, Isoun TT. Experimental Congo virus (Ib-AN 7620) infection in primates. Virologie 1975; 26: 33–37.

Federation of American Scientists (FAS). Crimean–Congo Hemorrhagic Fever and America's War on Terrorism—Update March 2002. < http://www.fas.org/ahead/disease/cchf/outbreak/2001afg.htm > . Accessed 13 December 2005.

Fisher-Hoch SP, McCormick JB, Swanepoel R, Van Middlekoop A, Harvey S, Kustner HG. Risk of human infections with Crimean–Congo hemorrhagic fever virus in a South African rural community. Am J Trop Med Hyg 1992; 47: 337–345.

Garcia S, Chinikar S, Coudrier D, Billecocq A, Hooshmand B, Crance JM, Garin D, Bouloy M. Evaluation of a Crimean–Congo hemorrhagic fever virus recombinant antigen expressed by Semliki forest suicide virus for IgM and IgG antibody detection in human and animal sera collected in Iran. J Clin Virol 2006; 35(2): 154–159.

Gear JH, Thomson PD, Hopp M, Andronikou S, Cohn RJ, Ledger J, Berkowitz FE. Congo–Crimean haemorrhagic fever in South Africa. Report of a fatal case in the Transvaal. S Afr Med J 1982; 62: 576–580.

Geisbert TW, Jahrling PB. Exotic emerging viral diseases: progress and challenges. Nat Med 2004; (Suppl 12): S110–S121.

Gligic A, Stamatovic L, Stojanovic R, Obradovic M, Boskovic R. The first isolation of the Crimean hemorrhagic fever virus in Yugoslavia. Vojnosanit Pregl 1977; 34: 318–321.

Goldfarb LG, Chumakov MP, Myskin AA, Kondratenko VF, Reznikova OY. An epidemiological model of Crimean hemorrhagic fever. Am J Trop Med Hyg 1980; 29: 260–264.

Gonzalez JP, Camicas JL, Cornet JP, Faye O, Wilson ML. Sexual and transovarian transmission of Crimean–Congo haemorrhagic fever virus in *Hyalomma truncatum* ticks. Res Virol 1992; 143: 23–28.

Gonzalez JP, Camicas JL, Cornet JP, Wilson ML. Biological and clinical responses of West African sheep to Crimean–Congo haemorrhagic fever virus experimental infection. Res Virol 1998; 149: 445–455.

Gonzalez JP, LeGuenno B, Guillaud M, Wilson ML. A fatal case of Crimean–Congo haemorrhagic fever in Mauritania: virological and serological evidence suggesting epidemic transmission. Trans R Soc Trop Med Hyg 1990; 84: 573–576.

Gonzalez JP, Wilson ML, Cornet JP, Camicas JL. Host-passage-induced phenotypic changes in Crimean–Congo haemorrhagic fever virus. Res Virol 1995; 146: 131–140.

Han L, Tang Q, Zhao X, Saijo M, Tao X. Serologic studies of Xinjiang hemorrhagic fever in Bachu county, 2001. Zhonghua Liu Xing Bing Xue Za Zhi 2002; 23: 179–181.

Hewson R, Chamberlain J, Mioulet V, Lloyd G, Jamil B, Hasan R, Gmyl A, Gmyl L, Smirnova SE, Lukashev A, Karganova G, Clegg C. Crimean–Congo haemorrhagic fever virus: sequence analysis of the small RNA segments from a collection of viruses world wide. Virus Res 2004; 102: 185–189.

Honig JE, Osborne JC, Nichol ST. Crimean–Congo hemorrhagic fever virus genome L RNA segment and encoded protein. Virology 2004; 321: 29–35.

Hoogstraal H. The epidemiology of tick-borne Crimean Congo hemorrhagic fever in Asia Europe and Africa. J Med Entomol 1979; 15: 307–417.

Jahrling PB. Viral hemorrhagic fevers. In: Medical Aspects of Chemical and Biological Warfare (Sidell FR, Takafuji ET, Franz DR, editors). Washington, DC: Office of the Surgeon General at TMM Publications, Borden Institute, Walter Reed Army Medical Center; 1997; pp. 591–602.

Jaureguiberry S, Tattevin P, Tarantola A, Legay F, Tall A, Nabeth P, Zeller H, Michelet C. Imported Crimean–Congo hemorrhagic fever (CCHF). J Clin Microbiol 2005; 43(9): 4905–4907.

Joubert JR, King JB, Rossouw DJ, Cooper R. A nosocomial outbreak of Crimean–Congo haemorrhagic fever at Tygerberg Hospital. Part III. Clinical pathology and pathogenesis. S Afr Med J 1985; 68: 722–728.

Karti SS, Odabasi Z, Korten V, Yilmaz M, Sonmez M, Caylan R, Akdogan E, Eren N, Koksal I, Ovali E, Erickson BR, Vincent MJ, Nichol ST, Comer JA, Rollin PE, Ksiazek TG. Crimean–Congo hemorrhagic fever in Turkey. Emerg Infect Dis 2004; 10: 1379–1384.

Kazakov SV, Karimov SK, Dernovoi AG, Durumbetov Ye, Askarov AM, Zhetibayev BK, Ospanov KS. Methodological approaches to the study of the epidemic process of Crimean hemorrhagic fever in the Moiunkum natural foci in the Zhambyl Region. Gig Epidemiol Immunol 2001; 1–2: 75–84.

Khan AS, Maupin GO, Rollin PE, Noor AM, Shurie HH, Shalabi AG, Wasef S, Haddad YM, Sadek R, Ijaz K, Peters CJ, Ksiazek TG. An outbreak of Crimean–Congo hemorrhagic fever in the United Arab Emirates, 1994–1995. Am J Trop Med Hyg 1997; 57: 519–525.

Kinsella E, Martin SG, Grolla A, Czub M, Feldmann H, Flick R. Sequence determination of the Crimean–Congo hemorrhagic fever virus L segment. Virology 2004; 321: 23–28.

Kolman JM. Some physical and chemical properties of Uukuniemi virus, strain Potepli-63. Acta Virol 1970; 14: 159–162.

Lvov DK, Leonova GN, Gromashevsky VL, Skvortsova TM, Shestakov VI, Belikova NP, Berezina LK, Gofman YP, Klimenko SM, Safonov AV, Sazonov AA, Zakaryan VA. Khasan virus, a new ungrouped bunyavirus isolated from *Haemaphysalis longicornis* ticks in the Primorie region. Acta Virol 1978; 22: 249–252.

Mardani M, Jahromi MK, Naieni KH, Zeinali M. The efficacy of oral ribavirin in the treatment of Crimean–Congo hemorrhagic fever in Iran. Clin Infect Dis 2003; 36: 1613–1618.

Marriott AC, Nuttall PA. Comparison of the S RNA segments and nucleoprotein sequences of Crimean–Congo hemorrhagic fever, Hazara, and Dugbe viruses. Virology 1992; 189: 795–799.

Martin ML, Lindsey-Regnery H, Sasso DR, McCormick JB, Palmer E. Distinction between *Bunyaviridae* genera by surface structure and comparison with Hantaan virus using negative stain electron microscopy. Arch Virol 1985; 86: 17–28.

Montgomery RE. On a tick-borne gastro-enteritis of sheep and goats occurring in British East Africa. J Comp Pathol 1917; 30: 28–58.

Nabeth P, Cheikh DO, Lo B, Faye O, Vall IO, Niang M, Wague B, Diop D, Diallo M, Diallo B, Diop OM, Simon F. Crimean–Congo hemorrhagic fever, Mauritania. Emerg Infect Dis 2004a; 10: 2143–2149.

Nabeth P, Thior M, Faye O, Simon F. Human Crimean–Congo hemorrhagic fever, Senegal. Emerg Infect Dis 2004b; 10: 1881–1882.

National Institute for Communicable Diseases (NICD), South Africa. Annual Report 2003; pp. 58–59.

National Institute for Communicable Diseases (NICD), South Africa. Epidemic prone disease surveillance table. Communicable Diseases Surveillance Bulletin, January 2005a; p. 2.

National Institute for Communicable Diseases (NICD), South Africa. Viral haemorrhagic fevers, Crimean–Congo haemorrhagic fever (CCHF). Communicable Diseases Communiqué, 4 April 2005b.

Nichol ST. Bunyaviruses. In: Fields Virology (Knipe DM, Howley PM, editors). Philadelphia: Lippincott, Williams and Wilkins; 2001; pp. 1603–1633.

Onishchenko GG. Infectious diseases in natural reservoirs: epidemic situation and morbidity in the Russian Federation and prophylactic measures. Zh Mikrobiol Epidemiol Immunobiol 2001; 3: 22–28.

Onishchenko GG, Markov VI, Merkulov VA, Vasil'ev NT, Berezhnoi AM, Androshchuk IA, Maksimov VA. Isolation and identification of Crimean–Congo hemorrhagic fever virus in the Stavropol territory. Zh Mikrobiol Epidemiol Immunobiol 2001; 6: 7–11.

Pak TP. Structure of the distribution area of Crimean hemorrhagic fever in Tadzhikistan. Mater 9 Simp Ekol Virus (Dushanbe, October 1975) 1975; 39–43. (In English, NAMRU3-T1131).

Pak TP, Kostyukov MA, Daniyarov OA, Bulychev VP. A combined focus of arbovirus infections in Tadzhikistan. Mater 9 Simp Ekol Virus (Dushanbe, October 1975) 1975; 38–39. (In English, NAMRU3-T1127).

Papa A, Bino S, Llagami A, Brahimaj B, Papadimitriou E, Pavlidou V, Velo E, Cahani G, Hajdini M, Pilaca A, Harxhi A, Antoniadis A. Crimean–Congo hemorrhagic fever in Albania, 2001. Eur J Clin Microbiol 2002a; 21: 603–606.

Papa A, Bozovi B, Pavlidou V, Papadimitriou E, Pelemis M, Antoniadis A. Genetic detection and isolation of Crimean–Congo hemorrhagic fever virus, Kosovo, Yugoslavia. Emerg Infect Dis 2002b; 8: 852–854.

Papa A, Christova I, Papadimitriou E, Antoniadis A. Crimean–Congo hemorrhagic fever in Bulgaria. Emerg Infect Dis 2004; 10: 1465–1467.

Papa A, Ma B, Kouidou S, Tang Q, Hang C, Antoniadis A. Genetic characterization of the M RNA segment of Crimean Congo hemorrhagic fever virus strains, China. Emerg Infect Dis 2002c; 8: 50–53.

Papadopoulos O, Koptopoulos G. Isolation of Crimean–Congo hemorrhagic fever (C-CHF) virus from *Rhipicephalus bursa* ticks in Greece. Acta Hell Microbiol 1978; 23: 20–28.

Peters CJ, Reynolds JA, Slone TW, Jones DE, Stephen EL. Prophylaxis of Rift Valley fever with antiviral drugs, immune serum, an interferon inducer, and a macrophage activator. Antiviral Res 1986; 6: 285–297.

ProMED-mail. Crimean–Congo hem. fever-Kazakhstan (south). 6 May 1999: 19990506.0749 <http://www.promedmail.org>. Accessed 2 May 2005.

ProMED-mail. Crimean–Congo hem. fever-United Arab Emirates. 22 February 2000a: 20000224.0249 <http://www.promedmail.org>. Accessed 13 December 2005.

ProMED-mail. Crimean–Congo hem. fever-UAE: Background (02). 25 February 2000b: 20000226.0263 <http://www.promedmail.org>. Accessed 13 December 2005.

ProMED-mail. Crimean–Congo hemorrhagic fever-Tajikistan. 7 July 2000c: 20000708.1142 <http://www.promedmail.org>. Accessed 13 December 2005.

ProMED-mail. Crimean–Congo hem. fever-Yugoslavia (Kosovo). 11 July 2000d: 20000711.1151 <http://www.promedmail.org>. Accessed 13 December 2005.

ProMED-mail. Hemorrhagic fever-Iraq (Arbil). 20 September 2000e: 20000921.1629 <http://www.promedmail.org>. Accessed 13 December 2005.

ProMED-mail. Crimean–Congo hem. fever-Kazakhstan (south). 4 May 2001: 20010504.0865 <http://www.promedmail.org>. Accessed 13 December 2005.

ProMED-mail. Crimean–Congo hemorrhagic fever-Namibia. 18 January 2002a: 20020120.3327 <http://www.promedmail.org>. Accessed 13 December 2005.

ProMED-mail. Crimean–Congo hemorrhagic fever-Iran ex Afghanistan. 6 June 2002b: 20020607.4430 <http://www.promedmail.org>. Accessed 13 December 2005.

ProMED-mail. Crimean–Congo hem. fever-Pakistan: suspected. 28 February 2003a: 20030228.0498 <http://www.promedmail.org>. Accessed 13 December 2005.

ProMED-mail. Crimean–Congo hem. fever-Russia (Stavropol). 18 July 2003b: 20030718.1768 <http://www.promedmail.org>. Accessed 13 December 2005.

ProMED-mail. Crimean–Congo hem. fever-Russia (Stavropol). 4 June 2004a: 20040610.1563 <http://www.promedmail.org>. Accessed 13 December 2005.

ProMED-mail. Crimean–Congo hem fever-Pakistan (Bal): suspected (04). 8 June 2004b: 20040608.1540 <http://www.promedmail.org>. Accessed 13 December 2005.

ProMED-mail. Crimean–Congo hemorrhagic fever-Pakistan (Bal) (05): suspected. 21 June 2004c: 20040621.1657 <http://www.promedmail.org>. Accessed 13 December 2005.

ProMED-mail. Crimean–Congo hem. fever-Serbia and Montenegro (Kosovo). 26 June 2004d: 20040626.1706 <http://www.promedmail.org>. Accessed 13 December 2005.

ProMED-mail. Crimean–Congo hem. fever-Kazakhstan (south). 4 July 2004e: 20040704.1793 <http://www.promedmail.org>. Accessed 13 December 2005.

ProMED-mail. Crimean–Congo hem. fever-Pakistan (Rawalpindi). 27 September 2004f: 20040927.2663 <http://www.promedmail.org>. Accessed 13 December 2005.

ProMED-mail. Crimean–Congo hemorrhagic fever, 2004-Iran. 5 February 2005a: 20050205.0397 <http://www.promedmail.org>. Accessed 13 December 2005.

ProMED-mail. Crimean–Congo hem. fever-Pakistan (Islamabad). 25 April 2005b: 20050425.1150 <http://www.promedmail.org>. Accessed 13 December 2005.

ProMED-mail. Crimean–Congo hem. fever-Russia (Stavropol). 1 May 2005c: 20050501.1214 <http://www.promedmail.org>. Accessed 13 December 2005.

ProMED-mail. Crimean–Congo hemorrhagic fever-Russia (Southern Federal District). 3 October 2005d: 20051003.2891 <http://www.promedmail.org>. Accessed 13 December 2005.

ProMED-mail. Crimean–Congo hem. fever-South Africa (Southern Cape). 11 October 2005e: 20051011.2963 <http://www.promedmail.org>. Accessed 13 December 2005.

ProMED-mail. Crimean–Congo hemorrhagic fever-Turkey (04) WHO. 9 August, 2006: 20060809.2230 <http://www.promedmail.org>. Accessed 29 September, 2006a.

ProMED-mail (2006b) Crimean–Congo hem. fever - Russia (Southern Federal District) (04). 10 August, 2006: 20060810.2242 <http://www.promedmail.org>. Accessed 29 September, 2006.

Pullikotil P, Vincent M, Nichol ST, Seidah NG. Development of protein-based inhibitors of the proprotein of convertase SKI-1/S1P: processing of SREBP-2, ATF6, and a viral glycoprotein. J Biol Chem 2004; 279: 17338–17347.

Rodriguez LL, Maupin GO, Ksiazek TG, Rollin PE, Khan AS, Schwarz TF, Lofts RS, Smith JF, Noor AM, Peters CJ, Nichol ST. Molecular investigation of a multisource outbreak of Crimean–Congo hemorrhagic fever in the United Arab Emirates. Am J Trop Med Hyg 1997; 57: 512–518.

Rybalko SI, Pankina MV, Kannegiser NI, Burlakova TS. Hemorrhagic fever in southern localities of Kazakhstan. Med Parazitol Parazit Bolezni 1963; 32: 619–620 (In English, NAMRU3-T154).

Saijo M, Tang Q, Shimayi B, Han L, Zhang Y, Asiguma M, Tianshu D, Maeda A, Kurane I, Morikawa S. Recombinant nucleoprotein-based serological diagnosis of Crimean–Congo hemorrhagic fever virus infections. J Med Virol 2005; 75: 295–299.

Saluzzo JF, Aubry P, McCormick J, Digoutte JP. Haemorrhagic fever caused by Crimean Congo haemorrhagic fever virus in Mauritania. Trans R Soc Trop Med Hyg 1985a; 79: 268.

Saluzzo JF, Digoutte JP, Camicas JL, Chauvancy G. Crimean–Congo haemorrhagic fever and Rift Valley fever in south-eastern Mauritania. Lancet 1985b; 1: 116.

Saluzzo JF, Digoutte JP, Cornet M, Baudon D, Roux J, Robert V. Isolation of Crimean–Congo haemorrhagic fever and Rift Valley fever viruses in Upper Volta. Lancet 1984; 1: 1179.

Schmaljohn CS, Hooper JW. *Bunyaviridae*: the viruses and their replication. In: Fields Virology (Knipe DM, Howley PM, editors). Philadelphia: Lippincott, Williams and Wilkins; 2001; pp. 1581–1602.

Schwarz TF, Nitschko H, Jager G, Nsanze H, Longson M, Pugh RN, Abraham AK. Crimean–Congo haemorrhagic fever in Oman. Lancet 1995; 346: 123.

Schwarz TF, Nsanze H, Longson M, Nitschko H, Gilch S, Shurie H, Ameen A, Zahir AR, Acharya UG, Jager G. Polymerase chain reaction for diagnosis and identification of distinct variants of Crimean–Congo hemorrhagic fever virus in the United Arab Emirates. Am J Trop Med Hyg 1996; 55: 190–196.

Scrimgeour EM, Mehta FR, Suleiman AJ. Infectious and tropical diseases in Oman: a review. Am J Trop Med Hyg 1999; 61: 920–925.

Semyatkovskaya ZV, Sudtdykova NK. On the clinical aspects of infectious hemorrhagic fever. Klin Med Moscow 1950; 28: 69–71.

Sheikh AS, Sheikh AA, Sheikh NS, Rafi US, Asif M, Afridi F, Malik MT. Bi-annual surge of Crimean–Congo haemorrhagic fever (CCHF): a five-year experience. Int J Infect Dis 2005; 9: 37–42.

Shepherd AJ, Swanepoel R, Leman PA, Shepherd SP. Comparison of methods for isolation and titration of Crimean–Congo hemorrhagic fever virus. J Clin Microbiol 1986; 24: 654–656.

Shepherd AJ, Swanepoel R, Leman PA, Shepherd SP. Field and laboratory investigation of Crimean–Congo haemorrhagic fever virus (Nairovirus, family *Bunyaviridae*) infection in birds. Trans R Soc Trop Med Hyg 1987; 81: 1004–1007.

Simpson DIH, Knight EM, Courtois GH, Williams MC, Weinbren MP, Kibukamusoke JW. Congo virus: a hitherto undescribed virus occurring in Africa. I. Human isolations-clinical notes. E Afr Med J 1967; 44: 87–92.

Smego Jr. RA, Sarwari AR, Siddiqui AR. Crimean–Congo hemorrhagic fever: prevention and control limitations in a resource-poor country. Clin Infect Dis 2004; 38: 1731–1735.

Suleiman MN, Muscat-Baron JM, Harries JR, Satti AG, Platt GS, Bowen ET, Simpson DI. Congo/Crimean haemorrhagic fever in Dubai. An outbreak at the Rashid Hospital. Lancet 1980; 2: 939–941.

Swanepoel R. Nairovirus infections. In: Exotic Viral Infections (Porterfield JS, editor). London: Chapman & Hall; 1995; pp. 285–293.

Swanepoel R, Gill DE, Shepherd AJ, Leman PA, Mynhardt JH, Harvey S. The clinical pathology of Crimean–Congo hemorrhagic fever. Rev Infect Dis 1989; 11(Suppl 4): 794–800.

Swanepoel R, Leman PA, Abbott JC. Epidemiology, diagnosis, clinical pathology and treatment of Crimean–Congo haemorrhagic fever (CCHF) in South Africa. In: VIIIth International Congress of Virology, Berlin 430 (abstract P70-003); 1990.

Swanepoel R, Leman PA, Burt FJ, Jardine J, Verwoerd DJ, Capua I, Bruckner GK, Burger WP. Experimental infection of ostriches with Crimean–Congo haemorrhagic fever virus. Epidemiol Infect 1998; 121: 427–432.

Swanepoel R, Shepherd AJ, Leman PA, Shepherd SP, McGillivray GM, Erasmus MJ, Searle LA, Gill DE. Epidemiologic and clinical features of Crimean–Congo hemorrhagic fever in southern Africa. Am J Trop Med Hyg 1987; 36: 120–132.

Swanepoel R, Shepherd AJ, Leman PA, Shepherd SP, Miller GB. A common-source outbreak of Crimean–Congo haemorrhagic fever on a dairy farm. S Afr Med J 1985; 68: 635–637.

Swanepoel R, Struthers JK, Shepherd AJ, McGillivray GM, Nel MJ, Jupp PG. Crimean Congo hemorrhagic fever in South Africa. Am J Trop Med Hyg 1983; 32: 1407–1415.

Tamura M, Asada H, Kondo K, Takahashi M, Yamanishi K. Effects of human and murine interferons against hemorrhagic fever with renal syndrome (HFRS) virus (Hantaan virus). Antiviral Res 1987; 8: 171–178.

Tang Q, Saijo M, Zhang Y, Asiguma M, Tianshu D, Han L, Shimayi B, Maeda A, Kurane I, Morikawa S. A patient with Crimean–Congo hemorrhagic fever serologically diagnosed by recombinant nucleoprotein-based antibody detection systems. Clin Diagn Lab Immun 2003; 10: 489–491.

Temonen M, Lankinen H, Vapalahti O, Ronni T, Julkunen I, Vaheri A. Effect of interferon-alpha and cell differentiation on Puumala virus infection in human monocyte/macrophages. Virology 1995; 206: 8–15.

Tignor GH, Hanham CA. Ribavirin efficacy in an *in vivo* model of Crimean–Congo hemorrhagic fever virus (CCHF) infection. Antiviral Res 1993; 22: 309–325.

Tkachenko EA, Butenko AM, Badalov ME, Chumakov MP. Results of remote revaccination against Crimean hemorrhagic fever. Tezisy 17 Nauchn Sess Inst Posvyashch Aktual Probl Virus Profilakt Virus Zabolev Moscow October 1972; 349. (In English, NAMRU3-T1058).

Tkachenko EA, Butenko AM, Badalov ME, Zavodova TI, Chumakov MP. Investigation of the immunogenic activity of killed brain vaccine against Crimean hemorrhagic fever. Tr Inst Polio Virusn Entsefalitov Akad Med Nauk SSSR 1971; 19: 119–129 (In English, NAMRU3-T931).

Tkachenko EA, Khanun K, Berezin VV. Serological investigation of human and animal sera in agar gel diffusion and precipitation (AGDP) test for the presence of antibodies of Crimean hemorrhagic fever and Grand Arbaud viruses. Mater 16 Nauchn Sess Inst Polio Virus Entsefalitov Moscow October 1969 [2] 1969; 2: 265. (In English, NAMRU3-T620).

USACHPPM. Health information operations (HIO) Update 25 July 2002. <http://chppm-www.apgea.army.mil/HIOupdate/>. Accessed 13 December 2005.

van de Wal BW, Joubert JR, van Eeden PJ, King JB. A nosocomial outbreak of Crimean–Congo haemorrhagic fever at Tygerberg Hospital. Part IV. Preventive and prophylactic measures. S Afr Med J 1985; 68: 729–732.

Vassilenko SM. Results of the investigation on etiology, epidemiologic features and the specific prophylactic of Crimean hemorrhagic fever (CHF) in Bulgaria. Abstr Inv Pap 9 Int Congr Trop Med Malar (Athens, October 1973) 1973; 1: 32–33.

Vassilenko SM, Vassilev TL, Bozadjiev LG, Bineva IL, Kazarov GZ. Specific intravenous immunoglobulin for Crimean–Congo haemorrhagic fever. Lancet 1990; 335: 791–792.

Watts DM, Ksiazek TG, Linthicum KJ, Hoogstraal H. Crimean–Congo hemorrhagic fever. In: The Arboviruses: Epidemiology and Ecology (Monath TP, editor). vol. II. Boca Raton, FL: CRC Press; 1989a; pp. 177–222.

Watts DM, Ussery MA, Nash D, Peters CJ. Inhibition of Crimean–Congo hemorrhagic fever viral infectivity yields *in vitro* by ribavirin. Am J Trop Med Hyg 1989b; 41: 581–585.

Williams MC, Tukei PM, Lule M, Mujomba E, Mukuye A. Virology: identification studies. Rep E Afr Virus Res Inst 1966 1967; 16: 24–26.

Williams RJ, Al-Busaidy S, Mehta FR, Maupin GO, Wagoner KD, Al-Awaidy S, Suleiman AJ, Khan AS, Peters CJ, Ksiazek TG. Crimean–Congo haemorrhagic fever: a seroepidemiological and tick survey in the Sultanate of Oman. Trop Med Int Health 2000; 5: 99–106.

Woodall JP, Williams MC, Simpson DIH, Ardoin P, Lule M, West R. The Congo group of agents. Rep E Afr Virus Res Inst (1963–1964) 1965; 14: 34–36.

World Health Organization (WHO). Crimean–Congo haemorrhagic fever in Afghanistan. Disease outbreaks reported, 8 May 1998 <http://www.who.int/csr/don/1998_05_08a/en/>. Accessed 13 December 2005.

World Health Organization (WHO). Crimean–Congo haemorrhagic fever (CCHF) in Kosovo-Update 5, 29 June 2001a <http://www.who.int/csr/don/2001_06_29e/en/>. Accessed 13 December 2005.

World Health Organization (WHO). Outbreak news. Wkly Epidemiol Rec 2001b; 76: 318.

Yashina L, Petrova I, Seregin S, Vyshemirskii O, Lvov D, Aristova V, Kuhn J, Morzunov S, Gutorov V, Kuzina I, Tyunnikov G, Netesov S, Petrov V. Genetic variability of Crimean–Congo haemorrhagic fever virus in Russia and Central Asia. J Gen Virol 2003a; 84: 1199–1206.

Yashina L, Vyshemirskii O, Seregin S, Petrova I, Samokhvalov E, Lvov D, Gutorov V, Kuzina I, Tyunnikov G, Tang YW, Netesov S, Petrov V. Genetic analysis of Crimean–Congo hemorrhagic fever virus in Russia. J Clin Microbiol 2003b; 41: 860–862.

Zarubinski VI, Klisenko GA, Kuchin VV, Timchenko VV, Shanoyan NK. Application of the indirect hemagglutination inhibition test for serological investigation of Crimean hemorrhagic fever focus in Rostov Oblast (in Russian). Sb Tr Inst Virus imeni D.I. Ivanovsky, Akad Med Nauk SSSR 1975; 2: 73–77. (In English, NAMRU3-T1145).

Emerging Viruses in Human Populations
Edward Tabor (Editor)
DOI 10.1016/S0168-7069(06)16013-9

Surveillance for Newly Emerging Viruses

David Buckeridge, Geneviève Cadieux

Department of Epidemiology, Biostatistics, and Occupational Health, Clinical and Health Informatics, McGill University, 1140 Pine Avenue West, Montreal, Quebec H3A 1A3, Canada

Introduction and background

Newly emerging infectious diseases will pose an increasing global health threat over the next 20 years. However, the future impact of infectious diseases will be heavily influenced by the degree of success of global and national efforts to create public health infrastructure with effective systems of surveillance and response (Institute of Medicine of the National Academies, 2003).

Goals of surveillance

Surveillance is a fundamental tool for public health, producing information to guide actions. Modern surveillance tends to follow health measures such as the incidence of a disease or syndrome or even the occurrence of health-related behaviors. There are many reasons for conducting surveillance, and the data collected and the approach taken to analyzing those data are both influenced by the overall goal of a surveillance system. In the context of newly emerging viruses, surveillance may be performed to detect disease outbreaks, to monitor the spread or development of ongoing outbreaks, to evaluate the effectiveness of disease control measures, or to identify the determinants of infection and disease.

   The focus of this chapter is on surveillance that will provide information useful for the detection of disease outbreaks due to newly emerging viruses. Surveillance systems aimed mainly at detection also provide information that may be useful for other purposes. The goal of detecting an outbreak of a newly emerging virus, however, places specific demands on the type of data collected and the types of analysis performed.

   The term 'newly emerging' virus is different from 'emerging virus' in that a newly emerging virus has not yet been isolated in the laboratory (Barrett et al.,

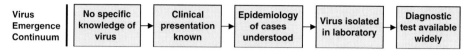

Fig. 1 Surveillance continuum for a newly emerging virus.

1998). Whether the virus has been isolated, and more importantly, whether a diagnostic test is available, have implications for surveillance. As a new virus becomes recognized (Fig. 1), or 'emerges,' it is initially recognized through the clinical presentation of infected individuals. Cases of an apparently novel infectious illness in humans will prompt epidemiological investigations and initiate efforts to isolate the causative agent. Once the agent has been isolated, effort often turns to development of methods for diagnosis. At some point in this progression, the virus is seen as an established cause of endemic or epidemic disease, and is no longer thought of as 'newly emerging.'

The distinction between 'newly emerging' and 'emerging' viruses is therefore important from the perspective of surveillance, because it determines what data a surveillance system can draw upon. For 'newly emerging viruses,' any case definition must rely on clinical and possibly epidemiological data because there are no recognized laboratory tests. Routine surveillance of laboratory test results is likely to be of little use in sounding the initial alarm in an outbreak due to a newly emerging virus. An exception might be if the newly emerging virus is genetically similar to an existing virus, to the extent that it can cross-react in an existing diagnostic test. However, laboratory testing will be useful for ruling out known viruses as the cause of illness, and ultimately to identify the virus. The surveillance system must follow data other than positive laboratory test results, such as reports of abnormal cases, or the incidence of non-specific symptoms, or syndromes that might occur following infection with a newly emerging virus.

This observation raises an important point, which is that the likelihood of identifying a newly emerging virus through surveillance will depend, among other factors, on the novelty and the severity of symptoms due to infection with the virus and the number of symptomatic cases. The surveillance approach that is most likely to detect an outbreak due to a newly emerging virus will vary with virus and outbreak characteristics. Depending on the combination of clinical presentation of those infected and the genotype of the virus (Fig. 2), different methods will be more or less efficient for early outbreak detection. Outbreaks of newly emerging viruses characterized by symptoms common to other infections already under surveillance may be detected by an existing surveillance system if the number infected is sufficiently large. Alternatively, infections with a newly emerging virus causing symptoms similar to another, known pathogen may be incorrectly attributed to the known pathogen, thereby obscuring the emerging epidemic. Genetic similarity to a known virus may hasten the identification of a newly emerging virus and the development of a diagnostic test as well as contribute to our understanding of its host range, natural reservoir, and transmission route.

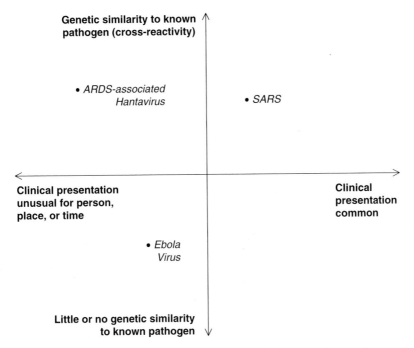

Fig. 2 Factors influencing the initial detection of outbreaks due to newly emerging viruses.

Relevant examples

The chronology of events surrounding the initial detection of two emerging viral disease, SARS-CoV and Hantavirus, illustrate how different approaches to surveillance contributed to the initial detection and early management of these outbreaks.

SARS

The emergence of severe acute respiratory syndrome (SARS) (Table 1; Brookes and Khan, 2005), caused by the SARS-CoV virus, was obscured because it appeared initially in the Chinese province of Guandong as cases of atypical pneumonia that were clinically similar to influenza and that occurred concurrently with an outbreak of avian influenza in chickens. The large number of cases and the circumstances similar to those of influenza outbreaks ensured that the SARS outbreak was detected, but the similarity of the clinical presentation to other diseases may have initially mislead public health officials about its etiology. Reports of an atypical pneumonia or influenza outbreak in China circulated as early as November 2002, disseminated via ProMED-mail (an Internet and email-based reporting and surveillance system), and picked up by the web-crawling surveillance system GPHIN (Global Public Health Intelligence Network, developed by Health Canada). The

Table 1

Timeline of SARS outbreak detection and virus identification (Brookes and Khan, 2005)

November 16, 2002	First known case of SARS occurs in Guandong Province, China
November 23, 2002	During a routine flu workshop in China, a participant informs the WHO Influenza Laboratory Network of a serious outbreak in Guandong, with high mortality and high involvement of health care staff
November 27, 2002	GPHIN (web-crawler developed by Health Canada) picks up rumors of avian influenza outbreak in mainland China
December 2002	Chinese Ministry of Health confirms outbreak of influenza B, now under control
February 10, 2003	An American infectious disease consultant receives an email from China concerning a rumor of closed hospitals and people dying due to an outbreak in Guangzhou. He posts the content of the e-mail on ProMED
	A relative of a former employee informs WHO of an epidemic involving over 100 fatalities in China. WHO contacts the Chinese Ministry of Health
February 11, 2003	The Chinese Ministry of Health in Beijing issues an official statement acknowledging an outbreak of atypical pneumonia dating back to November 2002 and involving 300 cases, of which 1/3 were health care workers
February 17, 2003	First SARS case introduced in Hong Kong
February 19, 2003	WHO issues an avian flu alert
February 26, 2003	First SARS case introduced in Vietnam
March 1, 2003	First SARS case introduced in Singapore
March 11, 2003	Outbreak of 'acute respiratory syndrome' among hospital workers in Hong Kong
March 13, 2003	SARS outbreak reaches Toronto
March 15, 2003	WHO confirms that SARS is a worldwide health threat, and that suspected cases have been identified in Canada, Indonesia, Philippines, Singapore, Thailand, and Vietnam
March 19, 2003	SARS spreads to the US, UK, Spain, Germany, and Slovenia
March 21, 2003	SARS coronavirus identified. Official identification announced on April 16
April 2003	PCR test to diagnose SARS from nasopharyngeal aspirate becomes available, followed by serological assay to diagnose SARS from blood sample

course of illness was rapid and its presentation severe; therefore the initial cases were not identified until infected persons sought the attention of health care professionals and a clinical assessment was made.

It was only when the outbreak spread beyond mainland China in February 2003 to hospital staff in Hong Kong that reliable information became available concerning the mysterious 'acute respiratory syndrome', allowing a novel etiology to be hypothesized. It was recognized that the disease was unlike influenza when numerous health care professionals treating SARS patients fell ill themselves. As more became known about the illness, syndromic surveillance (i.e., surveillance of cases identified on the basis of clinical symptoms, in this case fever and respiratory symptoms), contact tracing, and quarantine were implemented.

The virus was found to be a new coronavirus. Isolation of the virus did not occur initially, perhaps because the isolation of a coronavirus did not immediately raise suspicion because coronaviruses are commonly associated with milder respiratory illness. Laboratory-based surveillance did not become available until later in the outbreak, when diagnostic PCR and serology tests were developed. Population screening for SARS antibodies was instituted in some countries, with mixed results due to poor specificity of early versions of the tests.

Hantavirus

In contrast to the SARS outbreak, the May 1993 outbreak of acute respiratory distress syndrome (ARDS) in the Four Corners region of the western United States involved few cases and an unusual clinical presentation. According to many sources, the Four Corners epidemic would not have been detected, if not for one astute internist who saw a connection between an unusual death in his patient due to an acute respiratory syndrome, and the similar fatal illness of his fiancée. The illness was severe and the course rapid, therefore cases initially were identified only after infected persons sought medical attention. The internist sounded the alarm, alerting the state health department epidemiologist to a possible communicable disease outbreak; the epidemiologist launched a retrospective investigation to identify other similar recent cases, and instituted a mechanism for reporting suspected outbreak cases (Institute of Medicine of the National Academies, 2003).

Identification of the pathogen responsible for this outbreak was made easier and quicker because the virus was from a known virus family, and antibodies to the new virus cross-reacted with known viruses in the same family. The CDC's viral pathogens branch tested the clinical specimens received from Four Corners against antibodies for every known virus, and the test was positive for Hantavirus.

Hantaviruses had been discovered during the Korean War (1951–1954). Although they were known to cause renal impairment, they had never been associated with respiratory illness. Mice were known to be a reservoir for hantaviruses, so rodents were trapped in Four Corners and tested. PCR techniques were used to identify the deer mouse as the reservoir of Hantavirus in this outbreak.

Surveillance methodology and approaches to surveillance

The process of surveillance

All approaches to surveillance share some common principles. While some of the underlying methods used in public health surveillance have evolved considerably in

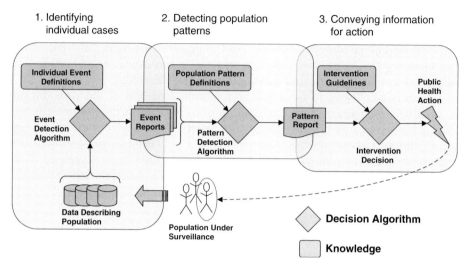

Fig. 3 The process of surveillance. Critical points in this process include the detection of events in individuals (e.g., a diagnosis of measles), the identification of patterns in the population (e.g., a rapid rise in incidence in a geographic location), and the incorporation of information about identified patterns into decisions about interventions. (For colour version: see Colour Section on page 357).

recent years, the general approach to surveillance has remained relatively constant. At a fundamental level, surveillance aims to (1) identify individual cases, (2) detect population patterns in identified cases, and then (3) convey information to decision-makers about population health patterns (Fig. 3).

Identification of individual cases

The definition of a case for a surveillance system (Fig. 3, Step 1) has important implications for the design and performance of the system. In settings where a surveillance system is intended to follow cases of a well-understood disease, it may be possible to make the case definition highly specific. For example, public health agencies in many developed countries conduct routine surveillance for communicable diseases such as measles. Definitions of cases in these systems tend to rely upon highly specific diagnostic tests. As a result, communicable disease surveillance systems tend to rely upon data from laboratory testing as opposed to data from clinical examinations (Koo and Wetterhall, 1996).

However, in many surveillance settings, it is not possible to rely on diagnostic tests as central components of a case definition. Worldwide surveillance for polio is an example in which, despite the existence of a specific diagnostic test, the case definition refers to a syndrome ('flaccid paralysis') as opposed to a laboratory test result (Kohler et al., 2002). Clinical data are used for the polio case definition because, in many countries, laboratory testing for polio is not readily available and because the clinical definition is highly sensitive. Newly emerging viruses present another example of a situation where it is generally not possible to rely on a laboratory test for a case definition.

By definition, laboratory tests are not available for newly emerging viruses, so the case definition must focus on the clinical and epidemiological characteristics of disease. This is problematic, however, because newly emerging viruses may cause a variety of clinical presentations, depending on the characteristics of the virus and the host. In other words, the specific characteristics of a case are not known in advance when developing a surveillance system to detect newly emerging viruses. One approach to this problem is not to define cases in advance, but instead to monitor information sources (e.g., the World Wide Web, posts to electronic discussion boards, etc.) for reports of unusual cases that could be due to a newly emerging virus. However, if used, case definitions must be broad enough to ensure that the surveillance system will be sufficiently sensitive. In this setting, the cost of increased sensitivity is reduced specificity. In other words, to ensure that a case definition will identify cases of infection from a newly emerging virus, we must accept that the definition will also pick up cases of disease due to other causes.

Detection of population patterns among cases of the disease

The detection of population patterns (Fig. 3, Step 2) among cases generally refers to the detection of *unexpected* patterns in the incidence of cases. Surveillance analysts are interested usually in detecting an unexpected increases in overall incidence or an increase in incidence in a population subgroup or in a geographic region. There is a close relationship between the characteristics of the case definition and the detection of population patterns. When a case definition is highly specific, a large proportion of identified cases will be true cases and there will be very little 'noise' in the signal at the population level. When the signal is strong, it is easier to detect unexpected patterns. If the historical variation in the incidence rate of measles, for instance, is low, then an increased incidence of positive test results for measles virus infection should be detected relatively easily. Accordingly, the methods used to search prospectively for outbreaks using communicable disease surveillance data tend to be straightforward: mainly observation and statistical methods (Stroup et al., 1993; Hutwagner et al., 1997). However, the necessity for high sensitivity in the case definition for newly emerging viruses tends to result in low specificity.

Another potential source of 'noise' is the normal variation in the incidence of cases. In general, the greater this baseline normal variation, the more difficult it will be to detect an unexpected increase in the incidence. At one extreme, if no cases are expected under normal conditions, then the occurrence of a single case may be sufficient to trigger further action. For example, one case of hemorrhagic fever in a developed country is probably sufficient to attract notice. However, when cases present with more commonly encountered symptoms, a few cases may not be distinguished from the baseline incidence of those symptoms. For example, influenza-like symptoms due to a newly emerging disease agent might not attract notice.

In situations where an increase is observed in the incidence of cases with non-specific symptoms, appropriate public health action may be delayed (Duchin, 2003; Pavlin, 2003).

The public health response

The public health response is determined by the communicability and severity of the disease, and the susceptibility of the population. With a newly emerging virus, there are likely to be many unknown aspects about both the public health threat and potentially effective intervention measures. The cautious approach is to assume that the public health threat is serious, and, until the transmission dynamics are known, to use generic control measures such as isolation of infected cases and quarantine of exposed individuals.

Surveillance settings and mandates

An appreciation of the fundamental issues of surveillance is important, but it is also important to realize that surveillance occurs in a context that includes the geographic setting of the surveillance system and the mandate of the surveillance organization. Often the data collected through regional surveillance systems are transmitted to national systems, which provide a broader perspective and allow identification of disease outbreaks that span adjacent regions. The National Notifiable Disease Surveillance System (NNDSS) in the United States is an example of this model (Koo and Wetterhall, 1996). The communication between national and international systems generally involves aggregate data. The SARS outbreak in 2002–2003 provides examples of this cooperation as well as the role of political considerations, in terms of the initial detection in China, and the ongoing management of the outbreak in Canada.

Organizations conducting surveillance have differing mandates for data collection and for intervention. In most countries, the government has the legal authority and mandate to maintain public health, and this includes both surveillance and intervention to control disease outbreaks. However, the authority to conduct surveillance is often mandated in terms of known diseases; the surveillance to detect newly emerging diseases may not be explicitly described. This may pose practical problems for public health authorities as they attempt to develop surveillance systems, especially if the systems require clinical data whose use may be restricted by law. Similarly, the communication of surveillance information between countries and to international agencies may not be clearly permitted by law or policy in some countries. The Global Outbreak Alert and Response Network (GOARN), coordinated by the World Health Organization (WHO), was established in 1997 and formalized in 2000 to address issues of international cooperation in the face of outbreaks of emerging infectious diseases (Heymann, 2004).

Types of surveillance

The appropriateness of a surveillance method for an emerging virus is determined to a large extent by the specificity of the case definition (Fig. 4). Any surveillance system searching for new viruses must follow cases with unusual presentations or must follow the incidence of non-specific syndromes. Once the clinical presentation and epidemiology of a newly emerging virus are understood, this knowledge can be incorporated into a more specific case definition. Even greater specificity in the case definition can be achieved once the virus is isolated and diagnostic tests have been developed.

Initial detection and early stage surveillance

For unknown viruses or those early in emergence, the focus of surveillance can follow either of two approaches. One is 'information surveillance', by which information about disease outbreaks is sought on the Internet or through other sources. The other is syndromic surveillance, which follows pre-diagnostic data generated when individuals use health care services.

Information surveillance. The Internet has enabled novel approaches to collecting public health data, both passively and actively. Passive approaches rely on submission of disease reports, usually via e-mail, to a single location; active approaches involve searches of the Internet for posted information about disease outbreaks. These systems conduct 'information surveillance', in that they follow information about outbreaks, as opposed to relying on the case definitions traditionally used in disease surveillance. One system that has been used is ProMED-mail, which relies on both submission of outbreak reports and manual review of Internet sources, and the resulting information is reviewed by experts who then disseminate their conclusions. Another system, GPHIN, relies on active computer search of the

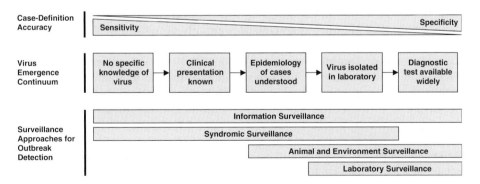

Fig. 4 The continuum of emergence for a virus showing the change in the sensitivity and specificity of the case definition for surveillance, and the appropriate approaches to surveillance, at different points along the continuum.

Internet for reports of disease outbreaks. Both of these systems have successfully identified recent outbreaks of newly emerging viruses, but neither approach to surveillance has been the subject of a rigorous peer-reviewed evaluation.

The Program for Monitoring Emerging Diseases (ProMED) and ProMED-mail: The Program for Monitoring Emerging Diseases (ProMED) was founded in 1993, and an e-mail list for sharing news about emerging diseases (ProMED-mail) was created in the following year (Madoff and Woodall, 2005). ProMED-mail now has > 32,000 subscribers in more than 150 countries, and it has developed into a mature system for receiving, analyzing, and disseminating information about newly described or unknown diseases and epidemics (Madoff, 2004). More than 20 staff members around the world search the Internet and traditional media daily for disease information and file reports on relevant findings. Spontaneous reports can also be submitted electronically to ProMED, and approximately 30 spontaneous reports of disease activity are received each day. Each report is reviewed by an editor and in many cases by a subject expert, and approximately seven reports and accompanying editorial comments are posted each day through e-mail lists and on the website. Posted reports are also stored in an archival database for future reference.

ProMED-mail relies in part on a community of interested individuals to submit information about unusual disease activity, and on a small group of experts to analyze this information and disseminate reports of interest. In terms of the surveillance process (Fig. 3), ProMED-mail does not operate with specific case definitions. Events of interest for ProMED-mail are defined loosely as 'newly described or unknown diseases, epidemics and outbreaks and diseases emerging in new areas or populations' (Madoff, 2004). Dissemination is rapid and broad, without political oversight or interference. This approach to surveillance is likely to be sensitive, rapid, and reasonably specific due to the expert analysis.

The Global Public Health Intelligence Network (GPHIN): The Global Public Health Intelligence Network (GPHIN) was initially developed in 1998 by Health Canada in partnership with the WHO for the collection, filtering and sorting, and review of emerging disease information. In the collection step, automated software is used to search the Internet for selected disease-specific words. An average of 8000–10,000 items of interest per month are identified in this way. In the filtering and sorting step, irrelevant and duplicate information are discarded, and each relevant item is categorized. In the review step, 9000 pieces of information are reviewed each month and posted on the Internet. The most recent version of the GPHIN software, placed into service in 2004, can process information in Arabic, English, French, Russian, Chinese, and Spanish. GPHIN is now operated by WHO Epidemic and Pandemic Alert and Response (EPR) in collaboration with Health Canada, and provides approximately 40% of the information that WHO receives about disease outbreaks.

In terms of the surveillance process model (Fig. 3), the keywords and word arrangements used to identify potentially relevant information are essentially the case definitions in GPHIN. These case definitions are highly sensitive but not very specific, and so retrieved information must be filtered, first automatically, and then manually. The events of interest to GPHIN are also quite broad, including not only infectious disease outbreaks, but also illnesses related to consumer products, radiation, food and water, and other causes. The filtering and human review steps in GPHIN correspond to the analysis step in the surveillance process.

While ProMED-mail and GPHIN can both be thought of as approaches to 'information surveillance', their differences are noteworthy. Neither system uses a case definition in the traditional sense, but GPHIN does use a pre-defined set of terms to identify information of potential interest. A precisely specified list of terms is required by GPHIN because it is an automated system. In contrast, ProMED-mail does not specify in detail what constitutes relevant information, and this degree of precision is not required because ProMED-mail relies on humans to identify and submit information. As a consequence of their different approaches to data collection, GPHIN collects more information than ProMED-mail, but it also collects more irrelevant information, which subsequently must be filtered. In both systems, the final assessment of relevance is manual.

From a management perspective, GPHIN is operated by governmental and international public health agencies, while ProMED-mail is operated by a non-governmental organization. As a result, information posted through ProMED-mail is not subject to any political review. In practice, however, the two systems are linked; since ProMED-mail posts information on a website, this information is included in that collected by GPHIN on the Internet. In addition, individuals may submit to ProMED-mail relevant information identified by the GPHIN website. Thus, in many ways these two approaches to information surveillance are complementary. The main strength of GPHIN is the breadth and volume of information that it can consider, whereas the main strengths of ProMED-mail are its expert analysis of information, and independence from governmental supervision. Both systems have performed well in identifying recent outbreaks due to newly emerging viruses, including the SARS outbreak in 2002–2003.

Syndromic surveillance. Advances in the electronic capture of health data have led to surveillance using data generated through the routine administration of health care services. This practice is known as 'syndromic surveillance' because cases are defined in terms of non-specific administrative codes or conditions, which can be thought of as syndromes (Mandl et al., 2004). Although using syndromes for case definitions has been practiced for many years, this 'syndromic surveillance' is novel in that it relies on the automated capture, transmission, and analysis of non-specific patterns of information in pre-diagnostic health data. For example, many syndromic surveillance systems follow administrative data from emergency room visits. The records are automatically obtained from hospital records and forwarded to a public health agency, automatically grouped into designated 'syndromes' such as 'respiratory disease' or 'gastrointestinal disease', and then analyzed to look for unexpected increases in the number of visits.

Rapid development of syndromic surveillance systems has occurred as a result of developing preparedness to detect episodes of bioterrorism, and the systems are equally useful for detecting emerging viruses (Institute of Medicine of the National Academies, 2003). The US Centers for Disease Control and Prevention (CDC) has supported demonstration projects in syndromic surveillance (Yih et al., 2004), and is developing an operational system to monitor several data sources, including emergency department visits, laboratory test orders, and pharmaceutical pre- scriptions (Loonsk, 2004; United States Government Accountability Office, 2005). A variety of other systems are also being operated by governmental and non- governmental organizations in the US (Lombardo et al., 2003; Wagner et al., 2003; Heffernan et al., 2004), in the United Kingdom (Cooper et al., 2004), and in Canada.

It is difficult to establish the utility of different types of syndromic surveillance systems because of the variation in data characteristics across locations. Data from early disease events, such as sales of over-the-counter pharmaceuticals and calls to telephone-based medical triage systems, offer promise due to their timeliness and the prevalence of these responses to symptoms. However, these data contain little specific clinical information, and outbreak signals are likely to be masked by con- siderable noise. For these reasons, many syndromic surveillance systems now rely on more specific data such as records of visits to emergency departments. Ideally, many available data sources would be used simultaneously, but further research is needed to identify the optimal approach to combining information from multiple types of data within single surveillance systems.

In terms of the framework for surveillance (Fig. 3), the case definition used in syndromic surveillance is usually a set of codes or keywords that correspond to a syndrome, and grouping of records into syndromes is usually conducted automat- ically. Outbreak detection algorithms consider the chronology of different syn- dromes (Buckeridge et al., 2005a), but some researchers have examined the use of algorithms that search for outbreaks over geographic space (Kulldorff et al., 2005), and other covariates found in medical records, such as age and gender (Wong et al., 2003). The link of surveillance systems of these types to public health decision- making is variable, and many public health agencies are still determining the best policy for the follow-up of alarms that are often non-specific (Duchin, 2003; Pavlin, 2003).

The main argument for conducting syndromic surveillance rests on the assump- tion that this approach to surveillance will detect a disease outbreak more rapidly than other surveillance systems. Because syndromic surveillance systems follow data from events that occur before diagnosis, it is assumed that they will detect outbreaks earlier because the incidence of pre-diagnostic events, such as purchase of over-the-counter medications, will increase before the incidence of diagnoses will increase. In general, these assumptions may hold true under some conditions, but not under other conditions. The limited research on these systems suggests that the results are affected by the clinical course of the disease, the number of individuals exposed, the type of data source monitored, whether an applicable routine test is positive in the disease, and the outbreak detection algorithm used (Buehler et al., 2003; Reis et al., 2003; Stoto et al., 2004; Buckeridge et al., 2005b). Syndromic surveillance is likely to be more rapid than clinical detection in detecting an outbreak when the clinical symptoms mimic an existing disease with a low incidence, when a clinical data source is being monitored, and when there is no routine diagnostic test for the disease. This is a conceivable scenario for the initial presentation of a newly emerging virus, and so it is reasonable to expect that syndromic surveillance systems may be useful in the initial detection of an outbreak due to a newly emerging virus.

Intermediate stage surveillance

Once public health personnel know more about the epidemiology and genetics of an emerging virus, additional surveillance approaches become feasible. One such approach, surveillance of animals and the environment, capitalizes on knowledge about the epidemiology of the virus to identify when and where human infection is likely to occur. A second approach, surveillance of laboratory test results, makes use of results from diagnostic testing to follow with high specificity the development of an epidemic or endemic disease.

Surveillance of animals and the environment. Many emerging viruses cause zoonotic diseases. Once a newly emerging virus is understood to have a vertebrate animal host, and the vector of transmission has been identified, it may be informative to conduct surveillance of the animal hosts of the disease, of the vector, or even the habitat of the animal host or vector. For example, researchers have found that the spatial and temporal patterns of human dengue virus infections follow known entomological risk factors (Tran et al., 2004). Other researchers have observed the same phenomenon with West Nile virus (WNV), for which deaths among birds and the distribution of habitats suitable for adult mosquitoes have both been shown to correlate well with virus-positive mosquito samples and the occurrence of human infections (Eidson et al., 2001; Brownstein et al., 2002; Mostashari et al., 2003). In fact, surveillance of these factors are now a component of many programs for WNV surveillance.

Laboratory-based surveillance. After diagnostic methods are available, surveillance of positive laboratory tests becomes possible. This approach to surveillance is likely to be highly specific, but it will identify only those cases that are tested at laboratories participating in the surveillance system. Automated surveillance of positive laboratory test results (Effler et al., 1999) and monitoring the incidence of emerging pathogens through laboratory methods (Bravata et al., 2004) can be a highly effective form of surveillance.

Ongoing surveillance

Surveillance, in practice, capitalizes on different approaches at different points in the emergence of a virus (Fig. 3).

West Nile virus

WNV was first isolated and identified in 1937, in samples from a febrile person in the West Nile district of Uganda. Prior to 1999, the virus was found only in the Eastern Hemisphere, with wide distribution in Africa, Asia, the Middle East, and Europe. In late summer 1999, the US documented its first domestically acquired human cases of West Nile encephalitis (Anderson et al., 1999; Briese, 1999; Jia et al., 1999; Lanciotti et al., 1999; Nash et al., 2001). The WNV epidemic of 2002 was the largest epidemic of WNV meningoencephalitis on record, and the largest recognized arboviral meningoencephalitis epidemic ever recorded in the Western Hemisphere. Significant human disease activity was recorded in Canada for the first time, in the Caribbean basin, and in Mexico. A program of surveillance is now in place for WNV detection in North America using data from human, avian, equine, and mosquito samples.

Human surveillance: Health care providers report all probable and confirmed cases of WNV infection to designated health authorities. In the absence of WNV activity in an area, passive surveillance is used for the reporting of hospitalized cases of encephalitis, and for patients who test positive for IgM antibodies to WNV. In areas with known WNV activity, active surveillance may take place, in which (1) public health professionals contact physicians in appropriate specialties and hospital infection control staff on a regular basis to inquire about patients with potential arboviral infections, and (2) laboratory-based surveillance is implemented to identify CSF specimens meeting sensitive but non-specific criteria for arboviral infections. Special surveillance projects can be used to supplement WNV surveillance, including the Emerging Infections Network of the Infectious Diseases Society of America (IDSA EIN), Emergency Department Sentinel Network for Emerging Infections (EMERGEncy ID NET), Unexplained Deaths and Critical Illnesses Surveillance of the Emerging Infections Programs (EIP), and the Global Emerging Infections Sentinel Network of the International Society of Travel Medicine (GeoSentinel). In addition, blood banks in the United States routinely screen all donated blood for WNV using PCR.

Avian surveillance: While most birds survive WNV infection, mortality in a wide variety of bird species has been a hallmark of WNV activity in North America. Avian mortality due to WNV is a sensitive indicator of ongoing enzootic transmission, such that public health agencies can use bird mortality to track effectively the spread of WNV. Avian morbidity and mortality surveillance includes the reporting and analysis of dead bird sightings, and the submission of selected birds for WNV testing. Detection of seroconversion in sentinel live-captive chickens or free-ranging birds can also be used for surveillance.

Equine surveillance: Among large land mammals, horses are particularly susceptible to WNV infection. Horses appear to be important sentinels of WNV epizootic activity and human risk, at least in some geographic regions. Veterinarians, veterinary service agencies, and state agriculture departments are essential partners in any surveillance activities involving equine WNV disease.

Mosquito surveillance: Surveillance of mosquitoes is the primary tool for quantifying the intensity of virus transmission in an area. WNV is transmitted principally by *Culex* spp. mosquitoes, though greater than 36 species of mosquitoes can be infected with WNV. In areas where WNV has never been detected, mosquito surveillance focuses on establishing which mosquito species are present, and how many are in the area. In areas where WNV has been detected, mosquitoes are collected and tested for WNV.

SARS

Health Canada's GPHIN system first recognized the outbreak of atypical pneumonia emerging in southern China, later identified as SARS and later shown to be caused by the coronavirus, SARS-CoV. During the 2003 SARS outbreak, surveillance relied heavily on passive reporting by health care providers of suspected and confirmed cases, active contact tracing, and active syndromic surveillance of quarantined contacts. Some countries also conducted serological screening of large segments of the population.

Since the end of the 2003 outbreak, SARS surveillance has focused on (1) persons with a potential epidemiologic link who are hospitalized with severe respiratory illness, (2) clusters of severe respiratory illness, (3) persons with laboratory evidence of SARS-CoV infection, and (4) in Canada, where there is joint surveillance for human cases of SARS and avian influenza, persons with laboratory confirmed influenza A (serotype H5N1) or other novel influenza virus infection. As more is learned about the natural reservoir, host species, and transmission of SARS-CoV, SARS surveillance will likely expand to include surveillance of host animal species. Global SARS surveillance uses GPHIN technology, passive reporting of laboratory-confirmed cases to WHO as well as special studies of SARS-CoV infection in areas at increased risk of reemergence.

Implications for future policy, practice, and research

The convergence of human disease ecologies resulting from increasing globalization is thought to be a driving force behind emerging viral diseases (Barrett et al., 1998).

Outbreaks arising in distant countries can be exported by jet travel, making it imperative that global and local outbreak detection and response be closely interrelated. Improved global infectious disease surveillance is needed to ensure adequate local outbreak detection and response (Institute of Medicine of the National Academies, 2003; United States Government Accountability Office, 2004). Improvement of global surveillance should focus on building surveillance capacity in many countries, especially in resource-poor regions (United States Government Accountability Office, 2004), establishing networks of expertise (The SARS Commission, 2004; World Health Organization, 2003), and improving case reporting to the WHO, permitting the issuance of timely alerts to prevent international spread (World Health Organization, 2003).

Many governments also seek to improve domestic surveillance through better case and contact reporting by health care professionals (Institute of Medicine of the National Academies, 2003; The SARS Commission, 2005), and through enhanced coordination between different government agencies at national and local levels (The SARS Commission, 2004, 2005; United States Government Accountability Office, 2004, 2005). Astute clinicians can be the first line of defense for identifying emerging viral threats, but many health care providers do not understand their potential role as a source of valuable disease data (Institute of Medicine of the National Academies, 2003). Solutions to enhance timeliness, accuracy, and completeness of disease reporting by health care providers include the development of secure, web-based reporting, implementation of automated laboratory reporting, and standardization and consolidation of local reporting systems (United States Government Accountability Office, 2004, 2005; The SARS Commission, 2005).

There is also a need to explore innovative systems of surveillance, such as those incorporating remote sensing, and automated systems of syndrome surveillance (Institute of Medicine of the National Academies, 2003). Careful evaluation of novel surveillance systems should be conducted to determine their accuracy and effectiveness (United States Government Accountability Office, 2004). Because the majority of emerging infectious diseases are zoonoses (Institute of Medicine of the National Academies, 2003), vector-borne and zoonotic disease surveillance and control should be improved (Institute of Medicine of the National Academies, 2003; United States Government Accountability Office, 2004). Significant improvements could be achieved by using robust models for predicting and preventing vector-borne and zoonotic diseases, and by adding veterinary laboratories to laboratory surveillance networks (Institute of Medicine of the National Academies, 2003).

References

Anderson JF, Andreadis TG, Vossbrinck CR, Tirrell S, Wakem EM, French RA, Garmendia AE, Van Kruiningen HJ. Isolation of West Nile virus from mosquitoes, crows, and a Cooper's hawk in Connecticut. Science 1999; 286: 2331.

Barrett JB, Kuzawa CW, Mcdade T, Armelagos GJ. Emerging and re-emerging infectious diseases: the third epidemiologic transition. Annu Rev Anthropol 1998; 27: 247.

Bravata DM, Mcdonald KM, Smith WM, Rydzak C, Szeto H, Buckeridge DL, Haberland C, Owens DK. Systematic review: surveillance systems for early detection of bioterrorism-related diseases. Ann Intern Med 2004; 140: 910–922.

Briese T. Identification of a Kunjin/West Nile-like flavivirus in brains of patients with New York encephalitis. Lancet 1999; 354: 1650.

Brookes T, Khan OA. Behind the Mask: How the World Survived SARS. Washington, DC: American Public Health Association; 2005.

Brownstein JS, Rosen H, Purdy D, Miller JR, Merlino M, Mostashari F, Fish D. Spatial analysis of West Nile virus: rapid risk assessment of an introduced vector-borne zoonosis. Vector Borne Zoonotic Dis 2002; 2: 157–164.

Buckeridge DL, Burkom H, Campbell M, Hogan WR, Moore AW. Algorithms for rapid outbreak detection: a research synthesis. J Biomed Inform 2005a; 38: 99–113.

Buckeridge DL, Switzer P, Owens D, Siegrist D, Pavlin J, Musen M. An evaluation model for syndromic surveillance: assessing the performance of a temporal algorithm. MMWR Morb Mortal Wkly Rep 2005b; 54(Suppl): 109–115.

Buehler JW, Berkelman RL, Hartley DM, Peters CJ. Syndromic surveillance and bioterrorism-related epidemics. Emerg Infect Dis 2003; 9: 1197–1204.

Cooper DL, Smith G, Baker M, Chinemana F, Verlander N, Gerard E, Hollyoak V, Griffiths R. National symptom surveillance using calls to a telephone health advice service—United Kingdom, December 2001–February 2003. MMWR Morb Mortal Wkly Rep 2004; 53(Suppl): 179–183.

Duchin JS. Epidemiological response to syndromic surveillance signals. J Urban Health 2003; 80: i115–i116.

Effler P, Ching-lee M, Bogard A, Ieong MC, Nekomoto T, Jernigan D. Statewide system of electronic notifiable disease reporting from clinical laboratories: comparing automated reporting with conventional methods. JAMA 1999; 282: 1845–1850.

Eidson M, Komar N, Sorhage F, Nelson R, Talbot T, Mostashari F, Mclean R. Crow deaths as a sentinel surveillance system for West Nile virus in the northeastern United States, 1999. Emerg Infect Dis 2001; 7: 615–620.

Heffernan R, Mostashari F, Das D, Karpati A, Kuldorff M, Weiss D. Syndromic surveillance in public health practice, New York City. Emerg Infect Dis 2004; 10: 858–864.

Heymann DL. Smallpox containment updated: considerations for the 21st century. Int J Infect Dis 2004; 8(Suppl 2): S15–S20.

Hutwagner LC, Maloney EK, Bean NH, Slutsker L, Martin SM. Using laboratory-based surveillance data for prevention: an algorithm for detecting Salmonella outbreaks. Emerg Infect Dis 1997; 3: 395–400.

Institute of Medicine of the National Academies. Microbial Threats to Health: Emergence, Detection, and Response. Washington, DC: The National Academies Press; 2003.

Jia XY, Briese T, Jordan I, Rambaut A, Chi HC, Mackenzie JS, Hall RA, Scherret J, Lipkin WI. Genetic analysis of West Nile New York 1999 encephalitis virus. Lancet 1999; 354: 1971.

Kohler KA, Hlady WG, Banerjee K, Francis P, Durrani S, Zuber PL. Predictors of virologically confirmed poliomyelitis in India, 1998–2000. Clin Infect Dis 2002; 35: 1321–1327.

Koo D, Wetterhall SF. History and current status of the National Notifiable Diseases Surveillance System. J Public Health Manag Pract 1996; 2: 4–10.

Kulldorff M, Heffernan R, Hartman J, Assuncao R, Mostashari F. A space-time permutation scan statistic for disease outbreak detection. PLoS Med 2005; 2: e59.

Lanciotti RS, Roehrig JT, Deubel V, Smith J, Parker M, Steele K, Crise B, Volpe KE, Crabtree MB, Scherret JH, Hall RA, Mackenzie JS, Cropp CB, Panigrahy B, Ostlund E, Schmitt B, Malkinson M, Banet C, Weissman J, Komar N, Savage HM, Stone W, Mcnamara T, Gubler DJ. Origin of the West Nile virus responsible for an outbreak of encephalitis in the northeastern United States. Science 1999; 286: 2333.

Lombardo J, Burkom H, Elbert E, Magruder S, Lewis SH, Loschen W, Sari J, Sniegoski C, Wojcik R, Pavlin J. A systems overview of the electronic surveillance system for the Early Notification of Community-Based Epidemics (ESSENCE II). J Urban Health 2003; 80: i32–i42.

Loonsk JW. Biosense—a national initiative for early detection and quantification of public health emergencies. MMWR Morb Mortal Wkly Rep 2004; 53(Suppl): 53–55.

Madoff LC. ProMED-mail: an early warning system for emerging diseases. Clin Infect Dis 2004; 39: 227–232.

Madoff LC, Woodall JP. The internet and the global monitoring of emerging diseases: lessons from the first 10 years of ProMED-mail. Arch Med Res 2005; 36: 724–730.

Mandl KD, Overhage JM, Wagner MM, Lober WB, Sebastiani P, Mostashari F, Pavlin JA, Gesteland PH, TReadwell T, Koski E, Hutwagner L, Buckeridge DL, Aller RD, Grannis S. Implementing syndromic surveillance: a practical guide informed by the early experience. J Am Med Inform Assoc 2004; 11: 141–150.

Mostashari F, Kulldorff M, Hartman JJ, Miller JR, Kulasekera V. Dead bird clusters as an early warning system for West Nile virus activity. Emerg Infect Dis 2003; 9: 641–646.

Nash D, Mostashari F, Fine A, Miller J, O'Leary D, Murray K, Huang A, Rosenberg A, Greenberg A, Sherman M, Wong S, Layton M, Campbell GL, Roehrig JT, Gubler DJ, Shieh WJ, Zaki S, Smith P. The outbreak of West Nile virus infection in the New York City area in 1999. N Engl J Med 2001; 344: 1807.

Pavlin JA. Investigation of disease outbreaks detected by "syndromic" surveillance systems. J Urban Health 2003; 80: i107–i114.

Reis BY, Pagano M, Mandl KD. Using temporal context to improve biosurveillance. Proc Natl Acad Sci USA 2003; 100: 1961–1965.

Stoto M, Schonlau M, Mariano L. Syndromic surveillance: is it worth the effort? Chance 2004; 17: 19–24.

Stroup DF, Wharton M, Kafadar K, Dean AG. Evaluation of a method for detecting aberrations in public health surveillance data. Am J Epidemiol 1993; 137: 373–380.

The SARS Commission. Interim Report: SARS and Public Health in Ontario. Canada; 2004.

The SARS Commission. Second Interim Report: SARS and Public Health Legislation. Canada; 2005.

Tran A, Deparis X, Dussart P, Morvan J, Rabarison P, Remy F, Polidori L, Gardon J. Dengue spatial and temporal patterns, French Guiana, 2001. Emerg Infect Dis 2004; 10: 615–621.

United States Government Accountability Office. Emerging Infectious Diseases: Review of State and Federal Disease Surveillance Efforts. Washington, DC; 2004.

United States Government Accountability Office. Information Technology: Federal Agencies Face Challenges in Implementing Initiatives to Improve Public Health Infrastructure. Washington, DC; 2005.

Wagner MM, Robinson JM, Tsui F-C, Espino JU, Hogan WR. Design of a national retail data monitor for public health surveillance. J Am Med Inform Assoc 2003; 10: 409–418.

Wong WK, Moore A, Cooper G, Wagner M. WSARE: what's strange about recent events? J Urban Health 2003; 80: i66–i75.

World Health Organization, World Health Report 2003; 2003.

Yih WK, Caldwell B, Harmon R, Kleinman K, Lazarus R, Nelson A, Nordin J, Rehm B, Richter B, Ritzwoller D, Sherwood E, Platt R. National bioterrorism syndromic surveillance demonstration program. MMWR Morb Mortal Wkly Rep 2004; 53(Suppl): 43–49.

Colour Section

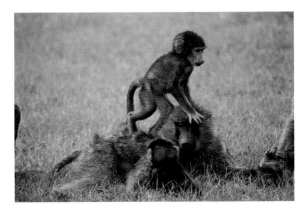

Plate 1 Non-human primates represent the origin of many important viral zoonoses, (See page 26).

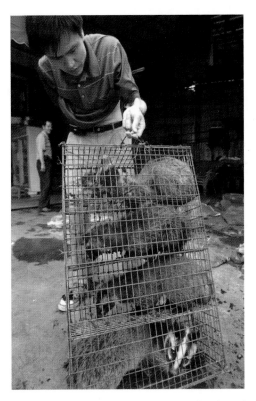

Plate 2 Animal markets represent a risk factor for transmission of various viral zoonoses, e.g. SARS. *Source*: Reuters/SCANPIX. (See page 32).

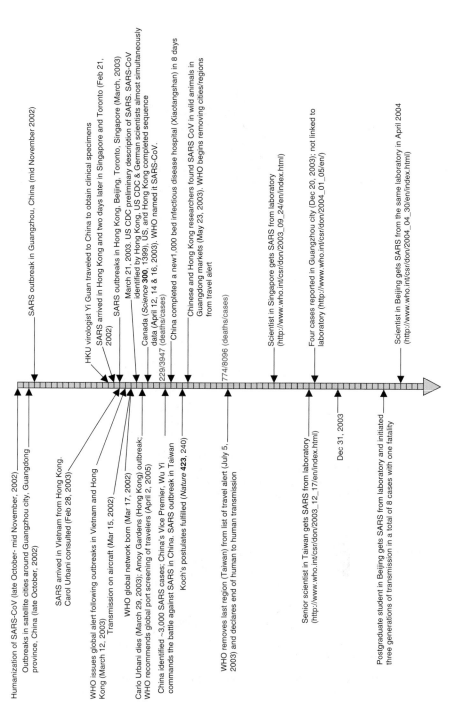

Plate 3 Timeline of the SARS epidemic. Major events are listed from top to bottom. Each interval in the arrow represents 1 week. For information on the first weeks of the epidemic in China, consult the book by Thomas Abraham, Twenty-First Century Plague. The Story of SARS. The Johns Hopkins University Press. Baltimore, Maryland, 2005. (See page 46).

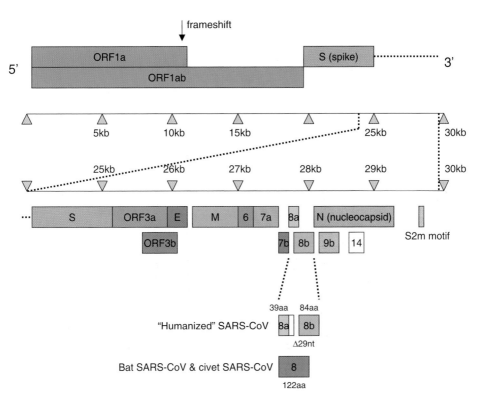

Plate 4 SARS-CoV genome organization. The genome organization is similar to other coronaviruses with respect to overall size, the relative positions of replicase, spike, envelope, membrane and nucleocapsid genes, and certain other features (see text for details). A 29-nucleotide stretch is deleted in the strain found in human isolates, as illustrated at the bottom. (See page 51).

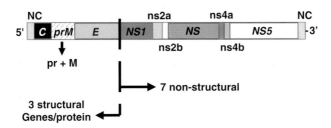

Plate 5 Genomic structure of WNV, showing 3 structural proteins, C-capsid, M-membrane, and E-envelope; and 7 nonstructural proteins (Petersen and Roehrig, 2001). (See page 134).

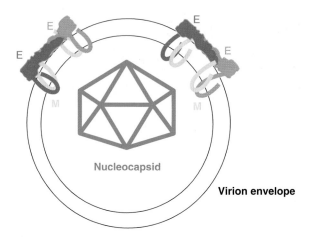

Plate 6 Flavivirus virion diagram. The single stranded RNA is enclosed in the nucleocapsid, which in turn is surrounded by an envelope containing E-glycoproteins (E) and integral membrane proteins (M) (Petersen and Roehrig, 2001). (See page 134).

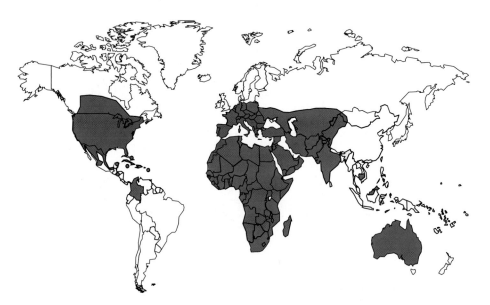

Plate 7 Approximate global distribution of West Nile virus. (See page 137).

Inoculation lesions

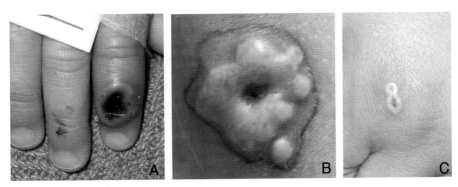

Dissemination lesions

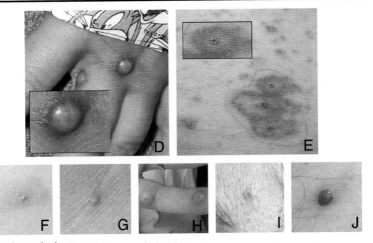

Evolution of primary lesions

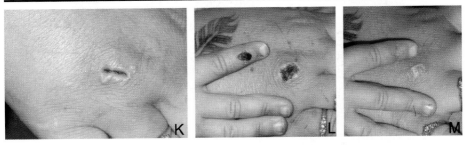

Plate 8 Cutaneous lesions of human monkeypox. The top panels show primary inoculation lesions at the site of a prairie dog bite (A) or scratch (B and C). The middle panels show the variation of the appearance of disseminated lesions of monkeypox ranging from smallpox-like (D) to varicella-like (E–J). The lower panels (K–M) document the progression of a primary lesion from the pustular stage through scarring. (See page 153).

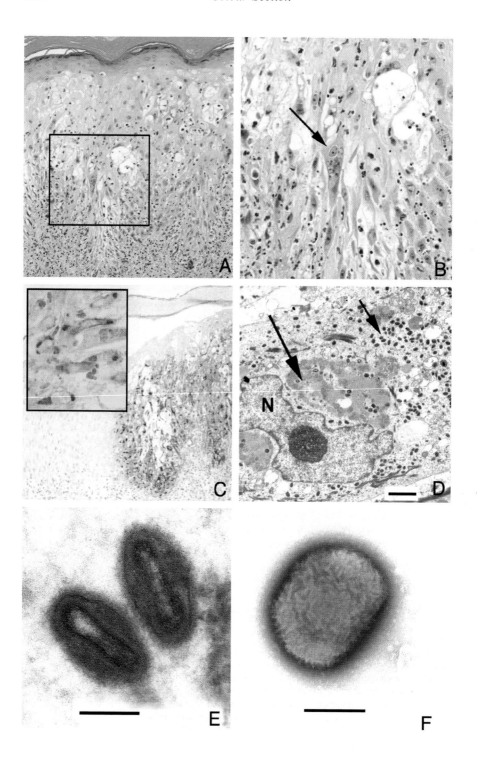

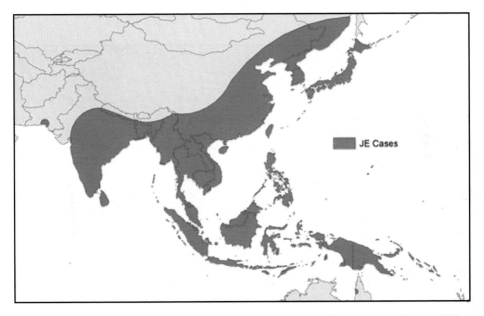

Plate 10 Map showing the distribution of JE cases (modified from CDC, Atlanta). (See page 215).

Plate 9 Histological, ultrastructural, and immunohistochemical appearance of MPV infection. Panel A: Scattered degenerating and necrotic keratinocytes are shown within the epidermis along with a moderate inflammatory cell infiltrate in the superficial dermis (hematoxylin and eosin). Panel B: Higher magnification of the boxed area shows multinucleated cells (long arrow) and eosinophilic viral inclusion bodies. Panel C: Strong immunoreactivity for orthopoxvirus antigen is present in the epidermis. Panel D: Transmission electron microscopy shows virions within the cytoplasm of a keratinocyte, including immature forms undergoing assembly (long arrow) and mature forms (short arrow). Panel E: High magnification shows the characteristic dumbbell-shaped inner core of poxviruses. Panel F: Negative staining of a virion from cell culture shows the brick-shaped particle with regularly spaced, threadlike ridges on the exposed surface. (See page 156).

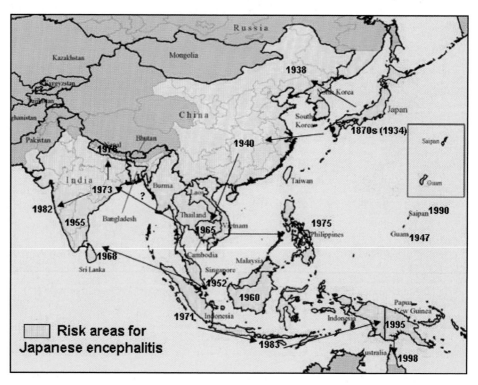

Plate 11 Map showing the temporal spread of JEV from the initial isolation in Japan. Modified from Solomon (2000). (See page 238).

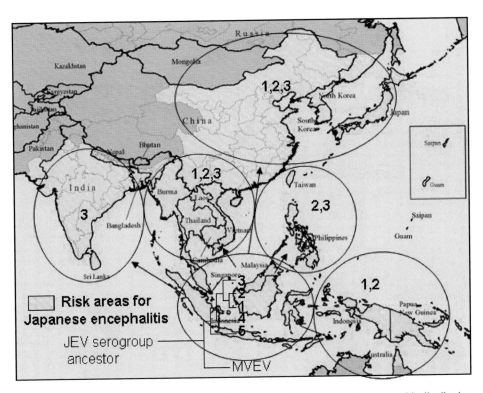

Plate 12 Map showing the possible origin and distribution of JEV, showing the geographic distribution of the genotypes. The ancestral virus is hypothesized to have given rise to genotype 4, and then to the other genotypes. A possible genotype 5, based on the Muar strain, would have been the earliest genotype if its sequence is confirmed. From Solomon and Winter (2004) and Solomon et al. (2003a). (See page 240).

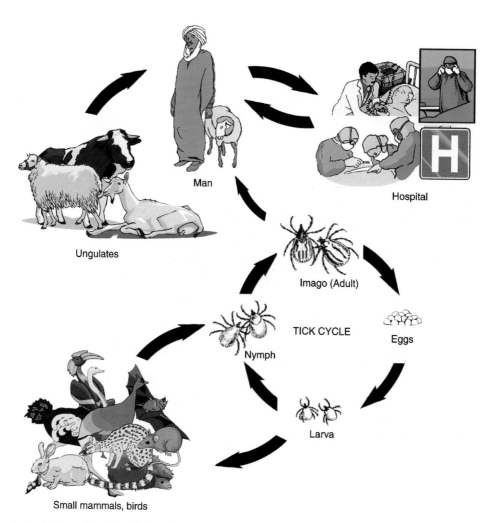

Plate 13 Example of CCHF virus circulation: transmission by the *Hyalomma marginatum rufipes* tick. (See page 307).

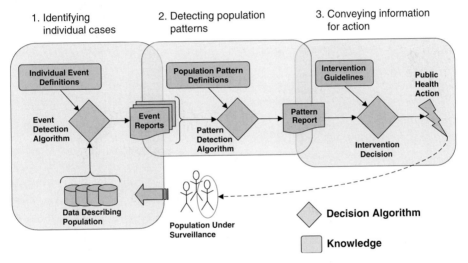

1. Identifying individual cases

2. Detecting population patterns

3. Conveying information for action

Individual Event Definitions

Population Pattern Definitions

Intervention Guidelines

Public Health Action

Event Detection Algorithm

Event Reports

Pattern Detection Algorithm

Pattern Report

Intervention Decision

Data Describing Population

Population Under Surveillance

Decision Algorithm

Knowledge

Plate 14 The process of surveillance. Critical points in this process include the detection of events in individuals (e.g., a diagnosis of measles), the identification of patterns in the population (e.g., a rapid rise in incidence in a geographic location), and the incorporation of information about identified patterns into decisions about interventions. (See page 330).

List of Contributors

Birgitta Åsjö
Center for Research in Virology
The Gade Institute, University of Bergen
The Bio-Building 5th floor, Jonas Lies vei 91
Bergen, N-5009, Norway

David Buckeridge
Clinical and Health Informatics Research Group
McGill University
1140 Pine Avenue
West Montreal, QC H3A1A3, Canada

Geneviève Cadieux
Clinical and Health Informatics Research Group
McGill University
1140 Pine Avenue
West Montreal, QC H3A1A3, Canada

Jan P. Clement
Hantavirus Reference Centre
Laboratory of Clinical and Epidemiological Virology
Rega Institute, Katholieke Universiteit Leuven
Minderbroedersstraat 10, B3000
Leuven, Belgium

Vincent P. Hsu
Clinical Performance Improvement and Infection Control
Florida Hospital
601 E. Rollins St.
Orlando, FL 32803, USA

Hilde Kruse
National Veterinary Institute
Department for Health Surveillance
Oslo, Norway

Ching-Juh Lai
Laboratory of Infectious Diseases
National Institute of Allergy and Infectious Diseases
National Institutes of Health
Bethesda, MD 20892, USA

John S. Mackenzie
Australian Biosecurity Cooperative Research Centre for
  Emerging Infectious Diseases
Curtin University of Technology
GPO Box U1987
Perth, WA6845, Australia

P. Maes
Hantavirus Reference Centre
Laboratory of Clinical and Epidemiological Virology
Rega Institute, Katholieke Universiteit Leuven
Minderbroedersstraat 10, B3000 Leuven
Belgium

Brian W.J. Mahy
National Center for Infectious Diseases
Centers for Disease Control and Prevention
Atlanta, GA 30333, USA

Pierre Nabeth
Institut Pasteur de Dakar
36 avenue Pasteur
BP 220, Dakar, Senegal

Robert Putnak
Division of Communicable Diseases and Immunology
Department of Virus Diseases
The Walter Reed Army Institute of Research
Silver Spring, MD 20910, USA

K.D. Reed
Emerging Infectious Disease Laboratory
Marshfield Clinic Research Foundation
1000 N. Oak Avenue
Marshfield, WI 54449, USA

David W. Smith
Division of Microbiology and Infectious Diseases
PathWest, Locked Bag 2009
Nedlands, WA6909, Australia

Theresa L. Smith
Division of Vector-Borne Infectious Diseases
National Center for Infectious Diseases
Centers for Disease Control and Prevention
Department of Health and Human Services
3150 Rampart Rd
Fort Collins, CO 80521, USA

Kanta Subbarao
Laboratory of Infectious Diseases
NIAID, NIH
Bldg 50, Room 6132, 50 South Drive
Bethesda, MD 20892, USA

Amorsolo L. Suguitan
Laboratory of Infectious Diseases
NIAID, NIH
Bldg 50, Room 6132, 50 South Drive
Bethesda, MD 20892, USA

Edward Tabor
Quintiles, Inc.
1801 Rockville Pike, Suite 300
Rockville, MD 20852, USA

Tommy R. Tong
Department of Pathology
Princess Margaret Hospital
Laichikok, Kowloon
Hong Kong, China

M. Van Ranst
Hantavirus Reference Centre
Laboratory of Clinical and Epidemiological Virology
Rega Institute, Katholieke Universiteit Leuven
Minderbroedersstraat 10, B3000 Leuven
Belgium

David T. Williams
Australian Biosecurity Cooperative Research Centre for
 Emerging Infectious Diseases
Curtin University of Technology
GPO Box U1987
Perth, WA6845, Australia

Index

Page numbers suffixed by t and f refer to Tables and Figures respectively.

accessory proteins, functions of 56, 180–1
acquired immunodeficiency syndrome (AIDS) 6,
    25, *see also* human immunodeficiency virus,
    type 1
    epidemic in Romania 27
acute respiratory distress syndrome (ARDS) 107,
    113, 161, 172, 191, 329
    risk factors, major 110
    therapeutic implications 62
adenovirus 70
adenovirus-based vaccines 118
adult T-cell leukemia (ATL) 27
Aedes aegypti 283
    dengue transmission by 270, 274
    resurgence of 275
    transmission efficiency 275
Aedes albopictus 19, 274
aerosols 17, 117, 157, 168
affinity tag technology, isotope-labeled 51
age-specific epidemic curves 103
agricultural practices
    influence of 21
    JEV infections and 233, 240, 241, *see also*
        vector control
airborne dissemination 47, 60
aircraft
    disinfection 241
    SARS transmission on 47
air-pollution haze 22
Alfuy virus (ALFV) 202
amplification reservoirs 48
amplifying hosts 22, 23, 138, 211, 223, 244
angiotensin II 62
angiotensin-converting enzyme 2 (ACE2) 31, 54,
    61, 66
animal host(s) 337
    animal–vector–human transmission cycles
        202
    control 241
    disease patterns in, active surveillance of 2
    markets, *see* zoonoses, transmission of
    movements 22
    of Sin Nombre virus 20
    reservoir 17, 34, 48, 187
    sentinel 119, 211, 339

surveillance of 337
virus introduction from 5
anti-apoptic protein, Bcl-xL 56
antibody-dependent enhancement (ADE)
    hypothesis 269, 281
antigenic drift 31, 100, 108, 116, 119, 204
antigenic shift 17, 30, 100
arboviruses 18, 240
ardeid birds 211, 213, 237, 239, 244
Arenaviruses 20
argasid ticks 300, 306
Asian tiger mosquito, *see Aedes albopictus*
avian influenza viruses 2, 24, *see also* influenza
    viruses
    antigenic drift in 119
    clinical characteristics in humans 110t
    H5N1 10, 17, 24, 31, 98
        detection of 109
        infection of humans by, direct 101
        limiting 119
        molecular and genetic characterization of
            human 108
        serologic studies of 112
        vaccines against, development of 117
    axonal neuropathy vs. demyelinating neuropathy,
        differentiating 141–2
    highly pathogenic avian influenza (HPAI)
        infections 98, 105, 108, 119
    mutations in 104
    poultry infections 105, 108
        vaccinated poultry 119
    replication in humans 102
    species barrier and 100
    transmission to humans 105
    treatment of 114
    vaccines 117

bacteria, larvicidal 241
Basic Reproductive Number (R0) 47
bat hendra virus 22
bats 21, 34, 71, 187, 193, 212, *see also* severe
    acute respiratory syndrome coronavirus
    (SARS-CoV): natural reservoir for
B-cell immortalization technique 67
Bcl-xL, anti-apoptic protein 56

Bill and Melinda Gates Foundation 216, 243
bioaerosol, reducing 47
bioinformatics software 53
biosafety level 2 (BSL-2) 154
biosafety level 3 (BSL-3) 117
biosafety level 4 (BSL-4) 192
biotope 167
birds
  ardeid 211, 213, 237, 239, 244
  bird-to-bird transmission 138
  Bubulcus ibis coromandus 239
  herons' migratory patterns, seasonal
    transmission and 215, 239
  migratory, role of 108
  Nankeen night heron (*Nycticorax caledonicus*)
    237
  waterfowl
    as natural reservoirs 99
    wild 24
blood transfusion 8
  WNV transmission by 139
bovine spongiform encephalopathy (BSE) 9
bovine-human parainfluenza virus (BHPIV3)
  68, 69
BSL-2, *see* biosafety level 2
BSL-3, *see* biosafety level 3
BSL-4, *see* biosafety level 4
Bunyaviridae family 19, 161, 300, 303
bushmeat 28

Cacipacore virus (CPCV) 202
case definition 326, 330, 335
  specificity in 333
caspase-dependent mechanism 56
cathepsin L inhibitors 67
cattle and goats, *see* Japanese encephalitis virus
  (JEV): human infection risk, predictor of
CCHV, *see* Congo–Crimean hemorrhagic fever
  (CCHF) virus
  gene influencing 205
cellular receptor 31, 181, 272, 273
Centers for Disease Control and Prevention
  (CDC) 44, 154, 336
Chandipura virus 229
chemical mediators 282
chemokines 57, 63, 110, 170
Chengdu Institute 243
chimerism 48
  chimeras, intertypic 285
chimpanzee 7, 18, 25, 33, 286
chordopoxvirus family 149
chorioretinitis, multifocal 141

choroid plexus 188
chronic fatigue syndrome 192
chymotrypsin-like protease 52
civets
  Himalayan palm 48
  palm civets 31, 32, 34, 88
climate changes 19, 194
Congo–Crimean hemorrhagic fever (CCHF) virus
  162, 299
  antibodies to 304
  circulation 307f
  diagnosis and isolation 310
  fatal outcomes 308, 312
  genetic variation 303
  geographical distribution 301t
  human-to-human transmission 308
  IgG and IgM antibodies to 311
  M gene 303
  phylogenetic tree 305f
  replication 309, 312
  reservoir 304
  treatment and prevention 311–13
  vectors of, principal 306
contact tracing 329, 339
coronavirus (*see also* SARS)
  classification 50
  discovery 31, 49, 329
  polymerase gene 44
  respiratory illness 329
variant Creutzfeldt-Jakob disease (vCJD) 9
cropping cycle 22
cross-species transmission 25, 29, 31, 34
  molecular biological evidence of 26
  propensity for 33
  risk for 28
C-type retroviruses 7
Culex mosquitoes 22, 138, 210, 229, 339
Culex tritaeniorhynchus 20, 213, 214
culinary culture 71
culling
  of pigs 22, 185
  of poultry 98
    in Hong Kong 108, 111
    treatment for workers 115
cytokines 57, 63, 110, 155, 282, 284
cytotoxic T-lymphocyte (CTL) vaccine 68

dead-end hosts and dead-end infections 18, 210,
  212, 244, 28, 138
deer mice, *see* hantavirus: infections
DEET (N,N-diethyl-meta-tolumide) 242
deforestation 20, 22, 28, 194, 241

Deltaretrovirus 7
dendritic cell-specific intercellular adhesion
    molecule-grabbing non-integrin (DC-SIGN)
    55, 273
dengue fever, short-term prevention of 286
dengue hemorrhagic fever (DHF) 172, 269, 277
    classification of, WHO guidelines for 278
    epidemic, first recorded 275
    mechanisms of 282
dengue shock syndrome (DSS) 62, 269, 277
    management, WHO guidelines for 283
    pathogenesis 280
dengue viruses 270
    detecting 269
    E gene phylogeny 205
    E protein 56, 70, 133, 203
    genome and replication 271
    immunization strategies 284
    isolation and propagation 273, 279
    pandemic status 275
    virulence 280
differential display priming 44
disease surveillance 279, 333, *see also* surveillance
    communicable 330
    disease outbreaks
        detection 325
        detection algorithms 336
        identification of 332
    global infectious 340
    H5N1 influenza 111
    henipaviruses 194
ditropic life cycle 306
drug use/abuse, intravenous 6, 27, 193, 209, 311
ducks 213
    influenza virus A H2 subtype circulation in 114
Dugbe virus 300

Ebola virus 20, 55
    wildlife reservoir of 34
encephalitis 23, 207
    acute 111
    cause of 224
    epidemics of 217, 230
    fatal 235
    late-onset 189, 192
    severe 151, 208, 212
    summer 219, 238
    symptoms of 140
    tick-borne 270, 273
encephalopathy 9, 277, 278
endocytosis, receptor-mediated 272
endosomal cathepsin L-mediated proteolysis 55

enzootic cycles 18, 134, 137, 150, 244, 274, 275,
    338
equine torovirus (EToV) 50

fibrinogen levels 31, 311
fish, larvivorous 241, 283
flaccid paralysis 209, 330, *see also* polio-like acute
    flaccid paralysis
flavivirus 22, 133, 270, *see also* West Nile Virus
    encephalitis 208
    genetic variation in 205
    HI antibodies and 278
    mosquito-borne 237
        encephalitic 201
    virion diagram 134f
flying foxes 22, 187, 194
fogging, chemical 283
Four Corners epidemic 329

Gambusia affinis 241
genetic changes, accumulation of 29, 30
genetic reassortment 2, 17, 30, 100, 108
    segmented/non-segmented 2, 50, 100
Global Outbreak Alert and Response Network
    (GOARN) 332
Global Public Health Intelligence Network
    (GPHIN) 334–5, 339
Guillain–Barré syndrome, WNV-associated 140,
    141

habitat, role of 2, 19, 20, 22, 71, 167, 194, 211,
    337
HAM/TSP, *see* human T-cell lymphotropic virus,
    type 1 (HTLV-1): associated myelopathy/
    tropical spastic paraparesis
hantavirus (HTV) 161–117, 329
    diagnosis 171
    infections 17, 19
    mortality rates 170
    pathogenic genotypes 164t
    person-to-person transmission 168
    phylogenetic tree 163f
    phylogeny and epidemiology 166
    rodent hosts 167
    serotypes 166
    transmission 168
    treatment 173
Hazara virus 300
Hendra virus
    amino acid homology with Nipah virus 180
    antibodies to, neutralizing 187
    epidemiology 182

human-to-human transmission 184
infection
    clinical features 189
    pathogenesis 188
natural reservoirs 187
outbreaks 182
phylogenetic tree 180f
transmission 184
treatment 193
Henipavirus 179
disease surveillance 194
features 181
geographical occurrence, 183t
person-to-person transmission 182
hepatitis C virus 8
hepatitis E virus (HEV) 18
hepatocellular carcinoma 8
hepatomegaly 277, 309
herd immunity 3, 217
herpes virus 6, 57, 155
heterotypic immunity 270, 271
highly active anti-retroviral therapy (HAART) 66
horses, 102, 138, 188, 212, 339, *see also* hosts:
    dead-end; hosts: intermediate
host(s)
    amplifying 22, 23, 138, 211, 221, 244
    animal 17
    dead-end 18, 138, 210, 244
    human 29, 59, 98, 161, 280
    intermediate 102, 179, 182, 187, *see also* pigs
    maintenance 211
    Nipah and Hendra viruses 182
    reservoir 230
    unconventional 109
    vertebrate 18, 211
human immunodeficiency virus, type 1 (HIV-1) 6
    emergent history 6, *see also* species jumping
    HIV-1 vs. HIV-2 25–7, 29, 34
metapneumovirus (hMPV) 45
papillomavirus 7
human T-cell lymphotropic virus, type 1 (HTLV-
    1) 7, 27
    associated myelopathy/tropical spastic
        paraparesis (HAM/TSP) 8, 27

influenza virus 101, *see also* avian influenza
    viruses
    1918 H1N1 virus 17, 97,103
        phylogenetic analysis 104
    antigenic variation 100
    Asian flu 17, 103
    contagiousness of 47

classification 30, 98
detection 109
formalin-inactivated vaccines 116, 242, 284
1968 H3N2 virus (Hong Kong flu) 17, 103
host(s) 17
    cell entry 64
    range 101
human infections 31
incubation period 109
live-attenuated vaccines 116-117
natural reservoirs 24, 100
pandemics 17, 97, 105
HA and NA proteins 99
reservoirs, natural 24
transmission 97
treatment and prevention 114–16
vaccines 116, *see also* antigenic drift; antigenic
    shift
virulence 103
    virulence determinants 106t
insect repellants 242, see also DEET
irrigation practices, *see* Japanese encephalitis
    virus (JEV): transmission initiation
    alternate wet and dry 241
ixodid ticks 300

Japanese encephalitis virus (JEV)
antigenic variation 204, 242
Beijing-1 strain 204
Biken Institute vaccine 221, 242
dengue antibody (pre-existing) 209
diagnosis 210
genomic variation 204
genotypic replacement 207
geographic range 215f
human infection risk, predictor of 212
Japanese encephalitis 22, 184
morphogenesis 203
phylogenetic groupings 206f
seasonal transmission, herons migratory
    patterns and 215
serological groups 202
spread 237, 238f, 240
surveillance hosts 212
transmission cycles 210
transmission initiation 220
vaccines 242–244

Khasan virus 300
Koutango virus (KOUV) 202
Kunjin virus 136, 202

larvicidal bacteria 241

marsupials 214, 244
Menangle virus 179, 187
meningitis 23, 182
  aseptic 209
molecular clock approach 25
molecular dating analysis 7
monkeypox virus (MPV) 24
  clades 150
  cutaneous lesions 153f
  diagnosis 154
  incubation period 152
  person-to-person transmission 150
  prevention 157
  rash 152
  serologic tests 155
  smallpox virus, distinguishing from 152
  smallpox vaccination , benefit of 154
  transmission 150
  vaccination 157
  virulent strain 151
morbilliviruses 182
mosquito
  dengue virus vector 274
  JEV vector 201, 213
  population build-up 22
  vector reduction 241
  WNV vector 138
Murray valley encephalitis virus (MVEV) 202
Nairovirus 300
National Notifiable Disease Surveillance System
  (NDSS) 332

Nipah virus
  amino acid homology with Hendra viruses 180
  CNS infection and encephalitis 185,189, 191
  epidemic 22
  epidemiology 182
  hematologic abnormalities 191
  mortality rate 192
  pathogenesis 188
  Malaysia outbreak vs. Bangladesh outbreak
    181, 186, 190
  natural reservoirs 187
  neutralizing antibodies 187
  outbreaks 184–186
  person-to-person transmission 185, 191
  phylogenetic tree 180f
  treatment 193
noroviruses 18
nucleoside analogue 6, 173

Orthomyxoviridae 98
Orthopoxvirus 149

paramyxoviruses 21
pathogenicity test, intravenous 105
phlebotomus flies (sand flies) 230
pigs 22, 182, 202, 210, 219, 243, see also hosts:
  intermediate
  culling 185
  farming 225, 241, 244
polio-like acute flaccid paralysis 209, see also
  flaccid paralysis
Program for Monitoring Emerging Diseases
  (ProMED)-mail 334
Program for the Appropriate Technology in
  Health (PATH) 218, 243
Pteropus fruit bat 182, 187
Puumala virus 19, 161

quasispecies 30, 53

rainfall, role of 216, 227
rat-bite fever (RBF) 172
reemergence 2, 71
rice cultivation 22, 211, 224, 241
  pesticides in 217, 220, 241
rickettsialpox 152
Romanomermis culicivorax 241
Rubulavirus 188

Saaremaa virus (SAAV) 166
St. Louis encephalitis virus (SLEV) 202
SARS-CoV, see severe acute respiratory
  syndrome coronavirus
severe acute respiratory syndrome coronavirus
  (SARS-CoV) 31
  clinical features 60
  emergence 48
  genome
    organization 51f
    stability of 53
  humanization 48, 71
  identification 64
  immune response to 63–4
  inactivation 69
  molecular evolution 58–9
  natural reservoir 49, see also bats
  outbreak detection 328t
  pneumonia pathology 61
  receptor-based entry 54
  replication 57
  severity factor 32

strains 59
surveillance 339
treatment 66
ultrastructure 50, 45f
simian foamy virus (SFV) 17, 28
simian immunodeficiency virus (SIV) 18,
  25
cpz recombination 33
phylogeny 33
Sin Nombre virus 20, 161
smallpox virus mortality 1
smallpox vs. MPV infection, distinguishing
  152
species jumping 7, 49, 68, 71, 101
superinfection 34
"superspreading events" 45
surveillance102, 119, *see also* disease surveillance
  and characterization 30
CCHFV 304, 309
dengue virus 276
goals 325–7
H5N1 avian influenza virus 109
hantavirus (HTV) 169
Hendra virus 189
Nipah virus 190
passive 151
process of 330f
Syndromic, see syndromic surveillance
WNV 140
syndromic surveillance 329, 333, 335

tick 299, 306
transmissible spongiform encephalopathies
  (TSEs) 9

Usutu virus (USUV) 202

variant Creutzfeldt-Jakob disease (vCJD) 9
variola virus 149

vectors
control 35, 241, 283, *see also* rice cultivation;
  agricultural practices, rice cultivation:
  pesticides in
densities 211, 220, 231
vector-borne diseases, dynamics of 19
temperature and transmission efficiency 275
viraemia 138, 172, 209, 244, 279, 311
viral load 52, 64, 119

weighted maximum parsimony method 306f
West Nile virus (WNV)
anterior myelitis, WNV-associated 140
avian mortality 338
categories of human infections 139
diagnosis 141–2
E-glycoprotein nucleic acid sequence data 135f
emergence 2, 23, 134, 338
genomic structure 134f
global distribution 137f
incubation period 140
prevention 139
surveillance 338
transmission 138, 139
treatment 142

Yaounde virus (YAOV) 202
yellow fever virus 19, 133, 202

zoonoses 15–35
epidemiology 18
historical aspects 16–17
prevention and control 34–5
transmission 32
zoonotic paramyxoviruses 179
zoonotic sylvan infection cycle 152
zoonotic transmission 25, 35, 186
zoonotic virus 48
transmission modes of 17–18